Heart Failure with Preserved Ejection Fraction

Editors

GEU-RU HONG
MANI A. VANNAN

HEART FAILURE CLINICS

www.heartfailure.theclinics.com

Consulting Editor
EDUARDO BOSSONE

Founding Editor
JAGAT NARULA

July 2021 • Volume 17 • Number 3

ELSEVIER

1600 John F. Kennedy Boulevard • Suite 1800 • Philadelphia, Pennsylvania, 19103-2899

http://www.theclinics.com

HEART FAILURE CLINICS Volume 17, Number 3
July 2021 ISSN 1551-7136, ISBN-13: 978-0-323-83538-1

Editor: Joanna Collett
Developmental Editor: Jessica Cañaberal

Heart Failure Clinics (ISSN 1551-7136) is published quarterly by Elsevier Inc., 360 Park Avenue South, New York, NY 10010-1710. Months of publication are January, April, July, and October. Business and editorial offices: 1600 John F. Kennedy Boulevard, Suite 1800, Philadelphia, PA 19103-2899. Periodicals postage paid at New York, NY, and additional mailing offices. Subscription prices are USD 277.00 per year for US individuals, USD 661.00 per year for US institutions, USD 100.00 per year for US students and residents, USD 300.00 per year for Canadian individuals, USD 684.00 per year for Canadian institutions, USD 315.00 per year for international individuals, USD 684.00 per year for international institutions, and USD 100.00 per year for Canadian and foreign students/residents. To receive student and resident rate, orders must be accompanied by name of affiliated institution, date of term, and the *signature* of program/residency coordinator on institution letterhead. Orders will be billed at individual rate until proof of status is received. Foreign air speed delivery is included in all *Clinics* subscription prices. All prices are subject to change without notice. **POSTMASTER:** Send address changes to *Heart Failure Clinics*, Elsevier Health Sciences Division, Subscription Customer Service, 3251 Riverport Lane, Maryland Heights, MO 63043. **Customer Service: 1-800-654-2452 (US and Canada). From outside of the US and Canada, call 314-447-8871. Fax: 314-447-8029. For print support, E-mail: JournalsCustomerService-usa@elsevier.com. For online support, E-mail: JournalsOnlineSupport-usa@elsevier.com.**

Reprints. For copies of 100 or more of articles in this publication, please contact the Commercial Reprints Department, Elsevier Inc., 360 Park Avenue South, New York, NY 10010-1710. Tel.: 212-633-3874; Fax: 212-633-3820; E-mail: reprints@elsevier.com.

Heart Failure Clinics is covered in *MEDLINE/PubMed (Index Medicus).*

Contributors

CONSULTING EDITOR

EDUARDO BOSSONE, MD, PhD, FCCP, FESC, FACC
Director, Division of Cardiology, AORN Antonio Cardarelli Hospital, Naples, Italy

EDITORS

GEU-RU HONG, MD, PhD
Professor, Division of Cardiology, Severance Cardiovascular Hospital, Yonsei University College of Medicine, Seoul, Republic of Korea

MANI A. VANNAN, MBBS, FACC, FAHA, FASE, MRCP (UK), MRCP (I)
Marcus Heart Valve Center, Structural and Valvular Center of Excellence, Piedmont Heart Institute, Atlanta, Georgia, USA

AUTHORS

YURAN AHN, MD
Division of Cardiology, Department of Internal Medicine, Seoul St. Mary's Hospital, College of Medicine, The Catholic University of Korea, Seoul, Republic of Korea

MANJULA G. ANANTHRAM, MBBS, FACC
Assistant Professor, Department of Internal Medicine, Division of Cardiology, University of Maryland, Baltimore, Maryland, USA

AHMET BARUTCU, MD
Associate Professor, Department of Cardiology, Onsekizmart University Medical Faculty, Canakkale, Turkey

TOR BIERING-SØRENSEN, MD, MPH, PhD
Associate Professor, Department of Biomedical Sciences, Faculty of Health and Medical Sciences, University of Copenhagen, Research Director, Cardiovascular Non-Invasive Imaging Research Laboratory, Department of Cardiology, Copenhagen University Hospital Gentofte, Copenhagen, Denmark

BARRY A. BORLAUG, MD
Department of Cardiovascular Medicine, Mayo Clinic, Rochester, Minnesota, USA

EDUARDO BOSSONE, MD, PhD, FCCP, FESC, FACC
Director, Division of Cardiology, AORN Antonio Cardarelli Hospital, Naples, Italy

CORENTIN BOURG, MD
University of Rennes, CHU Rennes, INSERM, LTSI–UMR 1099, Rennes, France

AHMET CELIK, MD
Professor, Department of Cardiology, Mersin University Medical Faculty, Mersin, Turkey

DONG-HYUK CHO, MD, PhD
Division of Cardiology, Department of Internal Medicine, Yonsei University Wonju College of Medicine, Gangwon-do, Republic of Korea

GIULIA CRISCI, MD
Department of Translational Medical Sciences, Federico II University, Naples, Italy

ANNA D'AGOSTINO, PhD
IRCCS SDN Nuclear and Diagnostic Research Institute, Naples, Italy

ROBERTA D'ASSANTE, PhD
Department of Translational Medical Sciences, Federico II University, Naples, Italy

MARIAROSARIA DE LUCA, MD
Department of Translational Medical Sciences, Federico II University, Naples, Italy

RADEK DEBIEC, MRCP(UK)
Department of Cardiovascular Sciences, University of Leicester, NIHR Biomedical Research Centre, Glenfield Hospital, Leicester, United Kingdom

ANITA DESWAL, MD, MPH
Department of Cardiology, The University of Texas MD Anderson Cancer Center, Houston, Texas, USA

ERWAN DONAL, MD, PhD
University of Rennes, CHU Rennes, INSERM, LTSI–UMR 1099, Rennes, France

MOHAMED ELTAYEB, MRCP(UK)
Department of Cardiovascular Sciences, University of Leicester, NIHR Biomedical Research Centre, Glenfield Hospital, Leicester, United Kingdom

YITING FAN, PhD
Department of Cardiology, Shanghai Chest Hospital, Shanghai Jiao Tong University, Shanghai, China

ELENA GALLI, MD, PhD
University of Rennes, CHU Rennes, INSERM, LTSI–UMR 1099, Rennes, France

STEPHEN S. GOTTLIEB, MD, FACC
Professor, Department of Internal Medicine, Division of Cardiology, University of Maryland, Baltimore, Maryland, USA

MARCO GUAZZI, MD, PhD
Heart Failure Unit, Cardiopulmonary Laboratory, University Cardiology Department, IRCCS Policlinico San Donato University Hospital, Milan, Italy

MUHAMMAD ZUBAIR ISRAR, PhD
Department of Cardiovascular Sciences, University of Leicester, NIHR Biomedical Research Centre, Glenfield Hospital, Leicester, United Kingdom

HAE OK JUNG, MD, PhD
Division of Cardiology, Department of Internal Medicine, Seoul St. Mary's Hospital, College of Medicine, The Catholic University of Korea, Seoul, Republic of Korea

MASAHIKO KATO, MD, PhD
Division of School of Health Science, Department of Pathobiological Science and Technology, Faculty of Medicine, Tottori University, Yonago, Japan

RAMANJIT KAUR, MD
Division of Cardiology, Department of Internal Medicine, McGovern Medical School, The University of Texas Health Science Center, Houston, Texas, USA

IN-CHEOL KIM, MD, PhD
Division of Cardiology, Department of Internal Medicine, Cardiovascular Center, Keimyung University Dongsan Hospital, Keimyung University School of Medicine, Daegu, Republic of Korea

MI-NA KIM, MD, PhD
Division of Cardiology, Department of Internal Medicine, Korea University Medicine, Korea University Anam Hospital, Seoul, Republic of Korea

WOJCIECH KOSMALA, MD, PhD
Cardiology Department, Wroclaw Medical University, Wroclaw, Poland

EFSTRATIOS KOUTROUMPAKIS, MD
Division of Cardiology, Department of Internal Medicine, McGovern Medical School, The University of Texas Health Science Center, Houston, Texas, USA

CHAN JOO LEE, MD, PhD
Division of Cardiology, Department of Internal Medicine, Severance Hospital, Yonsei University College of Medicine, Seoul, Republic of Korea

ALBERTO M. MARRA, MD, PhD
Department of Translational Medical Sciences, Federico II University, Naples, Italy

CIRO MAURO, MD
AORN A Cardarelli, Cardiac Rehabilitation Unit, Naples, Italy

NANDINI NAIR, MD, PhD
Professor, Department of Medicine, Texas Tech University Health Sciences Center, Lubbock, Texas, USA

EMMANUEL OGER, MD, PhD
University of Rennes, EA 7449 REPERES [Pharmacoepidemiology and Health Services Research], Rennes, France

KAZUNORI OMOTE, MD, PhD
Department of Cardiovascular Medicine, Mayo Clinic, Rochester, Minnesota, USA

SEONG-MI PARK, MD, PhD
Division of Cardiology, Department of Internal Medicine, Korea University Medicine, Korea University Anam Hospital, Seoul, Republic of Korea

SUNGHA PARK, MD, PhD
Division of Cardiology, Department of Internal Medicine, Severance Hospital, Yonsei University College of Medicine, Seoul, Republic of Korea

ALEX PUI-WAI LEE, MBChB, MD, FRCP, FACC, FESC
Laboratory of Cardiac Imaging and 3D Printing, Li Ka Shing Institute of Health Science, The Chinese University of Hong Kong, Division of Cardiology, Department of Medicine and Therapeutics, The Chinese University of Hong Kong, Hong Kong SAR, China

BRIGIDA RANIERI, PhD
IRCCS SDN Nuclear and Diagnostic Research Institute, Naples, Italy

SALVATORE REGA
Department of Translational Medical Sciences, Federico II University, Naples, Italy

ANDREA SALZANO, MD, PhD, MRCP(London)
IRCCS SDN Nuclear and Diagnostic Research Institute, Naples, Italy

MORTEN SENGELØV, MD
Department of Cardiology, Copenhagen University Hospital Gentofte, Copenhagen, Denmark, PhD student, Department of Biomedical Sciences, Faculty of Health and Medical Sciences, University of Copenhagen, Denmark

CHI YOUNG SHIM, MD, PhD
Division of Cardiology, Severance Cardiovascular Hospital, Yonsei University College of Medicine, Seoul, Republic of Korea

HIDEMI SORIMACHI, MD, PhD
Department of Cardiovascular Medicine, Mayo Clinic, Rochester, Minnesota, USA

IAIN B. SQUIRE, MD, FRCP
Department of Cardiovascular Sciences, University of Leicester, NIHR Biomedical Research Centre, Glenfield Hospital, Leicester, United Kingdom

TORU SUZUKI, MD, PhD, FRCP
Department of Cardiovascular Sciences, University of Leicester, NIHR Biomedical Research Centre, Glenfield Hospital, Leicester, United Kingdom

HEINRICH TAEGTMEYER, MD, DPhil
Division of Cardiology, Department of Internal Medicine, McGovern Medical School, The University of Texas Health Science Center, Houston, Texas, USA

OZGE OZDEN TOK, MD
Department of Cardiology, Memorial Bahcelievler Hospital, Istanbul, Turkey

MANI A. VANNAN, MBBS, FACC, FAHA, FASE, MRCP (UK), MRCP (I)
Marcus Heart Valve Center, Structural and Valvular Center of Excellence, Piedmont Heart Institute, Atlanta, Georgia, USA

JULIÁN VEGA-ADAUY, MD
Chilean Institute of Cardiac Imaging, Millennium Nucleus in Cardiovascular Magnetic Resonance, Cardio MR, Santiago de Chile, Chile

KAZUHIRO YAMAMOTO, MD, PhD
Department of Cardiovascular Medicine
and Endocrinology and Metabolism,
Faculty of Medicine, Tottori University,
Yonago, Japan

BYUNG-SU YOO, MD, PhD
Division of Cardiology, Department of
Internal Medicine, Yonsei University Wonju
College of Medicine, Gangwon-do, Republic
of Korea

JONG-CHAN YOUN, MD, PhD
Division of Cardiology, Department of Internal
Medicine, Seoul St. Mary's Hospital, College of
Medicine, The Catholic University of Korea,
Seoul, Republic of Korea

Contents

The current trends of prevalence, incidence, and mortality in heart failure with preserved ejection fraction are summarized. We describe the differences in the definitions of heart failure with preserved ejection fraction used in community-based studies, heart failure registries, and clinical trials. The worldwide prevalence of heart failure with preserved ejection fraction is approximately 2%; it is becoming the dominant form of heart failure owing to the aging population. The longitudinal trend of mortality in this disease is decreasing, and the risk of mortality is similar between heart failure with preserved ejection fraction and heart failure with reduced ejection fraction.

Heart failure with preserved ejection fraction (HFpEF) is a major public health problem that affects half of all patients with HF. It is rising in prevalence, is associated with high morbidity and mortality, and has very few effective treatments. HFpEF is currently understood as a heterogeneous syndrome originating from the interplay of cardiac and extracardiac abnormalities. The most important pathophysiology in patients with HFpEF is diastolic dysfunction, which presents with impairments in relaxation or increases in chamber stiffness that lead to an increase in left ventricular filling pressures at rest or during exercise that causes dyspnea.

The prevalence of heart failure with preserved ejection fraction (HFpEF) is increasing rapidly, and its prognosis is as poor as that of HF with reduced EF. Hypertension is an important risk factor involved in the pathophysiology of HFpEF. Although treatment of hypertension lowers the incidence of HF and is beneficial in patients with HFpEF, there is conflicting evidence on this topic. This article discusses the pathophysiological mechanisms linking hypertension with HFpEF and also the current evidence on the treatment of hypertension in patients with HFpEF.

Obese heart failure with preserved ejection fraction (HFpEF) is a distinct HFpEF phenotype. Sodium retention, high circulating neurohormone levels, alterations in energy substrate metabolism, group 3 pulmonary hypertension, pericardial restraint, and systemic inflammation are central pathophysiologic mechanisms. Confirming the diagnosis may be challenging and high suspicion is required. Reduction of visceral adipose tissue, via caloric restriction and/or bariatric surgery, may improve outcomes in obese HFpEF patients. Furthermore, mineralocorticoid receptor inhibition, neprilysin inhibition, and sodium-glucose cotransporter 2 inhibition can ameliorate the effects of adiposity on the cardiovascular system, allowing for promising new treatment targets for the obese HFpEF phenotype.

Heart failure with preserved ejection fraction (HFpEF) and chronic kidney disease (CKD) constitute a high-risk phenotype with significant morbidity and mortality and poor prognosis. Multiple proinflammatory comorbid conditions influence the pathogenesis of HFpEF and CKD. Renal dysfunction in HFpEF is a consequence of the complex interplay between hemodynamic factors, systemic congestion, inflammation, endothelial dysfunction, and neurohormonal mechanisms. In contrast to heart failure with reduced ejection fraction, there is a dearth of effective targeted therapies for HFpEF. Tailoring study design toward the different phenotypes and delving into their pathophysiology may be fruitful in development of effective phenotype-specific targeted pharmaceutical therapies.

It is generally considered that obstructive sleep apnea is a potential cause of heart failure (HF), and insomnia and central sleep apnea are results of HF. However, the number of reports describing the bidirectional relationship between sleep disorder and HF has increased. Sleep disorder may contribute to left ventricular diastolic dysfunction via left atrial overload, left ventricular remodeling, pulmonary hypertension, and atrial fibrillation, which lead to HF with preserved left ventricular ejection fraction. Overnight rostral fluid shift and lung congestion may lead to airflow obstruction in the upper pharynx and stimulate pulmonary irritant receptors, which induce hyperventilation and sleep disorder.

In this article, the definition; mechanisms; diagnostic strategies, including scoring systems; treatments; prognosis; and future perspectives in heart failure with preserved ejection fraction with atrial fibrillation, which are common comorbid conditions, are reviewed thoroughly.

Heart failure with preserved ejection fraction (HFpEF) is a clinical syndrome of shortness of breath and/or exercise intolerance secondary to elevated left ventricular filling pressures at rest or with exertion either as a result of primary diastolic dysfunction (primary HFpEF) or secondary to specific underlying causes (secondary HFpEF). In secondary HFpEF, early intervention of underlying valvular heart disease generally improves symptoms and prolongs survival. In primary HFpEF, there is increasing awareness of the existence and prognostic implications of secondary atrioventricular valve regurgitation. Further studies will clarify their mechanisms and the effectiveness of valvular intervention in this intriguing HFpEF subgroup.

Exercise intolerance represents a typical feature of heart failure with preserved ejection fraction (HFpEF), and is associated with a poor quality of life, frequent hospitalizations, and increased all-cause mortality. The cardiopulmonary exercise test is the best method to quantify exercise intolerance, and allows detection of the main mechanism responsible for the exercise limitation, influencing treatment and prognosis. Exercise training programs improve exercise tolerance in HFpEF. However, studies are needed to identify appropriate type and duration. This article discusses the pathophysiology of exercise limitation in HFpEF, describes methods of determining exercise tolerance class, and evaluates prognostic implications and potential therapeutic strategies.

Heart failure (HF) is an ongoing crisis reaching epidemic proportions worldwide. About 50% of HF patients have a preserved ejection fraction. Invasive hemodynamics have shown varied results in patients who have HF with preserved ejection fraction (HFpEF). This article attempts to summarize the importance of detecting pulmonary vascular remodeling in HFpEF using invasive hemodynamics. Incorporating newer invasive hemodynamic parameters such as diastolic pulmonary gradient, pulmonary arterial compliance, pulmonary vascular resistance, and pulmonary arterial pulsatility index may improve patient selection for studies used in defining advanced therapies and clinical outcomes. Profiling of patients using invasive hemodynamic parameters may lead to better patient selection for clinical research.

Noninvasive cardiac imaging by transthoracic echocardiography is among the first-line assessments in evaluation of heart failure patients with preserved ejection fraction (HFpEF). Although systolic function seems preserved by conventional measurers, important information is found through examination of the heart's hemodynamic profile through Doppler and novel echocardiographic measures. These measures aid in establishing the diagnosis of HFpEF and provide valuable prognostic information. Targets of interest include the left ventricle diastolic function, atrial structure and function, and right ventricular function including pulmonary pressures. Contemporary assessments of the hemodynamic profile attainable through echocardiography in HFpEF at rest are reviewed and future directions outlined.

describes currently recognized phenotypes of HFpEF and potential treatment strategies.

Phenomapping Heart Failure with Preserved Ejection Fraction Using Machine Learning Cluster Analysis: Prognostic and Therapeutic Implications 499

Elena Galli, Corentin Bourg, Wojciech Kosmala, Emmanuel Oger, and Erwan Donal

Heart failure with preserved ejection fraction (HFpEF) is characterized by a high rate of hospitalization and mortality (up to 84% at 5 years), which are similar to those observed for heart failure with reduced ejection fraction (HFrEF). These epidemiologic data claim for the development of specific and innovative therapies to reduce the burden of morbidity and mortality associated with this disease. Compared with HFrEF, which is due to a primary myocardial damage (eg ischemia, cardiomyopathies, toxicity), a heterogeneous etiologic background characterizes HFpEF. The authors discuss these phenotypes and specificities for defining therapeutic strategies that could be proposed according to phenotypes.

HEART FAILURE CLINICS

Preface

Heart Failure with Preserved Ejection Fraction: Current Opinion and Future Perspectives

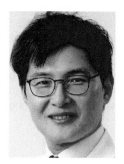

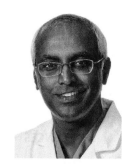

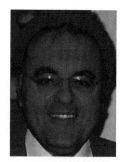

Geu-Ru Hong, MD, PhD

Mani A. Vannan, MBBS, FACC, FAHA, FASE, MRCP (UK), MRCP (I)

Eduardo Bossone, MD, PhD, FCCP, FESC, FACC

Editors

With the advancement of medical technology and an increase in the elderly population, the number of patients with heart failure (HF) is increasing significantly with a subsequent increase in the socioeconomic burden.[1] Approximately half of HF patients are known to have HF with preserved ejection fraction (HFpEF), linked to the rising life expectancy and various comorbidities, such as hypertension, diabetes mellitus, and chronic kidney disease.[2] Due to the fact that the left ventricular ejection fraction (LVEF) is maintained in HFpEF patients, the prognosis is often falsely thought to be better than those with heart failure with reduced ejection fraction (HFrEF). However, the mortality and acute exacerbation rate of HFpEF are reported to be similar to those of HFrEF, and readmission rates are equally high. Furthermore, HFpEF patients are known to have similar or worse quality of life compared with HFrEF patients.[3] At present, the concept of HFpEF is gradually evolving, and the pathophys-iologic mechanism of HFpEF is being revealed to be multifactorial and rather different from HFrEF. In particular, HFpEF is caused by complex interactions around the heart, vascular system, and surroundings and includes various interactions between the left ventricular size, contractile function, and autonomic imbalance.[4,5] Thus, it is unreasonable to characterize HFpEF with LVEF alone.

Although many clinical studies and advances in diagnostic imaging technology have revealed many details regarding the pathophysiology and cause of HFpEF, and the diagnosis rate has recently increased, the detection and management of these patients are still difficult in real clinical practice.[6] This is thought to be due to the fact that HFpEF is a complex heterogeneous syndrome originating from the interplay of cardiac (coronary microvascular and cardiomyocyte dysfunction) and extracardiac abnormalities (ie, systemic inflammation and skeletal muscle

Heart Failure Clin 17 (2021) xiii–xiv
https://doi.org/10.1016/j.hfc.2021.03.007
1551-7136/21/© 2021 Published by Elsevier Inc.

dysfunction).[7] While HFpEF is common and important in clinical practice, there is no definite optimal treatment, unlike HFrEF, which has firmly established appropriate standard treatment guidelines. The standard treatment of HF mainly focuses on neurohormonal modulators, such as renin-angiotensin blockers and beta-blockers, which reduce the mortality in HFrEF patients by inhibiting the remodeling of the left ventricle.[6] In contrast, the mortality and prognosis of HFpEF patients over the past 20 years have shown minimal improvement and is thought to be due to the fact that HFpEF is often accompanied by various other cardiovascular risk factors involving multiple pathologic mechanisms.[8,9] Thus, the treatment of HFpEF should be approached in a different manner according to its various phenotypes, and currently, clinical trials according to various treatment methods are taking place.[6,9]

This issue is deliberately designed to address the key pathophysiologic and clinical questions regarding HFpEF. The goal was to tackle the dilemma of how to optimally provide answers to important questions that arise in the real clinical world, including the diagnosis and treatment of HFpEF patients. In particular, we reviewed the current trend and clinical outcomes based on important clinical studies conducted so far on HFpEF as well as comorbidities commonly found in HFpEF patients, such as hypertension, obesity, renal dysfunction, sleep disorder, atrial fibrillation, and valvular heart diseases. We aimed to examine in detail various cardiac imaging modalities for noninvasive and accurate diagnosis of HFpEF patients with a wide range of clinical features, review recent up-to-date treatments, determine factors affecting the prognosis, as well as establish individualized treatment strategies. Given the importance of HFpEF, preparing for this issue was challenging. It is hoped this issue will be of value for every clinician who is involved in the care of HFpEF patients.

Geu-Ru Hong, MD, PhD
Division of Cardiology
Severance Cardiovascular Hospital
Yonsei University College of Medicine
50-1 Yonsei-Ro, Seodaemun-G
Seoul, Republic of Korea

Mani A. Vannan, MBBS, FACC, FAHA, FASE,
MRCP (UK), MRCP (I)
Marcus Heart Valve Center
Structural and Valvular Center of Excellence
Piedmont Heart Institute
95 Collier Road, Suite 2065
Atlanta, GA, 30309, USA

Eduardo Bossone, MD, PhD, FCCP, FESC, FACC
Division of Cardiology
Cardarelli Hospital
Via A. Cardarelli, 9
Naples 80131, Italy

E-mail addresses:
grhong@yuhs.ac (G.-R. Hong)
mvannan2560@gmail.com (M.A. Vannan)
ebossone@hotmail.com (E. Bossone)

REFERENCES

1. Own TE, Hodge DO, Herges RM, et al. Trends in prevalence and outcome of heart failure with preserved ejection fraction. N Engl J Med 2006;355:251–9.

2. Bhatia RS, Tu JV, Lee DS, et al. Outcome of heart failure with preserved ejection fraction in a population-based study. N Engl J Med 2006;355:260–9.

3. Dunlay SM, Roger VL, Redfield MM. Epidemiology of heart failure with preserved ejection fraction. Nat Rev Cardiol 2017;14:591–602.

4. Pfeffer MA, Shah AM, Borlaug BA. Heart failure with preserved ejection fraction: in perspective. Circ Res 2019;124:1598–617.

5. Shah SJ, Katz DH, Deo RC. Phenotypic spectrum of heart failure with preserved ejection fraction. Heart Failure Clin 2014;10:407–18.

6. Oktay AA, Shah SJ. Diagnosis and management of heart failure with preserved ejection fraction: 10 key lessons. Curr Cardiol Rev 2015;11:42–52.

7. Lewis GA, Shelbert EB, Williams SG, et al. Biological phenotypes of heart failure with preserved ejection fraction. J Am Coll Cardiol 2017;70:2186–200.

8. Shah SJ, Kitzman DW, Borlaug BA, et al. Phenotype-specific treatment of heart failure with preserved ejection fraction. A multiorgan roadmap. Circulation 2016;134:73–90.

9. Silverman DN, Shah SJ. Treatment of heart failure with preserved ejection fraction (HFpEF): the phenotype-guided approach. Curr Treat Options Cardiovasc Med 2019;21:20.

Current Prevalence, Incidence, and Outcomes of Heart Failure with Preserved Ejection Fraction

Dong-Hyuk Cho, MD, PhD, Byung-Su Yoo, MD, PhD*

KEYWORDS

- Heart failure with preserved ejection fraction • Epidemiology • Prevalence • Incidence • Outcome
- Mortality

KEY POINTS

- The definition of heart failure with preserved ejection fraction used in epidemiologic and clinical studies differs, and a simple, reliable definition is needed.
- Specific echocardiographic parameters including morphologic and diastolic functional parameters and biomarkers such as natriuretic peptide are used as multimodality diagnostic tools for epidemiologic studies regarding heart failure with preserved ejection fraction.
- The worldwide prevalence of heart failure with preserved ejection fraction is approximately 2% and varies based on study design, characteristics of the study population, and the definition of heart failure with preserved ejection fraction.
- Heart failure with preserved ejection fraction is becoming the dominant form of heart failure owing to the aging population.
- With limited studies, the longitudinal trend of mortality in heart failure with preserved ejection fraction is decreasing.

INTRODUCTION

Despite developments and improvements in treatment strategies, heart failure (HF) remains a significant socioeconomic burden and leads to individual health problems owing to its high mortality and readmission rates. The aging of the general population and the accompanying increase of cardiovascular comorbidities are considered to be the main causes of the increase in the incidence of HF, especially HF with preserved ejection (HFpEF), which has become the dominant form of HF.[1–4] However, the characteristics of HFpEF have been described in prospective clinical studies that investigate the efficacy of drugs in carefully selected populations. Research regarding the diagnosis and treatment of HFpEF is complicated by the heterogeneous forms of the condition. There is a lack of evidence-based treatment options with therapeutic effects. Therefore, identifying current trends from community-based and observational studies in addition to large-scale prospective clinical research is important for establishing treatment and prevention strategies.

Patients with HF are categorized as having HFpEF (an ejection fraction [EF] of $\geq$50%), HF with mid-range EF (EF of 40%–49%), and HF with reduced EF (HFrEF; EF of <40%).[2,5] Each type of HF has unique pathophysiological mechanisms, responses to medications, and epidemiologic characteristics. The purpose of this review

Division of Cardiology, Department of Internal Medicine, Yonsei University Wonju College of Medicine, Gangwon-do, Republic of Korea
* Corresponding author. Division of Cardiology, Department of Internal Medicine, Wonju College of Medicine, Yonsei University, 20, Ilsan- ro, Wonju, Gangwon-do 26426, South Korea (Republic of Korea).
E-mail address: yubs@yonsei.ac.kr

Heart Failure Clin 17 (2021) 315–326
https://doi.org/10.1016/j.hfc.2021.03.002
1551-7136/21/© 2021 Elsevier Inc. All rights reserved.

is to provide an overview of the epidemiology of HFpEF, focusing on the definition of HFpEF and current trends in prevalence, incidence, and outcomes.

DIAGNOSIS

Measuring an epidemic of HF has numerous challenges. Although HF is a heterogeneous clinical syndrome, the majority of epidemiologic studies depend on diagnostic codes for HF. Reliance on diagnostic codes is limited by several issues, including miscoding owing to reimbursement incentives and misdiagnoses by physicians. Previous studies have attempted to overcome the limitation of diagnostic codes using standardized criteria to diagnose HF (**Box 1**). The Framingham criteria, which are most commonly used to diagnose HF in epidemiologic and clinical studies, only includes clinical symptoms and signs and chest radiograph findings.[6] The Framingham criteria have good specificity but low sensitivity for HF and frequently miss patients with compensated HF without pulmonary congestion.

The epidemiologic study of HFpEF is more complex. First, the diagnosis of HFpEF is relatively new. In the 1980s and 1990s, the term diastolic HF was widely used; the term HFpEF has begun to rapidly replace diastolic HF during the last 2 decades,[7] rendering it difficult to study the longitudinal trends of HFpEF. In addition, there is no single diagnostic tool for HFpEF, and the threshold of the left ventricular (LV) EF and the definitions of structural remodeling and LV diastolic dysfunction differ in different studies (see **Box 1**). Despite these limitations, echocardiographic morphologic and functional parameters and brain natriuretic peptide (BNP) and N-terminal pro-BNP (NT-proBNP) are useful in the multimodality diagnosis of HFpEF.

New criteria, scoring models, and definitions for HFpEF have been suggested to overcome these limitations. The recent European Society of Cardiology (ESC) criteria for HFpEF include clinical symptoms and signs; echocardiographic findings for LV structure and function and left atrium structure; and elevated levels of natriuretic peptides.[2] The echocardiographic parameters of structural abnormalities and LV diastolic dysfunction and biomarkers that reflect the mechanical stretch of the myocardium (BNP and NT-proBNP) were added to the criteria. In the ESC criteria, delicate diastolic functional parameters such as early mitral tissue velocity (e') or the ratio of early diastolic mitral inflow velocity (E) to e' are used to detect ventricular relaxation abnormalities and elevated filling pressure, which are precursors of HFpEF.

The H2FPEF and HFA-PEFF scoring systems were developed to evaluate the probability of HFpEF in patients with a noncardiac origin of HF symptoms.[8,9] In the HFA-PEFF score, different cut-off values of natriuretic peptide are suggested for patients with sinus rhythm or atrial fibrillation. These scoring systems are useful for the diagnosis of HFpEF; however, further validation in community-based cohorts is needed to verify these scoring systems for use in epidemiologic studies.

The definitions of HFpEF used in landmark clinical trials are summarized in **Box 1**. In the CHARM-Preserved trial, clinical symptoms and an EF threshold of 40% were used for the diagnosis of HFpEF; no echocardiographic parameters or natriuretic peptide levels were used.[10] In the I-PRESERVE trial, echocardiographic LV hypertrophy and left atrial enlargement were added to the HFpEF criteria, and BNP levels were used for the definition of HFpEF in the TOPCAT trial.[11,12] In the PARAGON-HF trial, both echocardiographic parameters and natriuretic peptide levels were used to diagnose HFpEF; however, the broad echocardiographic criteria used in this study (septal or posterior wall thickness of ≥1.1 cm for LV hypertrophy) did not match those of the ESC criteria.[13] In the most recent clinical trial, EMPEROR-Preserved, both echocardiographic morphologic and functional parameters and levels of NT-proBNP were used to define HFpEF. The criteria of the EMPEROR-Preserved are clinically relevant and consistent with current practice guidelines.[14] The definition of HFpEF used in the EMPEROR-Preserved trial may be a landmark for future epidemiologic studies.

PREVALENCE

Based on community-based epidemiologic studies, the estimated prevalence of HF is approximately 1% to 2% of the general adult population. More than 20 community-based studies have reported the prevalence of overall HF.[1,15] Data regarding LVEF are essential to define HFpEF; therefore, few epidemiologic studies about HFpEF are available. The worldwide prevalence of HFpEF (based on 12 community-based studies) varies from 1.1% to 5.5% (**Fig. 1**).[16–27] Most of these studies were conducted in developed countries. Regardless of the location of the study, the prevalence of HFpEF increased with the age of the enrolled population; the prevalence of HFpEF was highest (5.5%) in a study conducted in the UK in which patients were aged more than 70 years,[17] and only 1.6% of patients in the EPICA study of Portugal, which enrolled patients more

Box 1
Definitions of HFpEF used in standardized criteria and clinical trials

Framingham criteria[5]

Major and minor symptoms and signs

Chest radiograph findings

No echocardiography and natriuretic peptide criteria

2016 ESC criteria[2]

Symptoms and sign

LVEF of $\geq$50% and $\geq$1 additional criteria:

1. LVMI of $\geq$115/95 g/m^2 (M/W) and/or LAVI of >34 mL/m^2

2. E/e' of $\geq$13 and a mean e' septal and lateral annulus of <9 cm/s

BNP of >35 pg/mL and/or NT-proBNP of >125 pg/mL

H2PEFP score[7]

Body mass index of >30 kg/m^2

Hypertension (the use of $\geq$2 antihypertensive medications)

Atrial fibrillation

Pulmonary hypertension (estimated PASP >35 mm Hg)

Age >60 years

Elevated filling pressure (E/e' >9)

HFA-PEFF score[8]

Functional major: septal e' of <7 cm/s or lateral e' of <10 cm/s or average E/e' of $\geq$15 or TR velocity $\geq$2.8 m/s

Functional minor: average E/e' 9 to 14, GLS greater than -16%

Morphologic major: LAVI 34 mL/m^2 or LVMI of $\geq$149/122 g/m^2 (M/W) and RWT of >0.42

Morphologic minor: LAVI 29 to 34 mL/m^2 or LVMI of >115/95 g/m^2 (M/W) or RWT >0.42 or LV wall thickness of $\geq$1.2 cm

Biomarker major: greater than 220 pg/mL or BNP 80 pg/mL (SR), of >660 pg/mL or BNP 240 pg/mL (AF)

Biomarker minor: of >125 to 220 pg/mL or BNP of 35 to 80 pg/mL (SR), 365 to 660 pg/mL or BNP 105 to 240 pg/mL (AF)

Major criteria: 2 points, minor criteria: 1 point

$\geq$5 points: HFpEF

CHARM-Preserved[9]

Symptoms

LVEF of $\geq$40%

No natriuretic peptide criteria

I-PRESERVE[10]

Symptoms and signs

LVEF of $\geq$45% and echocardiographic LVH or LAE

No natriuretic peptide criteria

TOPCAT[11]

Symptoms and signs

LVEF of $\geq$45%

De novo; no natriuretic peptide criteria, history of HF; BNP of $\geq$100 pg/mL and/or NT-proBNP of $\geq$360 pg/mL.

PARAGON-HF[12]

Symptoms and signs

LVEF of $\geq$45%, $\geq$1 additional criteria:

1. Septal or posterior wall thickness of $\geq$1.1 cm,

2. LA width of $\geq$3.8 cm or LA length of $\geq$5.0 cm or LA area of $\geq$20 cm^2 or LA volume of $\geq$55 mL or LA volume index of $\geq$29 mL/m^2

HF hospitalization; NT-proBNP of >200 pg/mL (SR) or of >200 pg/mL (AF), outpatients; NT-proBNP of >300 pg/mL (SR) or of >900 pg/mL (AF)

EMPEROR-preserved[13]

Symptoms and signs

LVEF of >40% and echocardiographic LVH or LAE or LV diastolic dysfunction

1. Septal or posterior wall thickness of $\geq$1.1 cm or LVMI of $\geq$115/95 g/m^2 (M/W)

2. LA width of $\geq$4.0 cm or LA length of $\geq$5.0 cm or LA area of $\geq$20 cm^2 or LA volume of $\geq$55 mL or LA volume index of $\geq$34 mL/m^2

3. mean E/e' of $\geq$13 and a mean e' septal and lateral annulus of <9 cm/s

NT-proBNP of >300 pg/mL (SR) or >900 pg/mL (AF)

Abbreviations: AF, atrial fibrillation; BNP, brain natriuretic peptide; E, early diastolic mitral inflow velocity; e', early mitral tissue velocity; GLS, global longitudinal strain; HFpEF, heart failure with preserved ejection fraction; LA, left atrium; LAE, left atrial enlargement; LAVI, left atrial volume index; LVEF, left ventricular ejection fraction; LVH, left ventricular hypertrophy; LVMI, left ventricular mass index; M/W, men/women; NP, natriuretic peptide; NT-proBNP, N-terminal pro-brain natriuretic peptide; PASP, pulmonary arterial systolic pressure; RWT, relative wall thickness; SR, sinus rhythm; TR, tricuspid regurgitation.

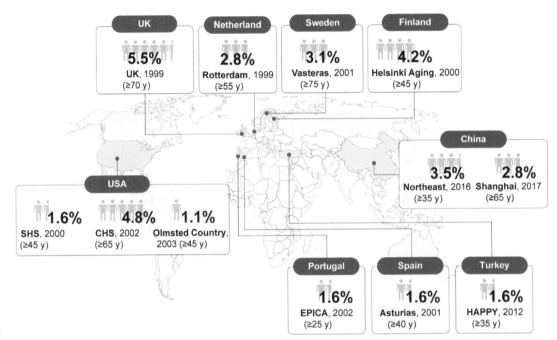

Fig. 1. Worldwide prevalence of HFpEF from community-based epidemiologic studies. The reported prevalence of HFpEF ranges from 1.1% to 5.5%. The prevalence increases with advancing age. This figure shows the results of community-based epidemiologic studies.[15–26] CHS, Cardiovascular Health Study; EPICA, Epidemiology of Heart Failure and Learning; HAPPY, Heart Failure Prevalence and Predictors in Turkey; SHS, Strong Heart Study.

than 25 years old, were diagnosed with HFpEF.[22] In the EPICA study, the prevalence of both HFpEF and HFrEF increased with age, although the prevalence of HFpEF increased more sharply than that of HFrEF.[22]

Fig. 2 illustrates the proportion of patients with HFpEF within all patients with HF in landmark community-based studies and HF registries.[28–35] HFpEF accounts for approximately 40% to 50% of HF in community-based studies. The proportion of HFpEF varies from 30.1% to 59.7% in HF registries. The selection bias of HF registries may affect the variability of the prevalence of HFpEF. Generally, the proportion of HFpEF was higher in community-based studies compared with that in HF registries.[36]

INCIDENCE

There are few community-based cohort studies that have reported the incidence of HFpEF (**Table 1**). Community-based cohort studies with echocardiographic evaluations were conducted in the United States (Framingham heart study,[37] Olmsted Country Study,[38] and the Multi-Ethnic Study of Atherosclerosis [MESA])[39] and the Netherlands (Prevention of Renal and Vascular End-stage Disease [PREVEND] study[40]). The annual incidence of HFpEF varied from 1.3 to 6.8

per 1000 persons. The incidence rate depended on the inclusion criteria, characteristics of the study population, and the study time frame.

Tsao and colleagues[41] pooled data from 2 longitudinal cohorts (the Cardiovascular Health Study and the Framingham Heart Study). The annual incidences of HFpEF from 1990 to 1999 and from 2000 to 2009 were 4.7 and 6.8 per 1000 persons, respectively. The incidence of HFpEF increases with age and depends on the baseline age of the cohort. The mean patient ages for 1990 to 1999 and 2000 to 2009 were 73 and 74 years, respectively, in the study analyzed by Tsao and colleagues.[41] The age of the study population may explain the relatively high incidence of HFpEF. In contrast, the age of patients in the PREVEND Study, which reported the lowest incidence rate of HFpEF (1.3 per 1000 persons), was 49.2 years. The annual incidence of HFpEF in the MESA study was 1.5 per 1000 persons, with a mean patient age of 62.5 years, although patients with established cardiovascular diseases were excluded.[41] These results suggest that underlying cardiovascular morbidities are associated with the development of HFpEF.

The Olmsted Country Study reported that the incidence of HF decreased from 3.2 per 1000 persons in 2000 to 2.2 per 1000 persons in 2010, which was a 37.5% decrease.[38] The incidences

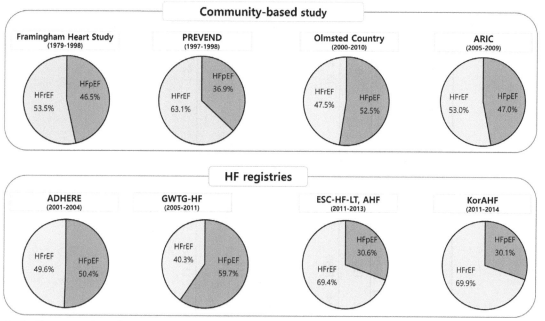

Fig. 2. The proportion of HFpEF in community-based and registry studies. The proportion of patients with HFpEF among all patients with HF varies according to the study design, time, and population. It is typically approximately 50%. ADHERE, Acute Decompensated Heart Failure National Registry; AHF, acute heart failure; ARIC, Atherosclerosis Risk in Communities Study; ESC-HF-LT, European Society of Cardiology-Heart Failure- Long Term; GWTG-HF, Get With The Guidelines–Heart Failure; KorAHF; Korean Acute Heart Failure; PREVEND, Prevention of Renal and Vascular Endstage Disease.

of HFpEF and HFrEF also decreased, though the decrease in the incidence of HFrEF (−45.1%) was greater than that of HFpEF (−27.9%). The proportion of HFpEF among all patients with HF substantially increased from 2000 to 2010. However, all of these studies were based in the United States. Studies including patients in Asia, Africa, and other regions are warranted.

RISK FACTORS AND COMORBIDITIES

The initial epidemiologic studies reported that older age and female sex are more common among patients with HFpEF compared with those with HFrEF.[22,42,43] Recent observational studies confirm these findings.[39,44] Therefore, older age and female sex are believed to be independent risk factors for the development of HFpEF. The greater susceptibility for coronary microvascular dysfunction in females may explain these results.[45] Ho and colleagues[46] developed risk prediction models for incident HFpEF and HFrEF based on pooled data from community-based studies including the Framingham Heart Study, the Cardiovascular Health Study, and the PREVEND Study. Older age was identified as an independent risk factor for HFpEF and HFrEF in the

multivariable analysis. Although sex was not identified as an independent risk factor for HFpEF, male sex was associated with a higher risk of HFrEF. Furthermore, in the Olmsted Country Study, the age-standardized annual incidence rate of HFpEF was similar between men and women, although the age-standardized annual incidence rate of HFrEF was higher in men compared with women.[38] The higher frequency of HFpEF among females that is, reported in observational studies may be due to the higher proportion of females in the elderly population. Data comparing the risks of race and ethnicity are limited. In the Atherosclerosis Risk in Communities (ARIC) Study, the age-adjusted hospitalization rate for HFpEF was highest in Black women, followed by Black men, White women, and White men.[44]

Hypertension is the most common cardiovascular risk factor observed in patients with HFpEF.[47,48] Hypertension-induced myocardial remodeling and increased LV filling pressures are thought to be the main mechanisms of the development of HFpEF.[49] However, Ho and colleagues reported that hypertension was associated with a higher risk of HFpEF and HFrEF. Patients with diabetes are more likely to have HF than patients

Table 1
Community-based cohort studies reporting the incidence of HFpEF

Author, Published year	Cohort	Country	Time Frame	Mean Patient Age, Years	Total Population	Population	HF (n)	HFpEF (n)	HFrEF (n)	Proportion of HFpEF (%)	Incidence (per 1000 Patient-years)
Ho et al, 2013[37]	Framingham heart Study	USA	1979–2008	60	6340	General	512	196	261	42.9	2.0
Gerber et al, 2015[38]	Olmsted[b]	USA	2000–2010	N/A	144,248	General, ≥65 y	2074	1089	985	52.5	M: 1.4→1.0, F: 1.7→1.3[a]
Tsao et al, 2018[41]	FHS + CHS	USA	1990–1999	73	8762	General	1367	309	491	38.6	4.7
			2000–2009	74	6455	General	1177	373	431	46.4	6.8
Brouwers et al, 2013[40]	PREVEND	Netherland	1997–2010	49.2	8592	General, ≥28 y	374	125	249	33.4	1.3[a]
Silverman et al, 2016[39]	MESA	USA	2000–2012[c]	62.5	6812	No CVD, ≥45 y	257	111	107	50.9	1.5[a]

Abbreviations: FHS + CHS, Framingham Heart Study and Cardiovascular Health Study; MESA, Multi-Ethnic Study of Atherosclerosis; PREVEND, Prevention of Renal and Vascular End-stage Disease.

[a] Incidence rate was calculated using incident HF, total population, and study period.
[b] Incidence rate of males (M) and females (F) from 2002 to 2010.
[c] The median of follow-up was 11.2 years from 2000.[39]

without diabetes.[50,51] Diabetes was reported to be independently associated with a greater risk of HFrEF, but not HFpEF in a community-based study.[46] The prevalence of obesity (defined by body mass index) was approximately 50% in patients with HFpEF and an increased body mass index was associated with a higher risk of both HFpEF and HFrEF.[37,46] In the pooled analysis of 4 community-based cohort studies, a higher body mass index and insulin resistance were associated with an increased risk of HFpEF compared with HFrEF.[52] These results suggest that obesity and cardiometabolic traits are potential pathways leading to HFpEF. Coronary artery disease (CAD) and myocardial infarction have been established as the main risk factors for the development of HFrEF.[1,2] The reported prevalence of CAD in patients with HFpEF varied from 20% to 53% in community-based studies,[19,53,54] and the reported prevalence was up to 76% in HF registries.[35,55] It has not been established whether CAD or comorbidities are the major contributor to the development of subclinical LV diastolic dysfunction. In patients with suspected angina, the severity of CAD was found to be independently associated with the presence of LV diastolic dysfunction, and the association was more prominent in women.[56] In the multivariable risk prediction model, previous CAD was independently associated with the incidence of HFpEF and HFrEF.[46]

QUALITY OF LIFE AND HOSPITALIZATION

In patients with HFpEF, the burden of clinical symptoms and physical inactivity impair quality of life (QOL). Patient-reported QOL (assessed with the Kansas City Cardiomyopathy Questionnaire) is closely associated with HF severity, BNP levels, functional class, and exercise capacity.[57] In the TOPCAT and PARAGON-HF trials, the QOL of patients with HFpEF was impaired.[58,59] Some studies have reported that the QOL is similarly impaired in patients with HFpEF and HFrEF, although a pooled analysis of data from the PARAGON-HF and PARADIGM-HF trials revealed that the QOL was worse in patients with HFpEF than in those with HFrEF, especially among female patients. After adjusting for confounding factors including age and sex, the Kansas City Cardiomyopathy Questionnaire score was not significantly different between patients with HFpEF and HFrEF.[59] Patients receiving sacubitril–valsartan and spironolactone had improved QOL compared with patients receiving a placebo, although cardiovascular mortality and hospitalization for HF were not improved in patients using these medications.[13,58]

Hospitalization is common among patients with HFpEF or HFrEF. LV function and QOL decrease after a diagnosis of HF. With each acute episode, myocardial injuries may contribute to progressive LV dysfunction, resulting in an increased risk of mortality.[60] The prevention of hospitalizations and readmissions is an important goal in the management of HF. In a community-based study, the annual hospitalization rate after a diagnosis of HF was 1.39 and 1.38 per person-year for patients with HFpEF and HFrEF, respectively.[38] In the study of hospitalized Medicare beneficiaries with HF, the 30-day readmission rate was high (23%) in patients with HFpEF and in those with HFrEF.[61] In the Olmsted Country Study, 34% of patients with HFpEF experienced hospitalizations for HF at least once over a mean follow-up of 4.7 years.[62] The reported hospitalization rate varies depending on the study population and design, and is generally lower in clinical trials than in community-based or registry studies. Among patients with HF receiving spironolactone in the TOPCAT trial, only 12.0% were hospitalized during a mean follow-up of 3 years.[12] In the PARAGON-HF, there were 690 hospitalizations for HF among 2407 patients who received sacubitril–valsartan over a median follow-up of 35 months.[13]

MORTALITY

The reported mortality in epidemiologic and clinical studies depends on the study design, population, and the definition of HFpEF.[63] The definition of HFpEF is highly variable in landmark studies. In general, the mortality rate of HFpEF in clinical trials was lower than that of observational studies (**Figs. 3** and **4**), because patients with a younger age and fewer underlying cardiovascular diseases were included in the clinical trials. For example, patients with cancer or end-stage chronic kidney disease were excluded from most clinical studies. The reported in-hospital mortality was 2.9% and 3.0% in the ADHERE and the GWTG-HF registries, respectively.[32,35] The 1-year mortality was reported as 29.0%, 33.9%, and 16.2% in the Olmsted Country Study, GWTG-HF registry, and KorAHF registry, respectively.[28,32,54]

Few studies have evaluated the longitudinal trends of mortality in patients with HFpEF. In the GWTG-HF registry, the in-hospital mortality significantly improved from 3.3% in 2005% to 2.4% in 2010.[64] **Fig. 4** compares the mortality rates reported in the landmark trials of HFpEF. The mortality in the CHARM-Preserved trial was 15.7% and that in the PARAGON-HF trial was 8.9%.[10–13] However, the various definitions of HFpEF used

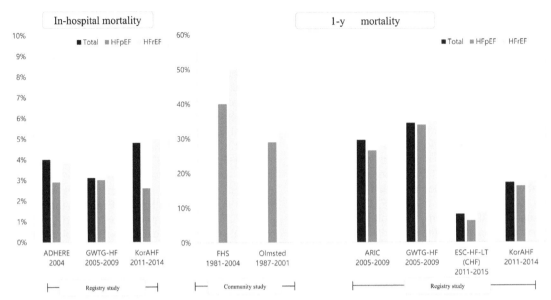

Fig. 3. Mortality of HF, HFpEF, and HFrEF. In most studies, the in-hospital and 1-year mortality rates of HFpEF were lower than those of HFrEF, although the differences were not significant. In the Olmsted Country Study, the mortality of patients with HFpEF was lower than that of patients with HFrEF. ADHERE, Acute Decompensated Heart Failure National Registry; ARIC, Atherosclerosis Risk in Communities Study; ESC-HF-LT, European Society of Cardiology-Heart Failure- Long Term; GWTG-HF, Get With The Guidelines–Heart Failure; FHS, Framingham Heart Study; KorAHF; Korean Acute Heart Failure; PREVEND, Prevention of Renal and Vascular Endstage Disease.

in clinical trials must be considered when interpreting the results.

Patients with any type of HF have higher mortality rates than patients without HF. The Early Framingham Heart Study reported that patients with HFpEF had an annual mortality rate of 8.7% and that participants without HF had an annual mortality rate of 3.0%.[64] However, comparisons of mortality between patients with HFpEF and those with HFrEF are inconsistent (see **Fig. 3**). In community-based studies, the

reported mortality was slightly higher in patients with HFrEF, although the differences between mortality in patients with HFpEF and in those with HFrEF were not significant.[42,43,65] In the Minneapolis study, the risk of mortality was lower in patients with HFpEF than that of patients with HFrEF.[66] The Olmsted Country Study reported that cardiovascular mortality was lower in patients with HFpEF and the noncardiovascular mortality was not different between patients with HFpEF and those with HFrEF.[38]

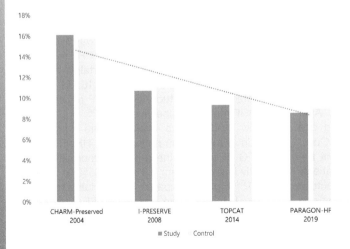

Fig. 4. The mortality of HFpEF in clinical trials. The mortality of the control group was 15.7% in the CHARM-Preserved trial and 8.9% in the PARAGON-HF trial. CHARM, Candesartan in Heart failure: Assessment of Reduction in Mortality and morbidity; I-PRESERVE, Irbesartan in Heart Failure with Preserved Ejection Fraction Study; PARAGON-HF, The Prospective Comparison of ARNI [angiotensin receptor–neprilysin inhibitor] with ARB [angiotensin-receptor blockers] Global Outcomes in HF with Preserved Ejection Fraction; TOPCAT, Treatment of Preserved Cardiac Function Heart Failure with an Aldosterone Antagonist.

FURTHER STUDIES

Recent studies have suggested that new echocardiographic parameters may be related to the prognosis of HFpEF. In an acute HF registry, global longitudinal strain measured by speckle-tracking echocardiography demonstrated greater prognostic value than LVEF.[67] Right ventricular function and pulmonary hypertension in HFpEF were also significant prognostic factors of HFpEF beyond LVEF.[68] Because HFpEF is a heterogeneous syndrome with diverse underlying pathophysiologic processes, diagnostic strategies including the use of multi-biomarker panels including natriuretic peptide, growth differentiation factor-15, galactin-3, and etc. may prove the usefulness in the diagnosis of HFpEF in the future.[69] Further epidemiologic studies with these emerging tools are needed to develop a simple and specific diagnostic tool for HFpEF.

SUMMARY

The reported prevalence of HFpEF is highly dependent on age and the underlying cardiovascular comorbidities of the study population. The establishment of effective preventative and treatment strategies for HFrEF has led to a decrease in the incidence of HFrEF. However, the proportion of patients with HFpEF among all patients with HF is increasing. HFpEF includes heterogeneous conditions, and the definition of HFpEF used in epidemiologic studies varies according to the study design and timeline. Therefore, the development of standard criteria for the definition of HFpEF to be used in epidemiologic studies is necessary. Emerging biomarkers and echocardiographic parameters may be useful tools to help overcome limitations of the current epidemiologic definitions of HFpEF. Last, previously reported epidemiologic studies are limited to developed Western countries and additional epidemiologic studies including patients of various races and ethnicities are required.

CLINICS CARE POINTS

- In the interpretation of epidemiologic studies, it is essential to understand the study population, study design, and definition of HFpEF.
- Although several epidemiologic studies used only clinical symptoms, signs, and LVEF, the current definition of HFpEF needs the multi-modality approach including biomarkers, echocardiographic morphologic and functional parameters.

- Because HFpEF is becoming the dominant form of HF owing to the aging population, clinicians should consider the high probability of HFpEF in the elderly with multiple comorbidities.

DISCLOSURE

The authors have no conflicts of interest to declare.

ACKNOWLEDGMENTS

This work was supported by the Research of Korea Disease Control and Prevention Agency (grant number 2019ER630300).

REFERENCES

1. Groenewegen A, Rutten FH, Mosterd A, et al. Epidemiology of heart failure. Eur J Heart Fail 2020;22(8): 1342–56.
2. Ponikowski P, Voors AA, Anker SD, et al. 2016 ESC Guidelines for the diagnosis and treatment of acute and chronic heart failure: the Task Force for the diagnosis and treatment of acute and chronic heart failure of the European Society of Cardiology (ESC) Developed with the special contribution of the Heart Failure Association (HFA) of the ESC. Eur Heart J 2016;37(27):2129–200.
3. Virani SS, Alonso A, Benjamin EJ, et al. Heart disease and stroke statistics-2020 update: a report from the American Heart Association. Circulation 2020;141(9):e139–596.
4. Andersson C, Vasan RS. Epidemiology of heart failure with preserved ejection fraction. Heart Fail Clin 2014;10(3):377–88.
5. Kim K-J, Cho H-J, Kim M-S, et al. Focused update of 2016 Korean Society of Heart Failure guidelines for the management of chronic heart failure. Int J Heart Fail 2019;1(1):4–24.
6. McKee PA, Castelli WP, McNamara PM, et al. The natural history of congestive heart failure: the Framingham study. N Engl J Med 1971;285(26):1441–6.
7. Pfeffer MA, Shah AM, Borlaug BA. Heart failure with preserved ejection fraction in perspective. Circ Res 2019;124(11):1598–617.
8. Reddy YNV, Carter RE, Obokata M, et al. A simple, evidence-based approach to help guide diagnosis of heart failure with preserved ejection fraction. Circulation 2018;138(9):861–70.
9. Pieske B, Tschope C, de Boer RA, et al. How to diagnose heart failure with preserved ejection fraction: the HFA-PEFF diagnostic algorithm: a consensus recommendation from the Heart Failure Association

(HFA) of the European Society of Cardiology (ESC). Eur Heart J 2019;40(40):3297–317.

10. Yusuf S, Pfeffer MA, Swedberg K, et al. Effects of candesartan in patients with chronic heart failure and preserved left-ventricular ejection fraction: the CHARM-Preserved Trial. Lancet 2003;362(9386): 777–81.

11. Massie BM, Carson PE, McMurray JJ, et al. Irbesartan in patients with heart failure and preserved ejection fraction. N Engl J Med 2008;359(23):2456–67.

12. Pitt B, Pfeffer MA, Assmann SF, et al. Spironolactone for heart failure with preserved ejection fraction. N Engl J Med 2014;370(15):1383–92.

13. Solomon SD, McMurray JJV, Anand IS, et al. Angiotensin-Neprilysin Inhibition in Heart Failure with Preserved Ejection Fraction. N Engl J Med 2019; 381(17):1609–20.

14. Anker SD, Butler J, Filippatos GS, et al. Evaluation of the effects of sodium-glucose co-transporter 2 inhibition with empagliflozin on morbidity and mortality in patients with chronic heart failure and a preserved ejection fraction: rationale for and design of the EMPEROR-Preserved Trial. Eur J Heart Fail 2019; 21(10):1279–87.

15. Dunlay SM, Roger VL, Redfield MM. Epidemiology of heart failure with preserved ejection fraction. Nat Rev Cardiol 2017;14(10):591–602.

16. Kupari M, Lindroos M, Iivanainen AM, et al. Congestive heart failure in old age: prevalence, mechanisms and 4-year prognosis in the Helsinki Ageing Study. J Intern Med 1997;241(5):387–94.

17. Morgan S, Smith H, Simpson I, et al. Prevalence and clinical characteristics of left ventricular dysfunction among elderly patients in general practice setting: cross sectional survey. BMJ 1999;318(7180): 368–72.

18. Mosterd A, Hoes AW, de Bruyne MC, et al. Prevalence of heart failure and left ventricular dysfunction in the general population; The Rotterdam Study. Eur Heart J 1999;20(6):447–55.

19. Devereux RB, Roman MJ, Liu JE, et al. Congestive heart failure despite normal left ventricular systolic function in a population-based sample: the Strong Heart Study. Am J Cardiol 2000;86(10):1090–6.

20. Cortina A, Reguero J, Segovia E, et al. Prevalence of heart failure in Asturias (a region in the north of Spain). Am J Cardiol 2001;87(12):1417–9.

21. Hedberg P, Lonnberg I, Jonason T, et al. Left ventricular systolic dysfunction in 75-year-old men and women; a population-based study. Eur Heart J 2001;22(8):676–83.

22. Ceia F, Fonseca C, Mota T, et al. Prevalence of chronic heart failure in Southwestern Europe: the EPICA study. Eur J Heart Fail 2002;4(4):531–9.

23. Gottdiener JS, McClelland RL, Marshall R, et al. Outcome of congestive heart failure in elderly persons: influence of left ventricular systolic function.

The Cardiovascular Health Study. Ann Intern Med 2002;137(8):631–9.

24. Redfield MM, Jacobsen SJ, Burnett JC Jr, et al. Burden of systolic and diastolic ventricular dysfunction in the community: appreciating the scope of the heart failure epidemic. JAMA 2003;289(2):194–202.

25. Degertekin M, Erol C, Ergene O, et al. [Heart failure prevalence and predictors in Turkey: HAPPY study]. Turk Kardiyol Dern Ars 2012;40(4):298–308.

26. Guo L, Guo X, Chang Y, et al. Prevalence and risk factors of heart failure with preserved ejection fraction: a population-based study in Northeast China. Int J Environ Res Public Health 2016;13(8):770.

27. Cui X, Zhou J, Jin X, et al. Prevalence and correlates of left ventricular diastolic dysfunction and heart failure with preserved ejection fraction in elderly community residents. Int J Cardiol 2017;227:820–5.

28. Cho JH, Choe WS, Cho HJ, et al. Comparison of characteristics and 3-year outcomes in patients with acute heart failure with preserved, mid-range, and reduced ejection fraction. Circ J 2019;83(2): 347–56.

29. Crespo-Leiro MG, Anker SD, Maggioni AP, et al. European Society of Cardiology Heart Failure Long-Term Registry (ESC-HF-LT): 1-year follow-up outcomes and differences across regions. Eur J Heart Fail 2016;18(6):613–25.

30. Gurwitz JH, Magid DJ, Smith DH, et al. Contemporary prevalence and correlates of incident heart failure with preserved ejection fraction. Am J Med 2013; 126(5):393–400.

31. Pandey A, Patel KV, Liang L, et al. Association of hospital performance based on 30-day risk-standardized mortality rate with long-term survival after heart failure hospitalization: an analysis of the get with the guidelines-heart failure registry. JAMA Cardiol 2018;3(6):489–97.

32. Powell-Wiley TM, Ngwa J, Kebede S, et al. Impact of body mass index on heart failure by race/ethnicity from the get with the guidelines-heart failure (GWTG-HF) registry. JACC Heart Fail 2018;6(3): 233–42.

33. Sharma A, Zhao X, Hammill BG, et al. Trends in non-cardiovascular comorbidities among patients hospitalized for heart failure: insights from the get with the guidelines-heart failure registry. Circ Heart Fail 2018; 11(6):e004646.

34. Tromp J, Teng TH, Tay WT, et al. Heart failure with preserved ejection fraction in Asia. Eur J Heart Fail 2019;21(1):23–36.

35. Yancy CW, Lopatin M, Stevenson LW, et al. Clinical presentation, management, and in-hospital outcomes of patients admitted with acute decompensated heart failure with preserved systolic function: a report from the Acute Decompensated Heart Failure National Registry (ADHERE) Database. J Am Coll Cardiol 2006;47(1):76–84.

36. Vaduganathan M, Michel A, Hall K, et al. Spectrum of epidemiological and clinical findings in patients with heart failure with preserved ejection fraction stratified by study design: a systematic review. Eur J Heart Fail 2016;18(1):54–65.

37. Ho JE, Lyass A, Lee DS, et al. Predictors of new-onset heart failure: differences in preserved versus reduced ejection fraction. Circ Heart Fail 2013; 6(2):279–86.

38. Gerber Y, Weston SA, Redfield MM, et al. A contemporary appraisal of the heart failure epidemic in Olmsted County, Minnesota, 2000 to 2010. JAMA Intern Med 2015;175(6):996–1004.

39. Silverman MG, Patel B, Blankstein R, et al. Impact of Race, Ethnicity, and Multimodality Biomarkers on the Incidence of New-Onset Heart Failure With Preserved Ejection Fraction (from the Multi-Ethnic Study of Atherosclerosis). Am J Cardiol 2016;117(9): 1474–81.

40. Brouwers FP, de Boer RA, van der Harst P, et al. Incidence and epidemiology of new onset heart failure with preserved vs. reduced ejection fraction in a community-based cohort: 11-year follow-up of PREVEND. Eur Heart J 2013;34(19):1424–31.

41. Tsao CW, Lyass A, Enserro D, et al. Temporal trends in the incidence of and mortality associated with heart failure with preserved and reduced ejection fraction. JACC Heart Fail 2018;6(8):678–85.

42. Lee DS, Gona P, Vasan RS, et al. Relation of disease pathogenesis and risk factors to heart failure with preserved or reduced ejection fraction: insights from the Framingham Heart Study of the National Heart, Lung, and Blood Institute. Circulation 2009; 119(24):3070–7.

43. Bursi F, Weston SA, Redfield MM, et al. Systolic and diastolic heart failure in the community. JAMA 2006; 296(18):2209–16.

44. Chang PP, Wruck LM, Shahar E, et al. Trends in Hospitalizations and Survival of Acute Decompensated Heart Failure in Four US Communities (2005-2014): ARIC Study Community Surveillance. Circulation 2018;138(1):12–24.

45. Crea F, Bairey Merz CN, Beltrame JF, et al. The parallel tales of microvascular angina and heart failure with preserved ejection fraction: a paradigm shift. Eur Heart J 2017;38(7):473–7.

46. Ho JE, Enserro D, Brouwers FP, et al. Predicting heart failure with preserved and reduced ejection fraction: the International Collaboration on Heart Failure Subtypes. Circ Heart Fail 2016;9(6).

47. Owan TE, Redfield MM. Epidemiology of diastolic heart failure. Prog Cardiovasc Dis 2005;47(5): 320–32.

48. Lam CS, Donal E, Kraigher-Krainer E, et al. Epidemiology and clinical course of heart failure with preserved ejection fraction. Eur J Heart Fail 2011; 13(1):18–28.

49. Nagueh SF, Smiseth OA, Appleton CP, et al. Recommendations for the evaluation of left ventricular diastolic function by echocardiography: an update from the American Society of Echocardiography and the European Association of Cardiovascular Imaging. Eur Heart J Cardiovasc Imaging 2016;17(12): 1321–60.

50. Seferovic PM, Petrie MC, Filippatos GS, et al. Type 2 diabetes mellitus and heart failure: a position statement from the Heart Failure Association of the European Society of Cardiology. Eur J Heart Fail 2018; 20(5):853–72.

51. Stewart Coats AJ. Common co-morbidities in heart failure–diabetes, functional mitral regurgitation and sleep apnoea. Int J Heart Fail 2019;1(1):25–41.

52. Savji N, Meijers WC, Bartz TM, et al. The Association of Obesity and Cardiometabolic Traits With Incident HFpEF and HFrEF. JACC Heart Fail 2018;6(8): 701–9.

53. Bhatia RS, Tu JV, Lee DS, et al. Outcome of heart failure with preserved ejection fraction in a population-based study. N Engl J Med 2006; 355(3):260–9.

54. Owan TE, Hodge DO, Herges RM, et al. Trends in prevalence and outcome of heart failure with preserved ejection fraction. N Engl J Med 2006; 355(3):251–9.

55. MacCarthy PA, Kearney MT, Nolan J, et al. Prognosis in heart failure with preserved left ventricular systolic function: prospective cohort study. BMJ 2003;327(7406):78–9.

56. Cho DH, Kim MA, Choi J, et al. Sex differences in the relationship between left ventricular diastolic dysfunction and coronary artery disease: from the Korean Women's Chest Pain Registry. J Womens Health (Larchmt) 2018;27(7):912–9.

57. Reddy YNV, Rikhi A, Obokata M, et al. Quality of life in heart failure with preserved ejection fraction: importance of obesity, functional capacity, and physical inactivity. Eur J Heart Fail 2020;22(6): 1009–18.

58. Lewis EF, Kim HY, Claggett B, et al. Impact of spironolactone on longitudinal changes in health-related quality of life in the treatment of preserved cardiac function heart failure with an aldosterone antagonist trial. Circ Heart Fail 2016;9(3):e001937.

59. Chandra A, Vaduganathan M, Lewis EF, et al. Health-related quality of life in heart failure with preserved ejection fraction: the PARAGON-HF Trial. JACC Heart Fail 2019;7(10):862–74.

60. Gheorghiade M, De Luca L, Fonarow GC, et al. Pathophysiologic targets in the early phase of acute heart failure syndromes. Am J Cardiol 2005;96(6A): 11G–7G.

61. Loop MS, Van Dyke MK, Chen L, et al. Comparison of length of stay, 30-day mortality, and 30-day readmission rates in Medicare patients with heart failure

and with reduced versus preserved ejection fraction. Am J Cardiol 2016;118(1):79–85.

62. Dunlay SM, Redfield MM, Weston SA, et al. Hospitalizations after heart failure diagnosis a community perspective. J Am Coll Cardiol 2009;54(18):1695–702.

63. Lee H-Y, Oh B-H. Paradigm shifts of heart failure therapy: do we need another paradigm? Int J Heart Fail 2020;2.

64. Steinberg BA, Zhao X, Heidenreich PA, et al. Trends in patients hospitalized with heart failure and preserved left ventricular ejection fraction: prevalence, therapies, and outcomes. Circulation 2012;126(1):65–75.

65. Vasan RS, Larson MG, Benjamin EJ, et al. Congestive heart failure in subjects with normal versus reduced left ventricular ejection fraction: prevalence and mortality in a population-based cohort. J Am Coll Cardiol 1999;33(7):1948–55.

66. Adabag S, Smith LG, Anand IS, et al. Sudden cardiac death in heart failure patients with preserved ejection fraction. J Card Fail 2012;18(10):749–54.

67. Park JJ, Park JB, Park JH, et al. Global Longitudinal Strain to Predict Mortality in Patients With Acute Heart Failure. J Am Coll Cardiol 2018;71(18):1947–57.

68. Ghio S, Guazzi M, Scardovi AB, et al. Different correlates but similar prognostic implications for right ventricular dysfunction in heart failure patients with reduced or preserved ejection fraction. Eur J Heart Fail 2017;19(7):873–9.

69. Tromp J, Khan MA, Klip IT, et al. Biomarker profiles in heart failure patients with preserved and reduced ejection fraction. J Am Heart Assoc 2017;6(4):e003989.

Pathophysiology of Heart Failure with Preserved Ejection Fraction

Jong-Chan Youn, MD, PhD[1], Yuran Ahn, MD[1], Hae Ok Jung, MD, PhD*

KEYWORDS

- Heart failure with preserved ejection fraction • Pathophysiology • Diastolic dysfunction
- Nondiastolic cardiac abnormality • Noncardiac abnormality

KEY POINTS

- HFpEF is increasing in prevalence, is associated with high morbidity and mortality, and has very few effective treatments.
- HFpEF is understood as a heterogeneous syndrome originating from the interplay of cardiac (central) and extracardiac (peripheral) abnormalities.
- The most important pathophysiology in patients with HFpEF is diastolic dysfunction. This may present with impairments in relaxation, increases in chamber stiffness, or both. These abnormalities lead to an increase in left ventricular filling pressures at rest or during exercise that causes dyspnea.
- In addition to diastolic dysfunction, patients with HFpEF display nondiastolic cardiac abnormalities including systolic dysfunction, pulmonary hypertension, right ventricular dysfunction, left atrial dysfunction, chronotropic incompetence, and noncardiac abnormalities including endothelial dysfunction, skeletal muscle abnormality, pulmonary disease, and renal dysfunction. The complex interplay of all of these pathophysiologic mechanisms is what drives symptoms and worsens outcome in HFpEF.

INTRODUCTION

Heart failure (HF) is an important cardiovascular disease because of its increasing prevalence, significant morbidity, high mortality, and rapidly expanding health care cost.[1] HF is a clinical syndrome characterized by distinct symptoms and signs, which is caused by structural and/or functional cardiac abnormalities.[1–4] Currently, the most common terminology for describing HF is based on left ventricular ejection fraction (LVEF). HF with normal LVEF (≥50%) is defined as HF with preserved ejection fraction (HFpEF), and HF with decreased LVEF (<40%) as HF with reduced ejection fraction (HFrEF).[1–4] Although there have

been steady developments regarding pharmacologic treatment for use in patients with HFrEF, no drugs have shown clear mortality benefits in patients with HFpEF.[5,6] Moreover, approximately half of the patients with specific signs and typical symptoms of HF have preserved LVEF. Therefore, HFpEF is one of the largest unmet clinical needs in the current cardiovascular medicine.[7–10]

TERMINOLOGY: DIASTOLIC DYSFUNCTION VERSUS DIASTOLIC HF VERSUS HEART FAILURE WITH PRESERVED EJECTION FRACTION

HFpEF is not equivalent to diastolic dysfunction.[10] Although several abnormalities in diastolic

Division of Cardiology, Department of Internal Medicine, Seoul St. Mary's Hospital, College of Medicine, The Catholic University of Korea, 222 Banpo-daero, Seocho-gu, Seoul 06591, Republic of Korea
[1] J.-C. Youn and Y. Ahn contributed equally to this article as first authors.
* Corresponding author.
E-mail address: hojheart@gmail.com

Heart Failure Clin 17 (2021) 327–335
https://doi.org/10.1016/j.hfc.2021.02.001
1551-7136/21/© 2021 Elsevier Inc. All rights reserved.

function form a major pathophysiologic basis for the development of the clinical syndrome of HFpEF, diastolic dysfunction and HFpEF are not synonymous. Diastolic dysfunction can be defined as a functional abnormality of diastolic relaxation, filling, or distensibility of the left ventricle (LV), regardless of whether the LVEF is preserved or reduced and whether the patient is symptomatic or not. Thus, diastolic dysfunction only refers to abnormal mechanical properties of the ventricle. HFpEF denotes the signs and symptoms of clinical HF in a patient with a preserved LVEF and diastolic dysfunction.

HFpEF and diastolic HF are not the same diagnostic terms.[7] In the 1980s and 1990s, the term "congestive HF" was widely used to encompass all those with the clinical signs and symptoms of HF across whole range of LVEF.[11] However, repeated observations that despite the same signs and symptoms, a proportion of those with HF with preserved systolic function led to the recognition that HF could also be the consequences of abnormalities in diastole, termed diastolic HF.[11] Since then, HFpEF and diastolic HF have been used interchangeably and confusedly for the past 20 years.[7] In principle, there are several alternative and complementary abnormalities in cardiac structure and function in HFpEF, including but not limited to diastolic dysfunction, thus favoring HFpEF terminology over diastolic HF.[12] Basic concepts of HFpEF compared with diastolic dysfunction and diastolic HF are shown in **Fig. 1**.

PATHOPHYSIOLOGY: DIASTOLIC DYSFUNCTION VERSUS NONDIASTOLIC ABNORMALITIES VERSUS NONCARDIAC ABNORMALITIES IN HEART FAILURE WITH PRESERVED EJECTION FRACTION

Although HFpEF was initially considered to be a hemodynamic disorder characterized by hypertension, cardiac hypertrophy, and diastolic dysfunction, it is now recognized to be a multisystem disorder involving the heart, lungs, kidneys, skeletal muscle, vascular system, and immune and inflammatory signaling.[13] Although diastolic dysfunction forms a major pathophysiologic basis for the development of the clinical syndrome of HFpEF, studies have shown that nondiastolic and noncardiac mechanisms also play an important role in the pathophysiology of HFpEF.[7,11–14] The heterogeneity of patient characteristics, organ-system involvement, and number of pathophysiological abnormalities that have been associated with established HFpEF support a multifactorial etiology in most patients.[15] Schematic pathophysiology of HFpEF, interplayed by central and peripheral mechanisms are shown in **Fig. 2**.

DIASTOLIC DYSFUNCTION IN HEART FAILURE WITH PRESERVED EJECTION FRACTION

LV filling pressure is a key index in the evaluation of pathophysiology, diagnosis, and treatment response of HFpEF. The elevation of LV filling pressure is the final product of diastolic dysfunctions including abnormal LV relaxation, LV stiffness, and poor compliance. The original assessment of LV filling pressure has been performed by the invasive cardiac catheterization. It is quite difficult to express LV filling pressure as a single value on the LV and left atrial (LA) pressure tracing because the pressures are easily fluctuated and LV filling is a complex process. Traditionally, cardiac catheterization–derived LV end-diastolic pressure (LVEDP), mean LV diastolic pressure, mean left atrial pressure (LAP), LV pre-A pressure, and pulmonary artery wedge pressure (PAWP) has been used interchangeably for an LV filling pressure (**Fig. 3**).[16,17]

Theoretically, mean LAP is the best parameter of LV filling pressure for determining dyspnea originated from pulmonary congestion because LV, LA, and pulmonary vein/capillary are interconnected in diastole. Because the placement of catheter in LA is too invasive, mean PAWP measured by balloon tip catheter on pulmonary artery has been widely used as a surrogate for mean LAP in clinical practice, and these 2 values are very closely consistent except at high LA pressure state.[17]

In contrast, LVEDP is the final diastolic pressure measured after LA contraction (A wave) just before systole, thus it is usually a higher than mean LA pressure or LV pre-A pressure. Because LVEDP can provide an estimate of LV end diastolic volume that means preload, the elevation of LVEDP means a state of comprehensive LV dysfunction. Elevation of LVEDP can be observed even in normal mean LAP, such as in poor LV compliance state. Thus LVEDP is a surrogate measure of LV preload and LV diastolic compliance. In a recent study, mean PAWP or LV pre-A pressure greater than 12 mm Hg, or LVEDP greater than 16 mm Hg were used interchangeably as abnormal LV filling pressures.[18] However, it should be noted that the different meanings between LVEDP and mean PAWP, unless the incorrect use of one term versus the other, can lead to erroneous conclusions on the relation between HF and patient symptoms.[19] The mean PAWP that integrates the atrial pressure tracing throughout systole and diastole provides a comprehensive measure of the hemodynamic

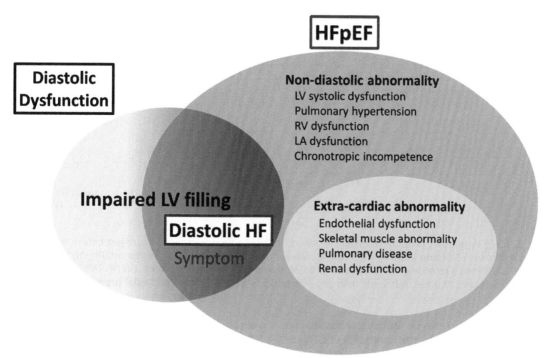

Fig. 1. Basic concepts of diastolic dysfunction, diastolic HF, and HFpEF.

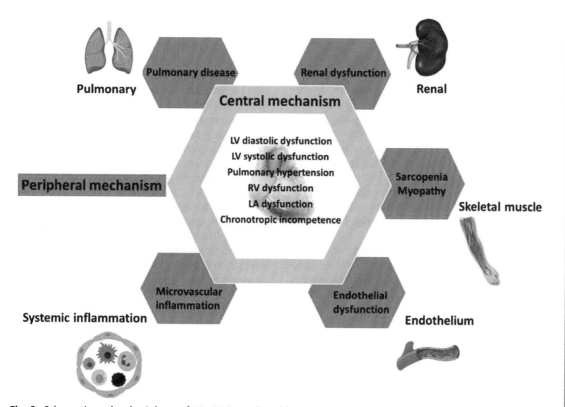

Fig. 2. Schematic pathophysiology of HFpEF, interplayed by central and peripheral mechanisms.

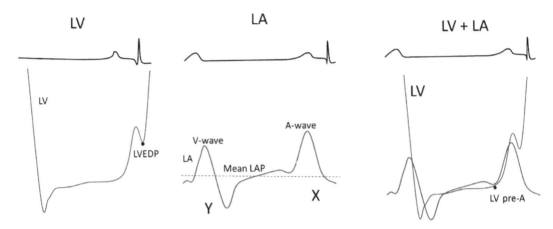

Fig. 3. (*Left*) LV diastolic pressure recording showing LVEDP, the final diastolic pressure just before systole. (*Middle*) LA pressure recording showing "V" and "A" waves marked along with Y and X descent. (*Right*) Simultaneous LV and LA pressure recording showing early and late transmitral pressure gradient. LVEDP: left ventricular end-diastolic pressure, LV pre-A: left ventricular pre-A pressure, Mean LAP: mean left atrial pressure.

burden imposed by the LA and LV compliance on the pulmonary circulation. In contrast, LVEDP provides only information about the LV compliance. The discrepancies between LVEDP and mean PAWP are particularly exaggerated in the presence of a large V-wave, as in mitral regurgitation, atrial fibrillation with poor atrial compliance, or stiff LA syndrome.[19,20] Because mean PAWP might be a better reflection of the cumulative hemodynamic impact of ventriculoatrial coupling and its compliance on the pulmonary circulation, it should be chosen in the evaluation of pulmonary hypertension associated with HFpEF.[20]

But the evaluation of LV filling pressure by cardiac catheterization is often not easy to perform in real clinical practice. Currently, echocardiography is the diagnostic method of choice for identifying patients with HFpEF because Doppler echocardiographic assessment has proved good accuracy to estimate LV filling pressure as well as ejection fraction, and moreover echocardiography can provide increased LV wall thickness and/or increased LA size as additive signs of increased filling pressures.[16,21,22]

Many studies have suggested the good correlation between echocardiography-derived E/e' (ratio of mitral early diastolic E velocity to average early diastolic e' velocity) and catheterization-derived LV filling pressure such as mean PAWP.[16,21,22] Average E/e' is the most feasible and reproducible index to predict the LV filling pressure. For example, average E/e' greater than 14 has high specificity for increased LV filling pressure, average E/e' less than 8 usually indicates normal LV filling pressure.[16] If LA volume index greater than 34 mL/m^2 and peak tricuspid regurgitation

velocity greater than 2.8 m/s are added to average E/e' greater than 14, the diagnostic accuracy for elevated LV filling pressure is increased.

CELLULAR AND MOLECULAR MECHANISMS OF DIASTOLIC DYSFUNCTION

Although HFpEF is a multifactorial, multiorgan disease, increased myocardial tissue stiffness is thought to play a key role in HFpEF pathophysiology. Increased LV chamber stiffness, as indicated by an upward-shifted and leftward-shifted LV end-diastolic pressure-volume relationship, is associated with worse outcomes in HFpEF and is caused by increased cardiomyocyte passive stiffness and myocardial fibrosis.[8] Underlying mechanisms include excitation–contraction coupling defects, sarcomere dysfunction, cyclic guanosine monophosphate (GMP)–protein kinase G (PKG) signaling deficiency, nitrosative–oxidative stress, microvascular insufficiency, inflammation, and mitochondrial and metabolic defects.[13] Among sarcomere dysfunction, titin, a giant sarcomere-spanning protein, is the main determinant of cardiomyocyte passive stiffness.[8,23,24] Titin-actin interactions are important for LV relaxation and several studies have shown that the stiffness of titin is elevated in HFpEF.[8,23,24] Stiffening is attributed to hypophosphorylation of titin that forms a molecular spring, which in turn is linked to depressed cyclic GMP-PKG activity.[13,23,24] Stiffer titin is correlated with reduced LV chamber compliance in diastole. Both in vitro and in vivo, activation of PKG or protein kinase A reversed these changes and improved muscle and LV chamber compliance.[13,23,24] Recently, genetic interventions revealed that increases or decreases in the stiffness of the titin spring region were associated with corresponding increases or decreases in LV diastolic stiffness.[8,25,26] Thus, titin could be a molecular target for improving LV diastolic dysfunction and symptoms in HFpEF.[8]

NONDIASTOLIC CARDIAC ABNORMALITIES IN HEART FAILURE WITH PRESERVED EJECTION FRACTION
Left Ventricular Systolic Dysfunction

While LVEF is normal in patients with HFpEF, LVEF is a poor and nonspecific index of contractile function. Studies evaluating load-independent myocardial contractile function have shown that there are decreases in systolic function in patients with HFpEF compared with age-matched healthy controls as well as asymptomatic hypertensive patients.[14,27] Inability to augment systolic function also begets and worsens diastolic reserve in HFpEF, by limiting elastic recoil and suction effects that normally facilitate filling. These relatively mild abnormalities in systolic function at rest become much more significant limitations during exercise, which further stresses an already compromised heart.[7,28] Prior studies have shown that the inability to augment cardiac output during exercise is related to poor systolic reserve, where contractile function cannot be augmented during stress in a normal fashion. This limits the ability to augment forward stroke volume and reduces cardiac output and end-organ perfusion.[7,28,29]

Pulmonary Hypertension

In the perspectives of HF specialist, pulmonary hypertension (PH) is one of the most important mechanism of dyspnea caused by HF. Elevated LV filling pressures from systolic dysfunction, diastolic dysfunction, atrial fibrillation, and/or valvular heart disease, can result in elevated pulmonary artery pressures. PH occurs in 60% to 80% of HF and has been known to be associated with high morbidity and mortality.[8,11,12,30] But the severity of PH in HF is highly variable, and contributing factors are not fully understood. Regardless of HFrEF or HFpEF, when PH develops in HF, the prognosis is quite poor.

On the other hand, in the perspective of PH specialists, PH due to left heart diseases means that pulmonary vascular changes have been developed in response to a backward transmission of filling pressures and has another name as group 2 PH.[31] PH due to left heart disease or group 2 PH can be defined as an increase in mean pulmonary arterial pressure (mean PAP) ≥25 mm Hg and

mean PAWP greater than 15 mm Hg as assessed by right heart catheterization (RHC).[32]

Traditionally, PH in HF has been also called a post-capillary PH because it can be developed in proportion to the pressure elevation of post-pulmonary capillary structures such as pulmonary vein, LA, or LV. If the precapillary pathologic changes or remodeling are added to post-capillary PH, it makes the prognosis more serious. In clinical practice, those conditions have been named isolated post-capillary PH (Ipc-PH or passive PH) and combined pre- and post-capillary PH (Cpc-PH, out-of-proportion PH). RHC of Ipc-PH shows an increase in mean PAP in proportion to the elevation of mean PAWP, normal diastolic pressure gradient (diastolic PAP – mean PAWP <7 mm Hg) and normal pulmonary vascular resistance (PVR<3 WU), whereas Cpc-PH can be diagnosed with mean PAP increases much more than the elevation of mean PAWP, increased diastolic pressure gradient ≥7 mm Hg, and/or PVR ≥3 WU.[31]

Guazzi and colleagues[30] compared HFpEF and HFrEF in the mechanisms to develop PH. We readily knew the differences in underlying etiologies and comorbidities between HFrEF and HFpEF. For example, typical patients with HFpEF have a phenotype as an old woman with obese and short stature, and more associated with diabetes mellitus, essential hypertension, LV hypertrophy, atrial fibrillation, and higher stiffness in major arteries and so forth. The investigators summarized that LA becomes stiffer earlier, atrial myopathy more susceptible to atrial fibrillation, more frequent functional MR, and vulnerable proinflammatory injury to pulmonary vasculatures may contribute to develop PH-HFpEF, especially Cpc-PH-HFpEF. Indeed, the frequency of Cpc-PH proved to be higher in HFpEF than HFrEF based on many retrospective analysis.[30–32]

Right Ventricular Dysfunction

Right ventricular (RV) dysfunction is common in HFpEF and longstanding PH leads to RV dysfunction, tricuspid regurgitation, and right-sided HF, which develops in approximately one-third of patients.[8,11,33–35] Similar to what is seen in the left side of the heart, there is also RV diastolic and systolic dysfunction in HFpEF.[34] RV dysfunction seems to develop more in patients with lower LVEF, with more severe PH, and in patients with atrial fibrillation. The presence of RV dysfunction is a potent marker of increased morbidity and mortality, independent of the severity of PH in HFpEF.[33–35] The development of RV dysfunction identifies patients with HFpEF with markedly increased risk of death and might be preventable through treatment of PH and associated risk factors.[11]

Left Atrial Dysfunction

Chronically elevated LV filling pressures promote LA remodeling and dysfunction, which contribute to increased burden of atrial fibrillation, worsening functional capacity, and increased mortality.[8] LA remodeling is central to the pathogenesis of both atrial fibrillation and HFpEF.[11,12,36–38] Whereas the LA in patients with HFrEF is typically enlarged with increased distensibility, LA reservoir function is diminished in patients with HFpEF. Accordingly, patients with HFrEF have larger LA volumes but lower peak LA pressures, whereas those with HFpEF have greater LA stiffness leading to relatively smaller LA volumes despite higher peak pressures.[36] The increases in LA pressures seen in HFpEF and atrial fibrillation may not be simply related to the retrograde transmission of LVEDPs, but instead reflect the hemodynamic consequences of the underlying atrial myopathy. Whereas the pulmonary wedge pressure is typically lower than the LV end-diastolic pressure in patients in sinus rhythm, the opposite is true in patients with left heart disease and atrial fibrillation.[36–38] Patients with HFpEF with LA dysfunction and atrial fibrillation are even more likely to also develop PH and right HF.[33,34]

Chronotropic Incompetence

Chronotropic incompetence is common in HFpEF and it contributes to reduced exercise capacity.[8,29,39,40] Cardiac output is equal to the product of stroke volume and heart rate, and the inability to augment heart rate with exercise, together with the known impairment in stroke volume reserve in HFpEF, greatly limits cardiac output responses to exercise in these patients.[29,39,40] However, the best way to define chronotropic incompetence in HFpEF and the risk and benefit of pharmacologic or nonpharmacologic (rate-adaptive pacing) intervention in these patients are largely unknown.[8]

NONCARDIAC ABNORMALITIES IN HEART FAILURE WITH PRESERVED EJECTION FRACTION
Endothelial Dysfunction

One potentially unifying mechanistic theory for central and peripheral abnormalities in HFpEF is comorbidity-driven systemic and microvascular inflammation, leading to oxidative stress, causing reduced nitric oxide (NO) bioavailability, impaired soluble guanylate cyclase activity, reduced GMP, and thus reduced PKG signaling.[8,41] Obesity,

insulin resistance, hypertension, and aging are frequently observed comorbidities in HFpEF that are closely associated with endothelial dysfunction.[41–44] Deranged NO–cyclic GMP-PKG signaling, driven by comorbidities and aging, may be the fundamental abnormality in HFpEF, resulting in a systemic inflammatory state and microvascular endothelial dysfunction.[8,11,15,45]

Aortic and conduit vessel stiffness is increased in HFpEF, leading to excessive blood pressure variability and greater arterial afterload mismatch, particularly during exercise.[7,10,11,29,46] The normal reduction in systemic vascular resistance with exercise is blunted in patients with HFpEF, and arterial stiffness is elevated, which leads to earlier arrival of reflected waves to the heart, increasing pulsatile arterial loading, which exacerbates LV remodeling, fibrosis, diastolic dysfunction, and pulmonary venous hypertension.[8]

Microvascular function is also impaired in the peripheral arteries, evidenced by impaired flow-mediated dilation during reactive hyperemia in HFpEF.[11,29] Endothelium-dependent vasodilation is impaired in HFpEF, and the presence and severity of endothelial dysfunction is associated with more severe HF symptoms, worse exercise capacity, and increased risk for HF hospitalization.[8,11,41,42]

Skeletal Muscle Abnormality

Recent studies have identified that skeletal muscle mass is reduced in HFpEF, beyond that which is observed with normal aging, and directly contributes to exercise limitation.[15] Skeletal muscle composition is also altered in HFpEF, with increased fatty infiltration and frank sarcopenia, even when total body weight is increased.[11] The ability to enhance oxygen extraction in skeletal muscle is impaired in HFpEF because of an inability to augment diffusional conductance for gas transfer within skeletal muscle, and an inability to improve oxygen utilization, likely at least in part because of mitochondrial dysfunction.[11,47] Although the pathogenesis of mitochondrial dysfunction in HFpEF is unclear, possible causes include chronic elevation of sympathetic tone, oxidative stress, and low-grade systemic inflammation.[47–49] Improvements in physical capacity noted with exercise training appear to be mediated not by the central mechanisms, but rather by improvement in peripheral mechanisms (improved microvascular and/or skeletal muscle function).[49,50]

Pulmonary Disease

Given the presence of elevated LV filling pressure in patients with HFpEF, pulmonary disease is unsurprisingly also common.[13] In some patients, there is a progressive increase in pulmonary vascular resistance in addition to passive elevation of LA pressures, referred to as combined precapillary and postcapillary PH or HFpEF with pulmonary vascular disease.[8] Pulmonary venous and small vessel intimal thickening and fibrosis are more severe than pulmonary arterial intimal thickening in patients with HFpEF, analogous to that seen in pulmonary venoocclusive disease.[8,51,52] Reduced alveolar capillary membrane conductance and pulmonary capillary blood volume are associated with a significant reduction in gas diffusion capacity at rest, which worsened to a robust reduction with exercise contributing to exertional intolerance.[13] Remodeling and pulmonary vasoconstriction limit the ability of the RV to transfer blood into the lungs as venous return increases, causing right-sided heart overload, heightened pericardial restraint, and compromised LV filling through enhanced ventricular interdependence.[8,51,52] The result is reduced stroke volume and, consequently, cardiac output. The right ventricle in patients with HFpEF can be particularly prone to the development of fibrosis with increased pulmonary vascular load.[13]

Renal Dysfunction

There is important bidirectional cross talk between the heart and kidney.[8,13,53] Although renal dysfunction is an important contributor to the development of HFpEF, venous congestion is also common in HFpEF and may contribute to worsening renal function.[8,13,53] Elevated renal vein pressure, particularly in the setting of low systemic blood pressure, can result in transglomerular gradient and thereby reduce kidney perfusion.[8] Renal venous hypertension may also impair renal function as a result of intrarenal congestion, which can further impede renal perfusion. Renal insufficiency is linked to elevated central venous pressures and therefore RV workload, contributing to RV failure, a major predictor of adverse outcomes in patients with HFpEF.[13] The underlying mechanisms between the bidirectional heart kidney relationships in HFpEF is not fully understood yet but clearly drive HFpEF pathophysiology.[8] Understanding the role of the kidney in determining why some patients with the myocardial substrate for HFpEF do not develop volume overload whereas others do could lead to improved strategies to prevent HFpEF and limit HF hospitalizations in patients with prevalent HFpEF.[8]

SUMMARY

HFpEF is a major public health problem, which affects half of all patients with HF. It is increasing in prevalence, is associated with high morbidity and mortality, and has very few effective treatments. HFpEF is one of the largest unmet clinical needs in current cardiovascular medicine. HFpEF is understood as a heterogeneous syndrome originating from the interplay of cardiac (central) and extracardiac (peripheral) abnormalities. The most important pathophysiology in patients with HFpEF is diastolic dysfunction, which presents with impairments in relaxation and/or increases in chamber stiffness. These abnormalities lead to an increase in LV filling pressures at rest or during exercise that causes dyspnea. In addition to diastolic dysfunction, patients with HFpEF display nondiastolic cardiac abnormalities including systolic dysfunction, PH, RV dysfunction, LS dysfunction, chronotropic incompetence, and noncardiac abnormalities, including endothelial dysfunction, skeletal muscle abnormality, pulmonary disease, and renal dysfunction. The complex interplay of all of these pathophysiologic mechanisms is what drives symptoms and worsens outcome in HFpEF.

CLINICS CARE POINTS

- HFpEF is not equivalent to diastolic dysfunction. Diastolic dysfunction only refers to abnormal mechanical properties of the ventricle, whereas HFpEF denotes the signs and symptoms of clinical HF in a patient with a preserved LVEF and diastolic dysfunction.

- HFpEF and diastolic HF are not the same diagnostic terms. There are several alternative and complementary abnormalities in cardiac structure and function in HFpEF, including but not limited to diastolic dysfunction, thus favoring HFpEF terminology over diastolic HF.

ACKNOWLEDGMENTS

This research was supported by the Basic Science Research Program through the National Research Foundation of Korea (NRF) funded by the Ministry of Science, ICT & Future Planning (NRF-2018R1C1B6005448). The funders had no role in study design, data collection and analysis, decision to publish, or preparation of the manuscript.

DISCLOSURE

The authors have nothing to disclose.

REFERENCES

1. Choi HM, Park MS, Youn JC. Update on heart failure management and future directions. Korean J Intern Med 2019;34(1):11–43.
2. Ponikowski P, Voors AA, Anker SD, et al. 2016 ESC Guidelines for the diagnosis and treatment of acute and chronic heart failure: The Task Force for the diagnosis and treatment of acute and chronic heart failure of the European Society of Cardiology (ESC) Developed with the special contribution of the Heart Failure Association (HFA) of the ESC. Eur Heart J 2016;37(27):2129–200.
3. Kim K-J, Cho H-J, Kim M-S, et al. Focused update of 2016 Korean Society of Heart Failure Guidelines for the Management of Chronic Heart Failure. Int J Heart Fail 2019;1(1):4–24.
4. Lee JH, Kim MS, Yoo BS, et al. KSHF guidelines for the management of acute heart failure: part II. Treatment of acute heart failure. Korean Circ J 2019; 49(1):22–45.
5. Lee H-Y, Oh B-H. Paradigm shifts of heart failure therapy: do we need another paradigm? Int J Heart Fail 2020;2(3):145–56.
6. Kim E-S, Youn J-C, Baek SH. Update on the pharmacotherapy of heart failure with reduced ejection fraction. Cardiovasc Prev Pharmacother 2020;2(4): 113–33.
7. Shim CY. Heart failure with preserved ejection fraction: the major unmet need in cardiology. Korean Circ J 2020;50(12):1051–61.
8. Shah SJ, Borlaug BA, Kitzman DW, et al. Research priorities for heart failure with preserved ejection fraction: national heart, lung, and blood institute working group summary. Circulation 2020;141(12):1001–26.
9. Kim MN, Park SM. Heart failure with preserved ejection fraction: insights from recent clinical researches. Korean J Intern Med 2020;35(3):514–34.
10. Yoon S, Eom GH. Heart failure with preserved ejection fraction: present status and future directions. Exp Mol Med 2019;51(12):1–9.
11. Pfeffer MA, Shah AM, Borlaug BA. Heart failure with preserved ejection fraction in perspective. Circ Res 2019;124(11):1598–617.
12. Nagueh SF. Heart failure with preserved ejection fraction: insights into diagnosis and pathophysiology. Cardiovasc Res 2021;117:999–1014.
13. Mishra S, Kass DA. Cellular and molecular pathobiology of heart failure with preserved ejection fraction. Nat Rev Cardiol 2021. https://doi.org/10.1038/s41569-020-00480-6.
14. Borlaug BA. The pathophysiology of heart failure with preserved ejection fraction. Nat Rev Cardiol 2014;11(9):507–15.
15. Zakeri R, Cowie MR. Heart failure with preserved ejection fraction: controversies, challenges and future directions. Heart 2018;104(5):377–84.
16. Nagueh SF, Smiseth OA, Appleton CP, et al. Recommendations for the evaluation of left ventricular diastolic function by echocardiography: an update from the American Society of Echocardiography and the European Association of Cardiovascular Imaging. J Am Soc Echocardiogr 2016;29(4):277–314.
17. Peverill RE. "Left ventricular filling pressure(s)" - Ambiguous and misleading terminology, best abandoned. Int J Cardiol 2015;191:110–3.
18. Andersen OS, Smiseth OA, Dokainish H, et al. Estimating left ventricular filling pressure by echocardiography. J Am Coll Cardiol 2017;69(15):1937–48.
19. Mascherbauer J, Zotter-Tufaro C, Duca F, et al. Wedge pressure rather than left ventricular end-diastolic pressure predicts outcome in heart failure with preserved ejection fraction. JACC Heart Fail 2017;5(11):795–801.
20. Reddy YNV, El-Sabbagh A, Nishimura RA. Comparing pulmonary arterial wedge pressure and left ventricular end diastolic pressure for assessment of left-sided filling pressures. JAMA Cardiol 2018;3(6):453–4.
21. Ommen SR, Nishimura RA, Appleton CP, et al. Clinical utility of Doppler echocardiography and tissue Doppler imaging in the estimation of left ventricular filling pressures: a comparative simultaneous Doppler-catheterization study. Circulation 2000; 102(15):1788–94.
22. Nagueh SF, Middleton KJ, Kopelen HA, et al. Doppler tissue imaging: a noninvasive technique for evaluation of left ventricular relaxation and estimation of filling pressures. J Am Coll Cardiol 1997; 30(6):1527–33.
23. Zile MR, Baicu CF, Ikonomidis JS, et al. Myocardial stiffness in patients with heart failure and a preserved ejection fraction: contributions of collagen and titin. Circulation 2015;131(14):1247–59.
24. Kruger M, Kotter S, Grutzner A, et al. Protein kinase G modulates human myocardial passive stiffness by phosphorylation of the titin springs. Circ Res 2009; 104(1):87–94.
25. Methawasin M, Strom JG, Slater RE, et al. Experimentally increasing the compliance of titin through RNA binding Motif-20 (RBM20) inhibition improves diastolic function in a mouse model of heart failure with preserved ejection fraction. Circulation 2016; 134(15):1085–99.
26. Methawasin M, Hutchinson KR, Lee EJ, et al. Experimentally increasing titin compliance in a novel mouse model attenuates the Frank-Starling mechanism but has a beneficial effect on diastole. Circulation 2014;129(19):1924–36.
27. Borlaug BA, Lam CS, Roger VL, et al. Contractility and ventricular systolic stiffening in hypertensive heart disease insights into the pathogenesis of heart failure with preserved ejection fraction. J Am Coll Cardiol 2009;54(5):410–8.

28. Borlaug BA, Kane GC, Melenovsky V, et al. Abnormal right ventricular-pulmonary artery coupling with exercise in heart failure with preserved ejection fraction. Eur Heart J 2016;37(43):3293–302.

29. Borlaug BA, Olson TP, Lam CS, et al. Global cardiovascular reserve dysfunction in heart failure with preserved ejection fraction. J Am Coll Cardiol 2010;56(11):845–54.

30. Guazzi M, Ghio S, Adir Y. Pulmonary hypertension in HFpEF and HFrEF: JACC review topic of the week. J Am Coll Cardiol 2020;76(9):1102–11.

31. Galie N, Humbert M, Vachiery JL, et al. 2015 ESC/ERS Guidelines for the diagnosis and treatment of pulmonary hypertension: The Joint Task Force for the Diagnosis and Treatment of Pulmonary Hypertension of the European Society of Cardiology (ESC) and the European Respiratory Society (ERS): Endorsed by: Association for European Paediatric and Congenital Cardiology (AEPC), International Society for Heart and Lung Transplantation (ISHLT). Eur Heart J 2016;37(1):67–119.

32. Vachiery JL, Tedford RJ, Rosenkranz S, et al. Pulmonary hypertension due to left heart disease. Eur Respir J 2019;53(1).

33. Mohammed SF, Hussain I, AbouEzzeddine OF, et al. Right ventricular function in heart failure with preserved ejection fraction: a community-based study. Circulation 2014;130(25):2310–20.

34. Melenovsky V, Hwang SJ, Lin G, et al. Right heart dysfunction in heart failure with preserved ejection fraction. Eur Heart J 2014;35(48):3452–62.

35. Gorter TM, van Veldhuisen DJ, Bauersachs J, et al. Right heart dysfunction and failure in heart failure with preserved ejection fraction: mechanisms and management. Position statement on behalf of the Heart Failure Association of the European Society of Cardiology. Eur J Heart Fail 2018;20(1):16–37.

36. Packer M, Lam CSP, Lund LH, et al. Interdependence of atrial fibrillation and heart failure with a preserved ejection fraction reflects a common underlying atrial and ventricular myopathy. Circulation 2020;141(1):4–6.

37. Kim M-N, Park S-M, Kim H-D, et al. Assessment of the left ventricular diastolic function and its association with the left atrial pressure in patients with atrial fibrillation. Int J Heart Fail 2020;2(1):55–65.

38. Casaclang-Verzosa G. Diastolic function assessment in atrial fibrillation conundrum. Int J Heart Fail 2020;2(2):115–7.

39. Brubaker PH, Kitzman DW. Chronotropic incompetence: causes, consequences, and management. Circulation 2011;123(9):1010–20.

40. Borlaug BA, Melenovsky V, Russell SD, et al. Impaired chronotropic and vasodilator reserves limit exercise capacity in patients with heart failure and a preserved ejection fraction. Circulation 2006; 114(20):2138–47.

41. Paulus WJ, Tschope C. A novel paradigm for heart failure with preserved ejection fraction: comorbidities drive myocardial dysfunction and remodeling through coronary microvascular endothelial inflammation. J Am Coll Cardiol 2013;62(4):263–71.

42. Shah SJ, Kitzman DW, Borlaug BA, et al. Phenotype-specific treatment of heart failure with preserved ejection fraction: a multiorgan roadmap. Circulation 2016;134(1):73–90.

43. Stewart Coats AJ. Common co-morbidities in heart failure – diabetes, functional mitral regurgitation and sleep Apnoea. Int J Heart Fail 2019;1(1):25–41.

44. Shen Q, Hiebert JB, Rahman FK, et al. Understanding obesity-related high output heart failure and its implications. Int J Heart Fail 2021;3.

45. Youn JC, Jung MK, Yu HT, et al. Increased frequency of CD4(+)CD57(+) senescent T cells in patients with newly diagnosed acute heart failure: exploring new pathogenic mechanisms with clinical relevance. Sci Rep 2019;9(1):12887.

46. Weber T. The role of arterial stiffness and central hemodynamics in heart failure. Int J Heart Fail 2020; 2(4):209–30.

47. Kumar AA, Kelly DP, Chirinos JA. Mitochondrial dysfunction in heart failure with preserved ejection fraction. Circulation 2019;139(11):1435–50.

48. Youn JC, Choi SW, Lee HS, et al. Prognostic value of leg muscle strength in acute heart failure syndrome. Med Sci Sports Exerc 2021;53(1):19–25.

49. Chun K-H, Kang S-M. Cardiac rehabilitation in heart failure. Int J Heart Fail 2021;3(1):1–14.

50. Haykowsky MJ, Brubaker PH, Stewart KP, et al. Effect of endurance training on the determinants of peak exercise oxygen consumption in elderly patients with stable compensated heart failure and preserved ejection fraction. J Am Coll Cardiol 2012;60(2):120–8.

51. Gorter TM, Obokata M, Reddy YNV, et al. Exercise unmasks distinct pathophysiologic features in heart failure with preserved ejection fraction and pulmonary vascular disease. Eur Heart J 2018;39(30): 2825–35.

52. Fayyaz AU, Edwards WD, Maleszewski JJ, et al. Global pulmonary vascular remodeling in pulmonary hypertension associated with heart failure and preserved or reduced ejection fraction. Circulation 2018;137(17):1796–810.

53. Unger ED, Dubin RF, Deo R, et al. Association of chronic kidney disease with abnormal cardiac mechanics and adverse outcomes in patients with heart failure and preserved ejection fraction. Eur J Heart Fail 2016;18(1):103–12.

Hypertension and Heart Failure with Preserved Ejection Fraction

Chan Joo Lee, MD, PhD, Sungha Park, MD, PhD*

KEYWORDS

- Antihypertensive agents • Blood pressure • Hypertension • Heart failure

KEY POINTS

- Hypertension increases the risk of heart failure (HF) by 2 to 3 folds and is the most common and important risk factor, especially for HF with preserved ejection fraction (HFpEF).
- Treatment of hypertension reduces the incidence of HF; although randomized clinical trials evaluating the efficacy of pharmacotherapy of hypertension in HFpEF are lacking, an initial combination of renin-angiotensin system inhibitors, diuretics, and spironolactone could be helpful.
- Although valsartan/sacubitril and spironolactone have failed to show an improvement in the outcomes in HFpEF patients, these drugs have shown a positive effect in a relatively low EF subgroup.

INTRODUCTION

There is a current epidemic of congestive heart failure (CHF) throughout the world, including Korea, where its current prevalence in adults is 1% to 3%.[1] The prevalence of HF in Korea increased from 0.75% in 2002 to 1.53% in 2013 and is estimated to increase to 3.35% by 2040.[2] HF is most commonly classified according to the left ventricular ejection fraction (LVEF) as follows: HF with reduced EF (<40%, HFrEF), HF with midrange EF (41–49%, HFmrEF), and HF with preserved EF (>50%, HFpEF). HFpEF develops in approximately 50% of cases of CHF and is associated with high mortality and morbidity. In a study of hospitalized patients with HF, both 1-year (32% vs 29%) and 5-year (68% vs 65%) mortality rates were slightly higher in HFrEF patients compared with those in HFpEF patients.[1,3] Hypertension is one of the common risk factors of HFpEF, and its treatment prevents the development of HF.[4] This article discusses the pathophysiological mechanisms linking hypertension with HFpEF, as well as the current evidence on the treatment of hypertension with HFpEF.

PATHOPHYSIOLOGICAL MECHANISMS LINKING HYPERTENSION AND HEART FAILURE WITH PRESERVED EJECTION FRACTION

In the Framingham Heart Study, hypertension antedated the development of HF in 91% of incident HF cases during 20 years, and the risk of HF was increased by two- and threefold in male and female hypertensive patients, respectively.[5,6] Classically, the paradigm of hypertension-induced HFpEF is hypertension-induced left ventricular (LV) hypertrophy, which results in left atrial remodeling and longitudinal systolic and diastolic dysfunctions, eventually resulting in clinical HF.[6] However, many cases of HFpEF do not conform to these classic paradigms. In an analysis of the Irbesartan in Heart Failure with Preserved Ejection Fraction Study (I-PRESERVE), the Candesartan in Heart failure: Assessment of Reduction in Mortality and morbidity (CHARM)-Preserved, and the Treatment of Preserved Cardiac Function Heart Failure with an Aldosterone Antagonist (TOPCAT) trial, approximately one-third to two-thirds of patients with HFpEF did not have LVH, and one-third to one-half of patients had normal left atrial size. Moreover, approximately

Division of Cardiology, Department of Internal Medicine, Severance Hospital, Yonsei University College of Medicine, 50-1 Yonsei-ro, Seodaemun-gu, Seoul 03722, Republic of Korea
* Corresponding author.
E-mail address: shpark0530@yuhs.ac

Heart Failure Clin 17 (2021) 337–343
https://doi.org/10.1016/j.hfc.2021.02.002
1551-7136/21/© 2021 Elsevier Inc. All rights reserved.

half of the patients had normal to mildly impaired LV diastolic function.[7–10] This might be because the pathophysiology of HFpEF is not a single uniform process but rather a manifestation of multiple, heterogeneous derangements involving myocardial and peripheral vascular function.[11] Moreover, there has been a shift in the proposed pathophysiology of HFpEF from that of isolated structural abnormality of the heart to that of multiorgan dysfunction, including the heart, because of an augmented systemic inflammation resulting from multiple comorbidities.[12] It has been proposed that multiple comorbidities, such as obesity, diabetes mellitus, hypertension, and chronic obstructive pulmonary disease, induce a proinflammatory state resulting in coronary microvascular endothelial dysfunction, reduced bioavailability of nitric oxide, reduced cyclic guanosine monophosphate, and reduced protein kinase G (PKG) activity in the cardiomyocytes. The low PKG activity results in the development of LV hypertrophy and increased LV stiffness.[13] This is supported by the fact that patients with hypertension and HFpEF, but not patients with isolated hypertension, have increased collagen-dependent and titin-dependent stiffness because of higher collagen deposition and changes in titin phosphorylation, which are characteristic changes observed in the myocardium of patients with HFpEF.[14]

Hypertension is characterized by increased arterial elastance (Ea) and LV end-systolic elastance (Ees). The increase in Ees to compensate for the elevated Ea will result in impaired LV contractile reserve during exertion or during episodes of increased afterload, which predisposes hypertensive patients to an increased risk of developing HF when exposed to an increased arterial pulsatile load.[15] In an analysis of 5960 participants of the Multiethnic Study of Atherosclerosis (MESA), hypertensive subjects with an elevated reflected wave magnitude had approximately 4 times the risk of developing cardiovascular events compared with normotensive subjects without an elevated reflected wave magnitude.[16] In addition, hypertensive HFpEF is characterized by multiple impairments of the cardiovascular functional reserve, such as exercise-induced increase in chronotropy, contractility, and peripheral vasodilatation, which may all act in synchrony to induce HF.[17]

TREATMENT OF HYPERTENSION IN HEART FAILURE WITH PRESERVED EJECTION FRACTION

Unlike HFrEF, randomized clinical trials have failed to demonstrate significant benefits of renin-angiotensin system (RAS) inhibitors, aldosterone antagonists, and sacubitril/valsartan in HFpEF.[8–10,18,19] Although the reason is unclear, it may be because of multiple comorbidities that are associated with HFpEF and the heterogeneous phenotypes of HFpEF. HFpEF is characterized by an association of multiple comorbidities, such as coronary artery disease, hypertension, diabetes mellitus, chronic kidney disease, obesity, and obstructive sleep apnea, which contribute to increasing the risk of non-HF-related morbidity and mortality.[20,21] Hence, treating comorbidities may be just as important as treating the HF itself and emphasized in the guideline.[22] Among the important comorbidities of HFpEF, hypertension is the most prevalent comorbidity and the most common risk factor and plays a critical role in the progression of HFpEF. Therefore, treatment of hypertension and maintaining BP below the treatment goal is essential. Both the latest American College of Cardiology (ACC)/American Heart Association (AHA) hypertension guideline and the European Society of Hypertension (ESH)/European Society of Cardiology (ESC) guideline recommend intensive BP lowering below 130/80 mm Hg for patients with HF.[23,24] However, despite the importance of hypertension in HFpEF, there have been no randomized clinical trials demonstrating the efficacy of hypertension treatment in HFpEF, as patients with HF are mostly excluded from hypertension trials. The case in the discussion is the Systolic Blood Pressure Intervention Trial (SPRINT), which excluded subjects with symptomatic HF or those with LVEF of less than 35%.[25] However, randomized clinical trials performed in hypertensive patients have clearly demonstrated the benefit of lowering BP in preventing HF. The SPRINT showed a 37% reduction in acute decompensated HF in the intensive treatment group.[26] The Hypertension in the Very Elderly Trial (HYVET), which enrolled elderly hypertensive patients (>80 years), showed a 64% reduction of HF incidence after a median follow-up of 2 years.[4] In a recent post-hoc analysis of the Prospective Comparison of ARNI with ARB Global Outcomes in HF With Preserved Ejection Fraction (PARAGON-HF) trial, a mean systolic BP of 120 to 129 mm Hg was associated with the lowest risk for the composite endpoint, cardiovascular mortality, total HF-related hospitalization, and myocardial infarction or stroke, thereby supporting the recommendations of intensive BP lowering in patients with HF.[27] The control of BP is important to reduce both HF aggravation and the incidence of myocardial infarction or stroke, considering the high prevalence of comorbidities associated with HFpEF. However, in a cohort study of elderly HFpEF patients with hypertension, a systolic BP of less than 130 mm Hg was not associated with a reduction in all-cause mortality, whereas a systolic BP of less than 120 mm Hg was associated with a higher risk of all-cause mortality compared with a systolic BP of greater than 130 mm Hg.[28] The causal relationship could not be evaluated, because it was not a randomized clinical trial. However, it suggests that a low BP may be associated with adverse events in HFpEF patients who are elderly or have multiple comorbidities. On the other hand, this may be because of a reverse causality phenomenon, as sicker HF patients will tend to have a lower BP. Therefore, further prospective studies are needed to evaluate the optimal BP in HFpEF patients.

Renin-Angiotensin System Inhibitors

Among the first-class anti-hypertensive drugs used in the treatment of hypertension, RAS inhibitors seem to be the obvious first choice considering their efficacy in HFrEF. Disappointingly, randomized clinical trials have not demonstrated a clear efficacy of RAS inhibitors in HEpEF, especially the CHARM-Preserve (candesartan vs placebo),[8] The Perindopril in Elderly People with Chronic Heart Failure Trial (perindopril vs placebo),[18] and I-PRESERVE (irbesartan vs placebo)[9] trials failed to demonstrate a significant reduction in the primary outcomes. Despite this, RAS inhibitors have clearly demonstrated efficacy in reducing LV hypertrophy and benefit for common comorbidities such as coronary heart disease and chronic kidney disease, and thus, are recommended as initial drugs of choice for hypertensive subjects with HFpEF unless contraindicated. In the TOPCAT trial, spironolactone did not significantly reduce the primary outcome compared with control. However, there was a significant reduction in HF-related hospitalization.[10] Moreover, when data from Russia and Georgia were excluded from the analysis, there was a significant reduction in the primary outcome.[29] Despite the negative results of the previously-mentioned trials, a post hoc analysis of the I-PRESERVE and the TOPCAT trials demonstrated significant interactions with the baseline N-terminal-pro hormone brain natriuretic peptide (NT-proBNP) levels; there was a significant benefit with irbesartan and spironolactone in patients with a lower baseline NT-proBNP levels.[30,31] It is worth noting that in a subgroup analysis of the I-PRESERVE trial,

patients with obesity, diabetes mellitus, dyslipidemia, and coronary artery disease had a significant reduction in the primary outcomes with irbesartan.[32] Similarly, in a subgroup analysis of the TOPCAT trial, spironolactone use was associated with a significant reduction of primary endpoints (hazard ratio: 0.75, 95% confidence interval [CI]: 0.59–0.95, P-value for interaction = .016) in a subgroup of patients with more functional impairment, obesity, diabetes mellitus, chronic kidney disease, and concentric LV hypertrophy.[33]

One of the common denominators of the previously mentioned findings is obesity. Patients with obesity-related HFpEF are characterized by NT-proBNP levels that are lower than expected from the filling pressure that is often below the traditional diagnostic threshold, overactivation of the renin-angiotensin-aldosterone system, and direct synthesis of aldosterone by adipocytes. Perhaps this may explain the benefits of irbesartan and spironolactone in obese HFpEF patients with relatively lower NT-proBNP levels.[34] When considering that HFpEF is an amalgam of heterogeneous phenotypes, clinical trials focusing on a more homogenous group of patients, such as those with obesity-associated HFpEF, may be needed in the future.[34]

Diuretics

Diuresis plays an important role in controlling BP, as well as improving symptoms of HF. Chlorthalidone is a thiazide-like diuretic that is effective in reducing the incidence of HF in hypertensive patients. In the Antihypertensive and Lipid-Lowering Treatment to Prevent Heart Attack Trial, chlorthalidone significantly reduced the risk of new-onset hospitalized HFpEF compared with lisinopril, amlodipine, and doxazosin.[35] When considering the initial combination treatment of hypertension with HFpEF, adding a RAS inhibitor with a diuretic (thiazide or thiazide-like/loop diuretic) and low-dose spironolactone to reduce hospitalization seems prudent with vigilant monitoring for hyperkalemia and acute kidney injury (**Fig. 1**).

Beta-Blockers

The efficacy of beta-blockers in HFpEF is not clear. In a meta-analysis of individual patient data of HF patients from 11 clinical trials, beta-blockers were found to reduce all-cause and cardiovascular mortality compared with placebo in all HF patients having sinus rhythm except in those with an LVEF of at least 50%.[36]

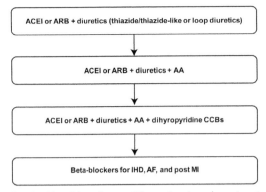

Fig. 1. Algorithm for anti-hypertensive drug treatment for HF with preserved ejection fraction (CCBs should be dihydropyridines). AA, aldosterone antagonist; ACEI, angiotensin converting enzyme inhibitors; AF, atrial fibrillation; ARB, angiotensin II receptor blockers; CCB, calcium channel blockers; IHD, ischemic heart disease; MI, myocardial infarction.

In a Swedish Doppler-echocardiographic study, which investigated the effects of carvedilol on diastolic function in HFpEF, carvedilol significantly improved the ratio of mitral peak velocity of early-to-late diastolic filling.[37] However, compared with placebo, carvedilol did not lead to an improvement in other markers of diastolic function. In addition, in the secondary analysis of the TOPCAT trial, beta-blocker use was associated with a higher risk of HF-related hospitalization in HFpEF patients with an LVEF of at least 50%.[38] Although beta-blockers are of clear benefit in patients with atrial fibrillation and ischemic heart disease, many patients with HFpEF have chronotropic incompetence, which may be aggravated by their use.[39] Therefore, beta-blockers should be used in HFpEF patients with underlying ischemic heart disease and atrial fibrillation and should be avoided in patients with chronotropic insufficiency.

Calcium Channel Blockers

Calcium channel blockers (CCBs) have excellent BP-lowering efficacy but tend to be less efficacious than diuretics in reducing the incidence of HF.[40] The guidelines for HF do not recommend the use of nondihydropyridine CCBs in symptomatic HFrEF patients because of their negative inotropic effects.[22] However, there is evidence that dihydropyridine CCBs, especially amlodipine and felodipine, are relatively safe in HEFrEF.[41,42] Therefore, adding a dihydropyridine CCB when BP is not controlled with RAS inhibitors and diuretics with or without spironolactone should be

considered with careful monitoring for the aggravation of HF symptoms. However, there are limited data on the benefits and risks of using CCBs in patients with HFpEF when diastolic dysfunction is a major concern rather than systolic dysfunction. In the Organized Program to Initiate Lifesaving Treatment in Hospitalized Patients with Heart Failure Registry, all-cause mortality, HF-related hospitalization, and all-cause hospitalization were compared between HFpEF patients who were prescribed CCBs at discharge from the hospital and those who were not. CCBs did not improve or worsen the clinical outcome, and this result was the same regardless of the type of the CCB used.[43]

Angiotensin Receptor Neprilysin Inhibitor

Lastly, although valsartan/sacubitril narrowly missed the primary endpoint in the PARAGON-HF trial, the door should not be closed for this important therapeutic armamentarium.[19] A recent subgroup analysis has shown benefits of valsartan/sacubitril in subjects with a relatively lower LVEF (<57%), women with HFpEF, and patients who were screened within 30 days of hospitalization for HF. Therefore, further research is needed to identify the subset of HFpEF patients who would benefit from valsartan/sacubitril. The benefit observed in subjects with a lower LVEF is an interesting finding as a similar interaction with LVEF was observed from a post hoc analysis of the TOPCAT trial. The analysis observed a significant interaction for the primary outcomes (P=.046) and HF-related hospitalization (P=.039), with a trend for stronger benefits of spironolactone at the lower range of LVEF.[44] Therefore, future trials are needed to determine the benefits of RAS inhibitors, valsartan/sacubitril, and spironolactone in patients with HFmrEF.

In conclusion, hypertension is both the most common risk factor and the most common co-morbidity associated with HFpEF. Optimal BP control is needed to reduce HF exacerbation, and to reduce other cardiovascular events, such as myocardial infarction or stroke. Although no specific treatment has shown to be beneficial in HFpEF patients, an initial combination of RAS inhibitors, diuretics, and spironolactone seems reasonable. Dihydropyridine CCBs should be added to achieve the target BP goal with due care not to exacerbate the symptoms of HF. Beta-blockers should be used when indicated with special consideration of avoiding these in subjects with chronotropic incompetence.

CLINICS CARE POINTS

- Hypertension is a common risk factor of HFpEF.

- Although it is a traditional paradigm that hypertension results in LV hypertrophy and left atrium remodeling, leading to clinical HF, there are multiple, heterogeneous derangements involving myocardial and peripheral vascular functions between hypertension and HFpEF.

- In HFpEF patients, SBP of 120 to 129 mm Hg appears to be associated with better prognosis, but attention should be paid to the adverse effects of intensive BP lowering in the elderly or patients with multiple comorbidities.

- It seems ideal to preferentially select RAS inhibitors, diuretics, and spironolactone for blood BP control in HFpEF patients, and beta-blocker or dihydropyridine CCBs should be used while closely monitoring whether HF symptoms worsen.

ACKNOWLEDGMENTS

None.

DISCLOSURE

The authors have nothing to declare. This work was supported by the National Research Foundation of Korea (NRF) grant funded by the Ministry of Science and ICT (NRF-2020R1C1C1013627) and was also supported by Basic Science Research Program through the NRF funded by the Ministry of Education (NRF-2017R1D1A1B03034053).

REFERENCES

1. Dunlay SM, Roger VL, Redfield MM. Epidemiology of heart failure with preserved ejection fraction. Nat Rev Cardiol 2017;14(10):591–602.

2. Lee JH, Lim NK, Cho MC, et al. Epidemiology of Heart Failure in Korea: present and future. Korean Circ J 2016;46(5):658–64.

3. Owan TE, Hodge DO, Herges RM, et al. Trends in prevalence and outcome of heart failure with preserved ejection fraction. N Engl J Med 2006; 355(3):251–9.

4. Beckett NS, Peters R, Fletcher AE, et al. Treatment of hypertension in patients 80 years of age or older. N Engl J Med 2008;358(18):1887–98.

5. Levy D, Larson MG, Vasan RS, et al. The progression from hypertension to congestive heart failure. JAMA 1996;275(20):1557–62.

6. Messerli FH, Rimoldi SF, Bangalore S. The transition from hypertension to heart failure: contemporary update. JACC Heart Fail 2017;5(8):543–51.

7. Lewis GA, Schelbert EB, Williams SG, et al. Biological phenotypes of heart failure with preserved ejection fraction. J Am Coll Cardiol 2017;70(17): 2186–200.

8. Yusuf S, Pfeffer MA, Swedberg K, et al. Effects of candesartan in patients with chronic heart failure and preserved left-ventricular ejection fraction: the CHARM-Preserved Trial. Lancet 2003;362(9386): 777–81.

9. Massie BM, Carson PE, McMurray JJ, et al. Irbesartan in patients with heart failure and preserved ejection fraction. N Engl J Med 2008;359(23):2456–67.

10. Pitt B, Pfeffer MA, Assmann SF, et al. Spironolactone for heart failure with preserved ejection fraction. N Engl J Med 2014;370(15):1383–92.

11. Borlaug BA. The pathophysiology of heart failure with preserved ejection fraction. Nat Rev Cardiol 2014;11(9):507–15.

12. Lam CSP, Voors AA, de Boer RA, et al. Heart failure with preserved ejection fraction: from mechanisms to therapies. Eur Heart J 2018;39(30):2780–92.

13. Paulus WJ, Tschöpe C. A novel paradigm for heart failure with preserved ejection fraction: comorbidities drive myocardial dysfunction and remodeling through coronary microvascular endothelial inflammation. J Am Coll Cardiol 2013;62(4):263–71.

14. Zile MR, Baicu CF, Ikonomidis JS, et al. Myocardial stiffness in patients with heart failure and a preserved ejection fraction: contributions of collagen and titin. Circulation 2015;131(14):1247–59.

15. Borlaug BA, Paulus WJ. Heart failure with preserved ejection fraction: pathophysiology, diagnosis, and treatment. Eur Heart J 2011;32(6):670–9.

16. Chirinos JA, Kips JG, Jacobs DR Jr, et al. Arterial wave reflections and incident cardiovascular events and heart failure: MESA (Multiethnic Study of Atherosclerosis). J Am Coll Cardiol 2012;60(21):2170–7.

17. Borlaug BA, Olson TP, Lam CS, et al. Global cardiovascular reserve dysfunction in heart failure with preserved ejection fraction. J Am Coll Cardiol 2010;56(11):845–54.

18. Cleland JG, Tendera M, Adamus J, et al. The perindopril in elderly people with chronic heart failure (PEP-CHF) study. Eur Heart J 2006;27(19): 2338–45.

19. Solomon SD, McMurray JJV, Anand IS, et al. Angiotensin-neprilysin inhibition in heart failure with preserved ejection fraction. N Engl J Med 2019; 381(17):1609–20.

20. Redfield MM. Heart failure with preserved ejection fraction. N Engl J Med 2016;375(19):1868–77.

21. Mentz RJ, Kelly JP, von Lueder TG, et al. Noncardiac comorbidities in heart failure with reduced versus preserved ejection fraction. J Am Coll Cardiol 2014;64(21):2281–93.

22. Ponikowski P, Voors AA, Anker SD, et al. 2016 ESC Guidelines for the diagnosis and treatment of acute and chronic heart failure: The Task Force for the Diagnosis and Treatment of Acute and Chronic Heart Failure of the European Society of Cardiology (ESC) developed with the special contribution of the Heart Failure Association (HFA) of the ESC. Eur Heart J 2016;37(27):2129–200.

23. Whelton PK, Carey RM, Aronow WS, et al. 2017 ACC/AHA/AAPA/ABC/ACPM/AGS/APhA/ASH/ASPC/NMA/PCNA guideline for the prevention, detection, evaluation, and management of high blood pressure in adults: a report of the American College of Cardiology/American Heart Association Task Force on Clinical Practice Guidelines. J Am Coll Cardiol 2018;71(19):e127–248.

24. Williams B, Mancia G, Spiering W, et al. 2018 ESC/ESH guidelines for the management of arterial hypertension. Eur Heart J 2018;39(33):3021–104.

25. Wright JT Jr, Williamson JD, Whelton PK, et al. A randomized trial of intensive versus standard blood-pressure control. N Engl J Med 2015;373(22):2103–16.

26. Upadhya B, Rocco M, Lewis CE, et al. Effect of intensive blood pressure treatment on heart failure events in the systolic blood pressure reduction intervention trial. Circ Heart Fail 2017;10(4):e003613.

27. Selvaraj S, Claggett BL, Böhm M, et al. Systolic blood pressure in heart failure with preserved ejection fraction treated with sacubitril/valsartan. J Am Coll Cardiol 2020;75(14):1644–56.

28. Faselis C, Lam PH, Zile MR, et al. Systolic blood pressure and outcomes in older patients with HFpEF and hypertension. Am J Med 2020 [e-pub ahead of print]. https://doi.org/10.1016/j.amjmed.2020.08.030.

29. Pfeffer MA, Claggett B, Assmann SF, et al. Regional variation in patients and outcomes in the Treatment of Preserved Cardiac Function Heart Failure With an Aldosterone Antagonist (TOPCAT) trial. Circulation 2015;131(1):34–42.

30. Anand IS, Claggett B, Liu J, et al. Interaction between spironolactone and natriuretic peptides in patients with heart failure and preserved ejection fraction: from the TOPCAT trial. JACC Heart Fail 2017;5(4):241–52.

31. Anand IS, Rector TS, Cleland JG, et al. Prognostic value of baseline plasma amino-terminal pro-brain natriuretic peptide and its interactions with irbesartan treatment effects in patients with heart failure and preserved ejection fraction: findings from the I-PRESERVE trial. Circ Heart Fail 2011;4(5):569–77.

32. Kao DP, Lewsey JD, Anand IS, et al. Characterization of subgroups of heart failure patients with preserved ejection fraction with possible implications for prognosis and treatment response. Eur J Heart Fail 2015;17(9):925–35.

33. Cohen JB, Schrauben SJ, Zhao L, et al. Clinical phenogroups in heart failure with preserved ejection fraction: detailed phenotypes, prognosis, and response to spironolactone. JACC Heart Fail 2020;8(3):172–84.

34. Packer M, Kitzman DW. Obesity-related heart failure with a preserved ejection fraction: the mechanistic rationale for combining inhibitors of aldosterone, neprilysin, and sodium-glucose Cotransporter-2. JACC Heart Fail 2018;6(8):633–9.

35. Davis BR, Kostis JB, Simpson LM, et al. Heart failure with preserved and reduced left ventricular ejection fraction in the antihypertensive and lipid-lowering treatment to prevent heart attack trial. Circulation 2008;118(22):2259–67.

36. Cleland JGF, Bunting KV, Flather MD, et al. Beta-blockers for heart failure with reduced, mid-range, and preserved ejection fraction: an individual patient-level analysis of double-blind randomized trials. Eur Heart J 2018;39(1):26–35.

37. Bergström A, Andersson B, Edner M, et al. Effect of carvedilol on diastolic function in patients with diastolic heart failure and preserved systolic function. Results of the Swedish Doppler-echocardiographic study (SWEDIC). Eur J Heart Fail 2004;6(4):453–61.

38. Silverman DN, Plante TB, Infeld M, et al. Association of β-blocker use with heart failure hospitalizations and cardiovascular disease mortality among patients with heart failure with a preserved ejection fraction: a secondary analysis of the TOPCAT trial. JAMA Netw Open 2019;2(12):e1916598.

39. Wang J, Fang F, Yip GW, et al. Importance of chronotropic response and left ventricular long-axis function for exercise performance in patients with heart failure and preserved ejection fraction. Int J Cardiol 2016;202:339–43.

40. Ettehad D, Emdin CA, Kiran A, et al. Blood pressure lowering for prevention of cardiovascular disease and death: a systematic review and meta-analysis. Lancet 2016;387(10022):957–67.

41. Packer M, O'Connor CM, Ghali JK, et al. Effect of amlodipine on morbidity and mortality in severe chronic heart failure. Prospective Randomized Amlodipine Survival Evaluation Study Group. N Engl J Med 1996;335(15):1107–14.

42. Cohn JN, Ziesche S, Smith R, et al. Effect of the calcium antagonist felodipine as supplementary

vasodilator therapy in patients with chronic heart failure treated with enalapril: V-HeFT III. Vasodilator-Heart Failure Trial (V-HeFT) Study Group. Circulation 1997;96(3):856–63.

43. Patel K, Fonarow GC, Ahmed M, et al. Calcium channel blockers and outcomes in older patients with heart failure and preserved ejection fraction. Circ Heart Fail 2014;7(6):945–52.

44. Solomon SD, Claggett B, Lewis EF, et al. Influence of ejection fraction on outcomes and efficacy of spirono-lactone in patients with heart failure with preserved ejection fraction. Eur Heart J 2016;37(5):455–62.

Obesity and Heart Failure with Preserved Ejection Fraction

Efstratios Koutroumpakis, MD[a], Ramanjit Kaur, MD[a],
Heinrich Taegtmeyer, MD, DPhil[a], Anita Deswal, MD, MPH[b],*

KEYWORDS

- Obesity • BMI • Heart failure with preserved ejection fraction

KEY POINTS

- Obesity is an established risk factor for the development of heart failure with preserved ejection fraction (HFpEF), with distinct pathophysiologic and phenotypic characteristics.
- Diagnosis of the obese HFpEF phenotype is challenging, and high clinical suspicion is required.
- Targeted therapies, including weight reduction and/or pharmacologic interventions, hold promise in improving clinical outcomes of HFpEF patients with obesity.

At present, heart failure with preserved ejection fraction (HFpEF) accounts for more than half of the heart failure (HF) diagnoses in the community.[1–3] Its prevalence has been increasing, although mortality rates have not changed over the past 2 decades.[4] Lack of effective treatments and failure to improve clinical outcomes are attributed to distinct pathophysiologic and phenotypic profiles within the broader spectrum of HFpEF, each of which might require its own therapeutic approach. Clinical investigations and experimental research in animal models have identified a causative association between HFpEF and obesity,[5,6] a syndrome with an alarming global increase in its prevalence.[7] Obesity-related HFpEF recently has been recognized as a unique and prevalent HFpEF phenotype.[8,9] Current knowledge on the pathophysiology, diagnosis, clinical outcomes, and available treatments of the obese HFpEF phenotype is summarized.

HEART FAILURE WITH PRESERVED EJECTION FRACTION PHENOTYPES

HFpEF is a collective term for a group of heterogeneous disease processes. This heterogeneity has contributed to the failure thus far to identify treatments that improve clinical outcomes in the group of HFpEF as a whole. Attempts have been made to classify patients with HFpEF, based on their phenotypic characteristics, as a means for more precise targeting of treatments.[8] Phenotypes based on predisposing factors, including the metabolic/obese phenotype, hypertensive phenotype, chronic kidney disease–related phenotype, and the coronary artery disease–related phenotype, among others, have been proposed.[8] Furthermore, phenotypes based on clinical presentation, including lung congestion, chronotropic incompetence, pulmonary hypertension, skeletal muscle weakness, and atrial fibrillation, also have been suggested.[8]

THE HEART FAILURE WITH PRESERVED EJECTION FRACTION OBESITY PHENOTYPE

Obesity is an established risk factor for HF, independent of other known risk factors, such as hypertension or diabetes.[5,6,10,11] A now classic analysis of 5881 participants in the Framingham Heart Study has revealed that, with each increase of 1 unit in body mass index (BMI), the risk of

---

[a] Division of Cardiology, Department of Internal Medicine, McGovern Medical School, The University of Texas Health Science Center, 6431 Fannin Street, MSB 1.220, Houston, TX 77030, USA; [b] Department of Cardiology, University of Texas MD Anderson Cancer Center, 1515 Holcombe Boulevard, Houston, TX 77030, USA
* Corresponding author.
E-mail address: ADeswal@mdanderson.org

Heart Failure Clin 17 (2021) 345–356
https://doi.org/10.1016/j.hfc.2021.02.003

developing HF increased 5% in men and 7% in women.[5] Overall, after adjusting for established risk factors, the risk of HF increased in a graded fashion with increasing BMI, and it was double in obese individuals (BMI $\geq$30 kg/m^2) compared with individuals with normal weight (BMI <25 kg/m^2).[5] Subsequently, a large meta-analysis of 23 prospective studies, including 647,388 participants, confirmed this association by reporting a relative risk of 1.41 for HF incidence and 1.26 for HF mortality for each 5-unit increment increase in BMI.[12]

Even though most studies traditionally have used BMI to define and quantify obesity, it has been recognized that BMI has several shortcomings when determining the association of obesity with HF. BMI is an expression of the total body weight and cannot differentiate between total body fat, muscle mass, or bone weight.[13] More importantly, BMI does not describe the pattern of fat distribution and the amount of biologically active adipose tissue, which counts more than total fat mass.[9,14–17] Accordingly, recent studies have shifted their focus on evaluating the association of central obesity, as expressed by waist circumference, or visceral adiposity, as assessed by computed tomography (CT) scan or magnetic resonance imaging with HF.[18] In their large meta-analysis, Aune and colleagues[12] reported a relative risk of 1.29 for HF incidence for each 10-cm increase in waist circumference or a 0.1-unit increase in waist-to-hip ratio. A study by Rao and colleagues[10] examined 1806 participants from the Multi-Ethnic Study of Atherosclerosis (MESA) cohort without baseline cardiovascular disease and reported that over a mean follow-up of 11 years, the adjusted hazard ratio (HR) for incident HFpEF was 1.59 (95% CI, 1.05–2.40) per 1-SD higher waist circumference, and 2.24 (95% CI, 1.44–3.49) per 1-SD higher visceral adipose tissue (VAT) area on CT (single CT slice at L2-L3 level). The HR for HFpEF was 1.66 (95% CI, 1.12–2.45) per 1-SD higher BMI. Even among overweight/obese adults (BMI $\geq$25 kg/m^2), VAT was strongly associated with HFpEF (HR 2.78 per 1-SD VAT; 95% CI, 1.62–4.76).[10] These findings underline the additional value of using VAT over BMI when examining the association of obesity with HF. Subcutaneous adipose tissue was not associated with the development of HF in that study.[10]

Although the large meta-analysis by Aune and colleagues[12] did not report any gender difference in the HF incidence overall, some HFpEF studies have reported a more profound association between visceral obesity and HFpEF in women than in men. In a case-control study of 105 HFpEF patients, age matched, sex matched, and BMI matched with 105 controls, VAT area measured by CT was 34% higher in women with HFpEF compared with women controls (186 cm^2 $\pm$ 112 cm^2 vs 139 cm^2 $\pm$ 72 cm^2, respectively; $P = .006$), whereas there was no significant difference in men.[19] Women with increased VAT area also developed 33% higher pulmonary capillary wedge pressure during exercise compared with women with normal VAT area (28 mm Hg, $\pm$ 10 mm Hg vs 21 mm Hg $\pm$ 10 mm Hg, respectively; $P = .001$). In contrast, exercise pulmonary capillary wedge pressure was similar in men with or without excess VAT.[19]

Obesity is highly prevalent in HFpEF patients.[5,8] Among 4109 individuals with HFpEF in the Irbesartan in Heart Failure with Preserved Ejection Fraction (I-PRESERVE) trial, 83% were either overweight or obese (42% with a BMI of 25–30 kg/m^2 and 41% with a BMI >30 kg/m^2).[20] Furthermore, a study using the Atherosclerosis Risk In Communities Study (ARIC) database demonstrated that among 1487 individuals who developed new HF, the majority (82%) were overweight or obese before their HF diagnosis (35% and 47%, respectively).[21] This study did not differentiate between incident HFpEF or HF with reduced ejection fraction (HFrEF).[21]

Obesity, however, is a more significant risk factor for the development of HFpEF than systolic dysfunction.[22] In a recent study, among 22,681 individuals followed for a median of 12 years, higher BMI was associated with an HR of 1.34 per 1 SD in BMI for development of HFpEF (95% CI, 1.24–1.45), as opposed to 1.18 for HFrEF (95% CI, 1.10–1.27).[22] In another study, investigators from the Mayo clinic evaluated the echocardiographic characteristics of 788 individuals over 4 years and reported a close association between weight and diastolic left ventricular (LV) stiffness after adjusting for arterial afterload.[23] Furthermore, the evaluation of 1806 participants from the MESA reported a significant association of increases in BMI, waist circumference, and VAT area with HFpEF but not with HFrEF.[10]

An important study by Obokata and colleagues[9] in 2017 reported a detailed characterization of cardiovascular structure, function, and reserve capacity in individuals with HFpEF and obesity, lending support to the obese HFpEF as a distinct HFpEF phenotype. The investigators did not distinguish between central/visceral and subcutaneous obesity. When compared with HFpEF patients without obesity (BMI <30 kg/m^2) and controls without HFpEF, however, patients with HFpEF and significant obesity (BMI $\geq$35 kg/m^2) demonstrated greater plasma volume expansion, increased biventricular remodeling, greater right ventricular dysfunction, worse exercise capacity, and impaired pulmonary vasodilation.[9] Furthermore, HFpEF patients with obesity demonstrated increased pericardial restraint and enhanced ventricular interaction, which further contributed to high intracardiac filling pressures.[9]

PATHOPHYSIOLOGY OF OBESE HEART FAILURE WITH PRESERVED EJECTION FRACTION

Central pathophysiologic abnormalities that have been proposed to contribute to the obese HFpEF phenotype include sodium retention, neurohormonal perturbations, alterations in energy substrate metabolism, group 3 pulmonary hypertension, pericardial restraint, and systemic inflammation (**Fig. 1**).[9,24]

Obesity has been associated with an abundance of renal tubular sodium transporters, overproduction of aldosterone, and the activation of the renin-angiotensin axis, leading to increased sodium reabsorption and plasma volume expansion.[25–28] Obesity also increases circulating catecholamine levels.[29,30] The increases in blood volume and blood pressure, and thus cardiac loading, in obesity lead to structural and functional alterations that contribute to HF.[9] As discussed previously, Obokata and colleagues[9] demonstrated that HFpEF subjects with obesity had greater estimated plasma volume, LV dilation and concentric remodeling, right ventricular enlargement, and increased chamber volume compared with nonobese HFpEF.

Furthermore, in individuals with obesity, there is a disruption of metabolic homeostasis and excess nutrient supply to the heart.[31,32] Myocardial cellular responses to excess glucose and free fatty acid uptake include dysregulated insulin signaling, impaired mitochondrial respiration, and reactive oxygen species formation.[31] This deleterious pathogenetic process is collectively is termed, *glucolipotoxicity*, and leads to impaired intracellular calcium cycling and, subsequently, LV diastolic dysfunction.[31,33,34]

Additionally, obstructive sleep apnea and obesity hypoventilation syndrome are prevalent in individuals with obesity.[35,36] They lead to hypoxia, acidosis, and subsequent development of group 3 pulmonary hypertension, right ventricular hypertrophy, and failure.[36] Furthermore, obesity often is associated with other comorbidities, such as hypertension and diabetes, which are drivers of HFpEF.[37]

The degree of obesity and adipose tissue location play essential roles in the pathophysiology of the obese HFpEF phenotype.[38,39] Specifically, epicardial fat increases pericardial restraint, enhances ventricular interaction, and increases intracardiac filling pressures in obese individuals with HFpEF.[9] In addition to its mechanical effects, epicardial fat acts as a metabolically active depot.

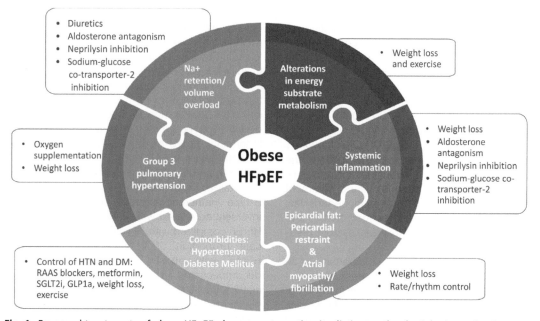

Fig. 1. Proposed treatments of obese HFpEF phenotype targeting its distinct pathophysiologic mechanisms. ASA, acetylsalicylic acid (aspirin); DM, diabetes mellitus; HTN, hypertension; GDMT, guideline-directed medical treatment; GLP1a, glucagon-like peptide-1 agonists; RAAS, renin-angiotensin-aldosterone system; SGLT2i, sodium-glucose co-trasporter-2 inhibitors.

Via the production and release of inflammatory cytokines, it can cause microvascular dysfunction and fibrosis of the underlying myocardium.[17] Electroanatomic remodeling and myopathy of the left atrium often lead to the development of atrial fibrillation, which further contributes to the pathogenesis and hemodynamic derangements of HFpEF in obesity.[40]

Lastly, in individuals with obesity, VAT transforms into a metabolically active state producing a wide array of proinflammatory adipokines.[11,41,42] Most prominent among the inflammatory markers is leptin.[11,41,42] The resultant systemic inflammatory response mediated by the metabolically active VAT has adverse effects on the structure and function of visceral organs and vasculature, resulting in increased arterial stiffness, microvascular and endothelial dysfunction, and tissue fibrosis, all representing key pathophysiologic characteristics of the HFpEF phenotype.[43,44] On the contrary, subcutaneous fat is metabolically quiet and not as important in HF development.[16,45]

DIAGNOSIS OF HEART FAILURE WITH PRESERVED EJECTION FRACTION WITH OBESITY

Establishing a diagnosis of HFpEF can be challenging, especially among euvolemic patients with unexplained dyspnea. Recent work by Reddy and colleagues[46] established noninvasive diagnostic criteria for HFpEF after studying 414 euvolemic patients with unexplained dyspnea, referred for invasive hemodynamic exercise testing. A weighted scoring system (H2FPEF score), ranging from 0 to 9, was developed based on 6 variables and subsequently validated in a separate test cohort of 100 patients.[46] For each score unit increase, the odds of HFpEF doubled (odds ratio [OR] 1.98; 95% CI, 1.74–2.30; $P<.0001$), whereas a score of 6 or more was associated with greater than 90% probability of HFpEF.[46] Obesity was 1 of the key score variables, adding 2 points to the total score. The rest of the variables include atrial fibrillation, age greater than 60 years, treatment with greater than or equal to 2 antihypertensives, echocardiographic E/e' ratio greater than 9, and echocardiographic pulmonary artery systolic pressure greater than 35 mm Hg.[46]

It seems simplistic to think that diagnosis of an obese HFpEF phenotype is equivalent to the presence of HFpEF and a BMI of greater than 30 kg/m². Although it may work in a large cohort, such a diagnostic approach has several limitations at the individual patient level (**Box 1**). First, BMI is an expression of the total body weight. It does not account for body composition and cannot

---

Box 1
Challenges with diagnosing the obese heart failure with preserved ejection fraction phenotype

BMI is not an accurate measure of visceral obesity.

Symptoms of dyspnea and edema in the setting of obesity are common even in the absence of HF.

Natriuretic peptides frequently are below diagnostic limits in obesity.

Echocardiographic assessment is technically limited in individuals with obesity.

---

differentiate between body fat, muscle mass, or bone weight.[13] Furthermore, what is more important than the total fat mass is the amount of biologically active adipose tissue and its distribution pattern.[14–16] For example, visceral (especially epicardial) fat is more significant than the accumulation of the metabolically silent subcutaneous fat.[9,16,17] As an extension to that, metabolically obese normal weight individuals can develop HFpEF, with characteristics similar to the obese HFpEF phenotype, but they would be misdiagnosed if they are evaluated merely based on their BMI.[47]

Another challenge with diagnosing HF, especially HFpEF, in obese individuals is that some symptoms and signs, such as dyspnea on exertion and edema, may be noted in individuals with obesity, even without HF. Furthermore, natriuretic peptide levels, a key diagnostic tool in HF, are lower in obese compared with nonobese patients. In an analysis of the ARIC study, of 12,230 individuals, 1861 developed incident HF during a median follow-up of 20.6 years.[48] Despite the increased risk of HF development in obesity, an inverse association was noted between baseline BMI and N-terminal pro–B-type natriuretic peptide (NT-proBNP) levels ($r = -0.10$).[48] In a separate analysis of the ARIC cohort, including 9820 individuals hospitalized with acutely decompensated HF, B-type natriuretic peptide (BNP) levels were inversely correlated with BMI and were higher in HFrEF compared with HFpEF patients.[49] A significant proportion of patients with adjudicated HFpEF with obesity presenting with acutely decompensated HF had BNP levels below diagnostic thresholds (14% of individuals with morbid obesity had BNP<100 pg/mL and 39% had BNP <200 pg/mL).[49] Another study of 159 patients with HFpEF also reported that 29% of the participants had BNP levels less than or equal to 100 pg/mL.[50] Normal BNP levels in the setting of

HFpEF were seen mostly among young, obese women. Spuriously normal or lower BNP levels in patients with HF have been attributed to enhanced natriuretic peptide degradation in fat tissue, alterations in sex hormones, and insulin resistance.[51–53]

Lastly, there are challenges related to technical limitations in obtaining accurate echocardiographic measurements in obese individuals, which add to the complexity of diagnosing the obese HFpEF phenotype. Considering the high prevalence of the obese HFpEF phenotype and the potential benefit that targeted therapies might have, a high level of suspicion and a thorough clinical and echocardiographic assessment of each patient with symptoms and signs of HF are recommended. If uncertainty with diagnosing HFpEF remains, an invasive diagnostic approach with assessment of hemodynamics at rest and with or without exercise during right heart catheterization should be pursued, as recommended by a recent consensus statement.[54]

CLINICAL OUTCOMES OF HEART FAILURE WITH PRESERVED EJECTION FRACTION PATIENTS WITH OBESITY AND THE OBESITY PARADOX

Surprisingly, obesity, at least as defined by BMI and waist-hip circumference, also has been associated in numerous studies with a protective effect on survival after the diagnosis of HF in general, a phenomenon known as the obesity paradox.[21,55] Previous work by the authors' group utilizing a national cohort of 2501 ambulatory veterans with HFpEF showed that overweight or obese patients had improved survival compared with their normal-weight counterparts.[56] Although not seen in the authors' study, other studies, such as a secondary analysis of the I-PRESERVE trial, suggested a U-shaped relationship of BMI with mortality, wherein severe obesity was not protective.[20] Furthermore, among 1487 individuals in the ARIC study, being overweight or obese before developing any HF had a positive association with survival, compared with a normal BMI (HR 0.72; 95% CI, 0.58–0.90; P = .004, and HR 0.70; 95% CI, 0.56–0.87; P = .001, respectively).[21] This finding suggests that the obesity paradox cannot be attributed simply to the weight loss and cachexia associated with advanced stages of HF.[21]

Trying to understand this relationship further, a subanalysis of the Treatment of Preserved Cardiac Function Heart Failure with an Aldosterone Antagonist (TOPCAT) trial revealed that, among 3310 patients with HFpEF, increased waist circumference was associated with increased all-cause mortality.[57] Although not confirmed by other studies, this may suggest that, even though BMI is associated with improved survival in HFpEF, waist circumference, which is a more direct marker of central adiposity, more accurately identifies patients at high risk for worse outcomes. This also emphasizes the limitations associated with the use of just BMI in the diagnosis of obese HFpEF. The obesity paradox, in this case, may be explained by the fact that a high BMI in some patients is associated with a greater lean mass (a surrogate for skeletal muscle mass), which drives greater cardiorespiratory fitness and a more favorable survival in HFpEF patients.[58] In contrast, waist circumference, which represents central obesity and is related more closely to visceral adiposity, is associated with worse clinical outcomes and increased all-cause mortality.[57] Additional explanations have been proposed to explain the obesity paradox.[21] It has been suggested that because HF is a catabolic state leading to cachexia, obese and overweight patients may have better outcomes because they have higher metabolic reserves.[59,60] Furthermore, obesity may alter the natural history of HF through neurohumoral pathways. Neutralization of bacterial lipopolysaccharides by higher levels of serum lipoproteins in obesity may attenuate the detrimental cytokine response in HF.[61,62] Production of soluble tumor necrosis factor (TNF) receptors by adipose tissue may serve as a reservoir for toxic circulating TNF.[63] Higher levels of circulating stem cells and decreased adiponectin levels and catecholamine response in obese individuals are other explanations proposed.[64–66] Additionally, early medical attention and earlier HF diagnosis among individuals with obesity in the setting of symptoms of dyspnea and edema exacerbated by obesity and/or higher prevalence of comorbidities, such as hypertension and diabetes, may contribute to a potential lead-time bias, giving a false impression of improved survival among HFpEF patients with obesity (**Box 2**).[21]

HFpEF in the setting of obesity also is associated with a higher risk of hospitalization and worse quality of life. The authors' study, comprising 2501 ambulatory patients with HFpEF, revealed the shorter time to HF hospitalization across all obesity classes compared with patients with normal BMI (overweight: adjusted HR 1.30; 95% CI, 0.88–1.90; obesity class I: HR 1.57; 95% CI, 1.05–2.34; obesity class II: HR 1.79; 95% CI, 1.15–2.78; and obesity class III: HR 1.96; 95% CI, 1.23–3.12).[56] A secondary analysis of the RELAX, NEAT-HFpEF, and INDIE-HFpEF trials, including 408 patients with chronic HFpEF,

---

Box 2
Proposed explanations of the obesity paradox

1. Higher lean mass in individuals with higher BMI

2. Higher metabolic reserve against the catabolic state of HF among individuals with obesity

3. Attenuation of detrimental cytokine response in HF through neutralization of bacterial lipopolysaccharides by higher levels of serum lipoproteins in obesity

4. Production of soluble TNF receptors by adipose tissue that serve as a reservoir for toxic circulating TNF

5. Higher levels of circulating stem cells in individuals with obesity

6. Decreased adiponectin levels in individuals with obesity

7. Beneficial effects related to renin-angiotensin-aldosterone blockade initiated earlier and at possibly higher doses for co-morbidities including hypertension

8. Lead-time bias

---

assessed by the Kansas City Cardiomyopathy Questionnaire and Minnesota Living with Heart Failure Questionnaire, revealed that the group of patients with the most inferior quality of life were the youngest, those with higher BMI, diabetes, and the lowest NT-proBNP levels.[67] After adjusting for age, sex, and BMI, poorer quality of life correlated with worse physical capacity and activity levels, assessed by peak oxygen consumption, 6-minute walk distance, and actigraphy.[67]

TARGETED TREATMENT OF THE OBESE HEART FAILURE WITH PRESERVED EJECTION FRACTION PHENOTYPE

Failure to identify effective treatments has sparked investigations into distinct pathophysiologic phenotypes within the broader spectrum of HFpEF. Initial treatments targeted to the obese HFpEF phenotype hold promise. These treatments focus on VAT reduction by pharmacologic and nonpharmacologic means and on attenuating the effects of adiposity on cardiovascular physiology (see **Fig. 1**).

Adipose Tissue Reduction

Caloric restriction and exercise

Dietary caloric restriction improves cardiac remodeling and LV diastolic function in both animal models and humans.[68,69] Meyer and colleagues[69] compared 25 individuals practicing caloric restriction with 25 age-matched and gender-matched controls, consuming Western diets, over a mean follow-up period of 6.5 years. The investigators reported a significant improvement in LV diastolic parameters in the caloric restriction group, as assessed by Doppler echocardiography.[69] Furthermore, blood pressure, serum C-reactive protein, TNF-α, and transforming growth factor $\beta 1$ levels were significantly lower among individuals adhering to caloric restriction.[69] The applicability and feasibility of these intense interventions in patients with established HFpEF, however, remain to be seen.

In a small clinical trial assessing caloric restriction and aerobic exercise in 100 obese patients with HFpEF, Kitzman and colleagues[70] reported improved exercise capacity, as measured by peak oxygen consumption, with either intervention, over the course of 20 weeks. The combination of caloric restriction with aerobic exercise had an additive effect.[70] Furthermore, LV mass and relative wall thickness decreased and the transmitral E/A ratio increased with diet.[70] A meta-analysis of 8 studies, including 436 HFpEF patients, most of whom were overweight or obese, reported that 12 weeks to 24 weeks of exercise training, in the form of walking or cycling, significantly improved peak exercise oxygen uptake, 6-minute walk distance, and quality of life in patients compared with controls.[71]

Bariatric surgery

Weight loss associated with bariatric surgery, but not with liposuction, may improve symptoms, quality of life, and hospitalization rates in HF patients with obesity.[72,73] In a study by Miranda and colleagues,[72] among 13 HF patients with severe obesity who underwent bariatric surgery, symptoms of exertional dyspnea, peripheral edema, and quality of life improved, compared with 6 similar control patients with HF treated conservatively, over a follow-up period exceeding 4 years. In a larger, self-controlled, case series study of 524 morbidly obese patients with HF, who underwent bariatric surgery, the rate of emergency room visits or hospitalization was significantly lower, 13 months to 24 months after surgery (9.9%; adjusted OR 0.57; $P = .003$), compared with prior to surgery (16.2%).[74] Neither of these retrospective observational studies, however, specifically evaluated patients with HFpEF.

In a prospective study by Leichman and colleagues,[75] 43 patients with morbid obesity underwent metabolic profiling, skeletal muscle biopsies, and resting echocardiograms at baseline, 3 months and 9 months after bariatric surgery; 42% of them had evidence of impaired LV relaxation on baseline tissue Doppler imaging.[75] A decrease in plasma leptin, restoration of insulin sensitivity and muscle metabolic derangements, and normalization of LV diastolic function were reported 9 months after bariatric surgery.[75] A follow-up study evaluating patients with clinically severe obesity, 2 years after bariatric surgery, showed a progressive decrease in ventricular wall thickness and LV mass index, despite plateaued weight-loss rates after the first 9 months from surgery.[76] It was proposed that this effect might be regulated by neurohumoral factors that potentially contribute to improved long-term survival.[76]

Furthermore, bariatric surgery also has been associated with the prevention of HF development in morbidly obese individuals. Within the Scandinavian Obesity Surgery Registry, comprising more than 25,000 individuals, gastric bypass surgery was associated with lower overall HF incidence compared with intensive lifestyle modification (HR 0.54; 95% CI, 0.36–0.82).[77]

Collectively, these findings support a potential beneficial effect of adipose tissue reduction by caloric restriction and bariatric surgery in HFpEF patients. The caution has been proposed, given multiple studies demonstrating the obesity paradox.[56] Only larger randomized controlled trials of targeted weight reduction in obese patients with HFpEF and long-term follow-up could establish the beneficial effect and safety of adipose tissue reduction in this patient population.

Attenuation of the Effects of Adiposity on Cardiovascular Physiology

Mineralocorticoid receptor antagonism

Given the abundance of renal tubular sodium transporters and elevated aldosterone levels in obese HFpEF patients,[26–28] aldosterone antagonists are a likely effective treatment.[24] Mineralocorticoid receptor antagonism in animal models decreases oxidative stress, cardiac inflammation, fibrosis, and intracardiac filling pressures.[78–80] Although clinical trials showing improvement in hard clinical outcomes of obese HFpEF patients are not yet available, aldosterone antagonists have been shown to improve serologic fibrosis markers and LV function in obese individuals.[81] The TOPCAT trial failed to show significant improvement in the primary composite outcome of cardiovascular death, aborted cardiac arrest, or HF hospitalization among 3445 patients with symptomatic HFpEF, treated with spironolactone versus placebo.[82] A secondary analysis of the TOPCAT trial suggested that HFpEF patients with obesity may respond better to spironolactone.[83] Future trials assessing the effect of aldosterone antagonists specifically in obese HFpEF patients are needed to confirm these observations.

Neprilysin and sodium-glucose transporter-2 inhibition

Obesity is associated with increased expression of the neutral endopeptidase neprilysin.[84] Neprilysin inhibitors augment the actions of endogenous natriuretic peptides, which are low in individuals with obesity, and suppress aldosterone.[85,86] Natriuretic peptides also exert lipolytic and anti-inflammatory effects, inhibit cardiac fibrosis, and promote capillary angiogenesis.[85,87–90] Based on these observations, neprilysin inhibition has been proposed as a potential targeted therapy in obese HFpEF.[24] A recent study in mice with obesity and metabolic heart disease showed striking improvements in diastolic dysfunction after treatment with sacubitril/valsartan compared with valsartan alone.[91] The PARAGON-HF trial, however, with 4822 HFpEF patients, treated with the neprilysin inhibitor sacubitril plus valsartan versus placebo, failed to meet the primary composite endpoint of HF hospitalization or cardiovascular death.[92] Failure to reveal benefits might be due to the diverse HFpEF population of the study. Individuals with morbid obesity (BMI >40 kg/m^2) were excluded from the trial, which might have contributed to a type II study error and failure to identify a beneficial effect of the medication class in obese HFpEF. Trials focusing specifically on the obese HFpEF phenotype are needed.

Lastly, inhibition of the sodium-glucose co-transporter-2 (SGLT2) is another promising treatment target in HFpEF patients with obesity. Inhibition of SGLT2 in animal models suppressed proinflammatory and profibrotic processes in the myocardium and reduced the amount of epicardial fat, ameliorating the development of HFpEF.[93–95] Large clinical trials in patients with type 2 diabetes mellitus at high risk for cardiovascular events reported a reduction in new-onset HF and HF hospitalizations with SGLT2 inhibitors.[96–99] Ongoing trials aim to evaluate the role of SGLT2 inhibitors on patients with HFpEF, with the completion of some of these trials expected soon.[100–102] Future trials and analyses focusing specifically on the obese HFpEF phenotype will be useful to establish the role of SGLT2 inhibition in this group of patients.

SUMMARY

Patients with HFpEF and obesity now are recognized as a distinct HFpEF phenotype with unique pathophysiology. Given the diagnostic challenges, a thorough assessment is required to identify those patients. Targeted therapies, including weight reduction and/or pharmacologic interventions, have demonstrated promising results in improving clinical outcomes of HFpEF patients with obesity. Future clinical trials focusing on the obese HFpEF phenotype are needed, not least because it represents the most prevalent of all the HFpEF phenotypes.

CLINICS CARE POINTS

- Patients with HFpEF and obesity now are recognized as having a distinct HFpEF phenotype with unique pathophysiology.

- Central pathophysiologic mechanisms of the obese HFpEF phenotype include systemic inflammation, sodium retention, high circulating neurohormone levels, alterations in energy substrate metabolism, group 3 pulmonary hypertension, pericardial restraint, and comorbidities of hypertension and diabetes.

- Diagnosis of the obese HFpEF phenotype is challenged by limitations associated with the use of BMI for quantification of adiposity, overlapping symptoms and signs with comorbidities, lower natriuretic peptide levels, and technical difficulties with obtaining accurate echocardiographic measurements.

- Reduction of VAT via caloric restriction and/or bariatric surgery attenuates the effects of adiposity on the cardiovascular system. Additionally, mineralocorticoid receptor inhibition, neprilysin inhibition, and SGLT2 inhibition are proposed treatment targets for the obese HFpEF phenotype.

DISCLOSURE

The authors have no conflicts of interest to disclose.

REFERENCES

1. Vasan RS, Larson MG, Benjamin EJ, et al. Congestive heart failure in subjects with normal versus reduced left ventricular ejection fraction: prevalence and mortality in a population-based cohort. J Am Coll Cardiol 1999;33(7):1948–55.
2. Devereux RB, Roman MJ, Liu JE, et al. Congestive heart failure despite normal left ventricular systolic function in a population-based sample: the Strong Heart Study. Am J Cardiol 2000;86(10):1090–6.
3. Kitzman DW, Gardin JM, Gottdiener JS, et al. Importance of heart failure with preserved systolic function in patients > or = 65 years of age. CHS Research Group. Cardiovascular Health Study. Am J Cardiol 2001;87(4):413–9.
4. Owan TE, Hodge DO, Herges RM, et al. Trends in prevalence and outcome of heart failure with preserved ejection fraction. N Engl J Med 2006;355(3):251–9.
5. Kenchaiah S, Evans JC, Levy D, et al. Obesity and the risk of heart failure. N Engl J Med 2002;347(5):305–13.
6. Carbone S, Mauro AG, Toldo S, et al. Diet-induced obesity HFpEF murine models. JACC Basic Transl Sci 2018;3(1):157.
7. González-Muniesa P, Mártinez-González M-A, Hu FB, et al. Obesity. Nat Rev Dis Primers 2017;3(1):17034.
8. Shah SJ, Kitzman DW, Borlaug BA, et al. Phenotype-specific treatment of heart failure with preserved ejection fraction: a multiorgan roadmap. Circulation 2016;134(1):73–90.
9. Obokata M, Reddy YNV, Pislaru SV, et al. Evidence supporting the existence of a distinct obese phenotype of heart failure with preserved ejection fraction. Circulation 2017;136(1):6–19.
10. Rao VN, Zhao D, Allison MA, et al. Adiposity and incident heart failure and its subtypes: MESA (Multi-Ethnic Study of Atherosclerosis). JACC Heart Fail 2018;6(12):999–1007.
11. Wannamethee SG, Shaper AG, Whincup PH, et al. Obesity and risk of incident heart failure in older men with and without pre-existing coronary heart disease: does leptin have a role? J Am Coll Cardiol 2011;58(18):1870–7.
12. Aune D, Sen A, Norat T, et al. Body mass index, abdominal fatness, and heart failure incidence and mortality: a systematic review and dose-response meta-analysis of prospective studies. Circulation 2016;133(7):639–49.
13. Liu P, Ma F, Lou H, et al. The utility of fat mass index vs. body mass index and percentage of body fat in the screening of metabolic syndrome. BMC Public Health 2013;13:629.
14. Britton KA, Massaro JM, Murabito JM, et al. Body fat distribution, incident cardiovascular disease, cancer, and all-cause mortality. J Am Coll Cardiol 2013;62(10):921–5.
15. Silva KR, Côrtes I, Liechocki S, et al. Characterization of stromal vascular fraction and adipose stem cells from subcutaneous, preperitoneal and visceral morbidly obese human adipose tissue depots. PLoS One 2017;12(3):e0174115.
16. Marinou K, Hodson L, Vasan SK, et al. Structural and functional properties of deep abdominal subcutaneous adipose tissue explain its association with insulin resistance and cardiovascular risk in men. Diabetes Care 2014;37(3):821–9.

17. Mazurek T, Zhang L, Zalewski A, et al. Human epicardial adipose tissue is a source of inflammatory mediators. Circulation 2003;108(20):2460–6.

18. Leichman JG, Aguilar D, King TM, et al. Improvements in systemic metabolism, anthropometrics, and left ventricular geometry 3 months after bariatric surgery. Surg Obes Relat Dis 2006;2(6):592–9.

19. Sorimachi H, Obokata M, Takahashi N, et al. Pathophysiologic importance of visceral adipose tissue in women with heart failure and preserved ejection fraction. Eur Heart J 2020. https://doi.org/10.1093/eurheartj/ehaa823.

20. Haass M, Kitzman DW, Anand IS, et al. Body mass index and adverse cardiovascular outcomes in heart failure patients with preserved ejection fraction: results from the Irbesartan in Heart Failure with Preserved Ejection Fraction (I-PRESERVE) trial. Circ Heart Fail 2011;4(3):324–31.

21. Khalid U, Ather S, Bavishi C, et al. Pre-morbid body mass index and mortality after incident heart failure: the ARIC Study. J Am Coll Cardiol 2014; 64(25):2743–9.

22. Savji N, Meijers WC, Bartz TM, et al. The association of obesity and cardiometabolic traits with incident HFpEF and HFrEF. JACC Heart Fail 2018;6(8): 701–9.

23. Wohlfahrt P, Redfield MM, Lopez-Jimenez F, et al. Impact of general and central adiposity on ventricular-arterial aging in women and men. JACC Heart Fail 2014;2(5):489–99.

24. Packer M, Kitzman DW. Obesity-related heart failure with a preserved ejection fraction: the mechanistic rationale for combining inhibitors of aldosterone, neprilysin, and sodium-glucose cotransporter-2. JACC Heart Fail 2018;6(8):633–9.

25. Bickel CA, Verbalis JG, Knepper MA, et al. Increased renal Na-K-ATPase, NCC, and beta-ENaC abundance in obese Zucker rats. Am J Physiol Renal Physiol 2001;281(4):F639–48.

26. Bentley-Lewis R, Adler GK, Perlstein T, et al. Body mass index predicts aldosterone production in normotensive adults on a high-salt diet. J Clin Endocrinol Metab 2007;92(11):4472–5.

27. Huby AC, Antonova G, Groenendyk J, et al. Adipocyte-derived hormone leptin is a direct regulator of aldosterone secretion, which promotes endothelial dysfunction and cardiac fibrosis. Circulation 2015; 132(22):2134–45.

28. Briones AM, Nguyen Dinh Cat A, Callera GE, et al. Adipocytes produce aldosterone through calcineurin-dependent signaling pathways: implications in diabetes mellitus-associated obesity and vascular dysfunction. Hypertension 2012; 59(5):1069–78.

29. Landsberg L, Young JB. Fasting, feeding and regulation of the sympathetic nervous system. N Engl J Med 1978;298(23):1295–301.

30. Reaven GM, Lithell H, Landsberg L. Hypertension and associated metabolic abnormalities–the role of insulin resistance and the sympathoadrenal system. N Engl J Med 1996;334(6):374–81.

31. Koutroumpakis E, Jozwik B, Aguilar D, et al. Strategies of unloading the failing heart from metabolic stress. Am J Med 2020;133(3):290–6.

32. Sharma S, Adrogue JV, Golfman L, et al. Intramyocardial lipid accumulation in the failing human heart resembles the lipotoxic rat heart. FASEB J 2004;18(14):1692–700.

33. Labbé SM, Grenier-Larouche T, Noll C, et al. Increased myocardial uptake of dietary fatty acids linked to cardiac dysfunction in glucose-intolerant humans. Diabetes 2012;61(11):2701–10.

34. Leichman JG, Aguilar D, King TM, et al. Association of plasma free fatty acids and left ventricular diastolic function in patients with clinically severe obesity. Am J Clin Nutr 2006;84(2):336–41.

35. Mokhlesi B, Tulaimat A, Faibussowitsch I, et al. Obesity hypoventilation syndrome: prevalence and predictors in patients with obstructive sleep apnea. Sleep Breath 2007;11(2):117–24.

36. Bozkurt B, Colvin M, Cook J, et al. Current diagnostic and treatment strategies for specific dilated cardiomyopathies: a scientific statement from the American Heart Association. Circulation 2016; 134(23):e579–646.

37. Paulus WJ, Tschöpe C. A novel paradigm for heart failure with preserved ejection fraction: comorbidities drive myocardial dysfunction and remodeling through coronary microvascular endothelial inflammation. J Am Coll Cardiol 2013;62(4):263–71.

38. Haykowsky MJ, Kouba EJ, Brubaker PH, et al. Skeletal muscle composition and its relation to exercise intolerance in older patients with heart failure and preserved ejection fraction. Am J Cardiol 2014;113(7):1211–6.

39. Haykowsky MJ, Nicklas BJ, Brubaker PH, et al. Regional adipose distribution and its relationship to exercise intolerance in older obese patients who have heart failure with preserved ejection fraction. JACC Heart Fail 2018;6(8):640–9.

40. Packer M. Disease-treatment interactions in the management of patients with obesity and diabetes who have atrial fibrillation: the potential mediating influence of epicardial adipose tissue. Cardiovasc Diabetol 2019;18(1):121.

41. Deswal A. Obesity, leptin, and incident heart failure. J Am Coll Cardiol 2011;58(18):1878–80.

42. Toth MJ, Gottlieb SS, Fisher ML, et al. Plasma leptin concentrations and energy expenditure in heart failure patients. Metabolism 1997;46(4):450–3.

43. Franssen C, Chen S, Unger A, et al. Myocardial microvascular inflammatory endothelial activation in heart failure with preserved ejection fraction. JACC Heart Fail 2016;4(4):312–24.

44. Weberruß H, Pirzer R, Böhm B, et al. Intima-media thickness and arterial function in obese and non-obese children. BMC Obes 2015;3:2.

45. Porter SA, Massaro JM, Hoffmann U, et al. Abdominal subcutaneous adipose tissue: a protective fat depot? Diabetes Care 2009;32(6):1068–75.

46. Reddy YNV, Carter RE, Obokata M, et al. A simple, evidence-based approach to help guide diagnosis of heart failure with preserved ejection fraction. Circulation 2018;138(9):861–70.

47. Voulgari C, Tentolouris N, Dilaveris P, et al. Increased heart failure risk in normal-weight people with metabolic syndrome compared with metabolically healthy obese individuals. J Am Coll Cardiol 2011;58(13):1343–50.

48. Ndumele CE, Matsushita K, Sang Y, et al. N-terminal Pro-brain natriuretic peptide and heart failure risk among individuals with and without obesity: the Atherosclerosis Risk in Communities (ARIC) Study. Circulation 2016;133(7):631–8.

49. Khalid U, Wruck LM, Quibrera PM, et al. BNP and obesity in acute decompensated heart failure with preserved vs. reduced ejection fraction: the Atherosclerosis Risk in Communities Surveillance Study. Int J Cardiol 2017;233:61–6.

50. Anjan VY, Loftus TM, Burke MA, et al. Prevalence, clinical phenotype, and outcomes associated with normal B-type natriuretic peptide levels in heart failure with preserved ejection fraction. Am J Cardiol 2012;110(6):870–6.

51. Lam CS, Cheng S, Choong K, et al. Influence of sex and hormone status on circulating natriuretic peptides. J Am Coll Cardiol 2011;58(6):618–26.

52. Chang AY, Abdullah SM, Jain T, et al. Associations among androgens, estrogens, and natriuretic peptides in young women: observations from the Dallas Heart Study. J Am Coll Cardiol 2007;49(1):109–16.

53. Khan AM, Cheng S, Magnusson M, et al. Cardiac natriuretic peptides, obesity, and insulin resistance: evidence from two community-based studies. J Clin Endocrinol Metab 2011;96(10):3242–9.

54. Pieske B, Tschöpe C, de Boer RA, et al. How to diagnose heart failure with preserved ejection fraction: the HFA-PEFF diagnostic algorithm: a consensus recommendation from the Heart Failure Association (HFA) of the European Society of Cardiology (ESC). Eur Heart J 2019;40(40):3297–317.

55. Padwal R, McAlister FA, McMurray JJ, et al. The obesity paradox in heart failure patients with preserved versus reduced ejection fraction: a meta-analysis of individual patient data. Int J Obes (Lond) 2014;38(8):1110–4.

56. Mandviwala TM, Basra SS, Khalid U, et al. Obesity and the paradox of mortality and heart failure hospitalization in heart failure with preserved ejection fraction. Int J Obes (Lond) 2020;44(7):1561–7.

57. Tsujimoto T, Kajio H. Abdominal obesity is associated with an increased risk of all-cause mortality in patients with HFpEF. J Am Coll Cardiol 2017;70(22):2739–49.

58. Carbone S, Lavie CJ. Disparate effects of obesity on survival and hospitalizations in heart failure with preserved ejection fraction. Int J Obes 2020;44(7):1543–5.

59. Anker SD, Ponikowski P, Varney S, et al. Wasting as independent risk factor for mortality in chronic heart failure. Lancet 1997;349(9058):1050–3.

60. Davos CH, Doehner W, Rauchhaus M, et al. Body mass and survival in patients with chronic heart failure without cachexia: the importance of obesity. J Card Fail 2003;9(1):29–35.

61. Rauchhaus M, Clark AL, Doehner W, et al. The relationship between cholesterol and survival in patients with chronic heart failure. J Am Coll Cardiol 2003;42(11):1933–40.

62. Rauchhaus M, Coats AJ, Anker SD. The endotoxin-lipoprotein hypothesis. Lancet 2000;356(9233):930–3.

63. Mohamed-Ali V, Goodrick S, Bulmer K, et al. Production of soluble tumor necrosis factor receptors by human subcutaneous adipose tissue in vivo. Am J Physiol 1999;277(6):E971–5.

64. Blogowski W, Serwin K, Budkowska M, et al. Clinical analysis of systemic and adipose tissue levels of selected hormones/adipokines and stromal-derived factor-1. J Biol Regul Homeost Agents 2012;26(4):607–15.

65. Kistorp C, Faber J, Galatius S, et al. Plasma adiponectin, body mass index, and mortality in patients with chronic heart failure. Circulation 2005;112(12):1756–62.

66. Weber MA, Neutel JM, Smith DH. Contrasting clinical properties and exercise responses in obese and lean hypertensive patients. J Am Coll Cardiol 2001;37(1):169–74.

67. Reddy YNV, Rikhi A, Obokata M, et al. Quality of life in heart failure with preserved ejection fraction: importance of obesity, functional capacity, and physical inactivity. Eur J Heart Fail 2020;22(6):1009–18.

68. Takatsu M, Nakashima C, Takahashi K, et al. Calorie restriction attenuates cardiac remodeling and diastolic dysfunction in a rat model of metabolic syndrome. Hypertension 2013;62(5):957–65.

69. Meyer TE, Kovács SJ, Ehsani AA, et al. Long-term caloric restriction ameliorates the decline in diastolic function in humans. J Am Coll Cardiol 2006;47(2):398–402.

70. Kitzman DW, Brubaker P, Morgan T, et al. Effect of caloric restriction or aerobic exercise training on peak oxygen consumption and quality of life in obese older patients with heart failure with preserved ejection fraction: a randomized clinical trial. JAMA 2016;315(1):36–46.

71. Fukuta H, Goto T, Wakami K, et al. Effects of exercise training on cardiac function, exercise capacity, and quality of life in heart failure with preserved ejection fraction: a meta-analysis of randomized controlled trials. Heart Fail Rev 2019;24(4):535–47.

72. Miranda WR, Batsis JA, Sarr MG, et al. Impact of bariatric surgery on quality of life, functional capacity, and symptoms in patients with heart failure. Obes Surg 2013;23(7):1011–5.

73. Klein S, Fontana L, Young VL, et al. Absence of an effect of liposuction on insulin action and risk factors for coronary heart disease. N Engl J Med 2004;350(25):2549–57.

74. Shimada YJ, Tsugawa Y, Brown DFM, et al. Bariatric surgery and emergency department visits and hospitalizations for heart failure exacerbation: population-based, self-controlled series. J Am Coll Cardiol 2016;67(8):895–903.

75. Leichman JG, Wilson EB, Scarborough T, et al. Dramatic reversal of derangements in muscle metabolism and left ventricular function after bariatric surgery. Am J Med 2008;121(11):966–73.

76. Algahim MF, Lux TR, Leichman JG, et al. Progressive regression of left ventricular hypertrophy two years after bariatric surgery. Am J Med 2010; 123(6):549–55.

77. Sundström J, Bruze G, Ottosson J, et al. Weight loss and heart failure: a nationwide study of gastric bypass surgery versus intensive lifestyle treatment. Circulation 2017;135(17):1577–85.

78. Youcef G, Olivier A, Nicot N, et al. Preventive and chronic mineralocorticoid receptor antagonism is highly beneficial in obese SHHF rats. Br J Pharmacol 2016;173(11):1805–19.

79. Bostick B, Habibi J, DeMarco VG, et al. Mineralocorticoid receptor blockade prevents Western diet-induced diastolic dysfunction in female mice. Am J Physiol Heart Circ Physiol 2015;308(9): H1126–35.

80. Bender SB, DeMarco VG, Padilla J, et al. Mineralocorticoid receptor antagonism treats obesity-associated cardiac diastolic dysfunction. Hypertension 2015; 65(5):1082–8.

81. Kosmala W, Przewlocka-Kosmala M, Szczepanik-Osadnik H, et al. Fibrosis and cardiac function in obesity: a randomised controlled trial of aldosterone blockade. Heart 2013;99(5):320–6.

82. Pitt B, Pfeffer MA, Assmann SF, et al. Spironolactone for heart failure with preserved ejection fraction. N Engl J Med 2014;370(15):1383–92.

83. Cohen JB, Schrauben SJ, Zhao L, et al. Clinical phenogroups in heart failure with preserved ejection fraction: detailed phenotypes, prognosis, and response to spironolactone. JACC Heart Fail 2020;8(3):172–84.

84. Schling P, Schäfer T. Human adipose tissue cells keep tight control on the angiotensin II levels in their vicinity. J Biol Chem 2002;277(50):48066–75.

85. Nakagawa H, Oberwinkler H, Nikolaev VO, et al. Atrial natriuretic peptide locally counteracts the deleterious effects of cardiomyocyte mineralocorticoid receptor activation. Circ Heart Fail 2014;7(5): 814–21.

86. Wang TJ, Larson MG, Levy D, et al. Impact of obesity on plasma natriuretic peptide levels. Circulation 2004;109(5):594–600.

87. Tamura N, Ogawa Y, Chusho H, et al. Cardiac fibrosis in mice lacking brain natriuretic peptide. Proc Natl Acad Sci U S A 2000;97(8):4239–44.

88. Polak J, Kotrc M, Wedellova Z, et al. Lipolytic effects of B-type natriuretic peptide 1-32 in adipose tissue of heart failure patients compared with healthy controls. J Am Coll Cardiol 2011;58(11): 1119–25.

89. Rydén M, Bäckdahl J, Petrus P, et al. Impaired atrial natriuretic peptide-mediated lipolysis in obesity. Int J Obes (Lond) 2016;40(4):714–20.

90. Del Ry S, Cabiati M, Martino A, et al. High concentration of C-type natriuretic peptide promotes VEGF-dependent vasculogenesis in the remodeled region of infarcted swine heart with preserved left ventricular ejection fraction. Int J Cardiol 2013; 168(3):2426–34.

91. Croteau D, Qin F, Chambers JM, et al. Differential effects of sacubitril/valsartan on diastolic function in mice with obesity-related metabolic heart disease. JACC Basic Transl Sci 2020;5(9):916–27.

92. Solomon SD, McMurray JJV, Anand IS, et al. Angiotensin–neprilysin inhibition in heart failure with preserved ejection fraction. N Engl J Med 2019; 381(17):1609–20.

93. Yagi S, Hirata Y, Ise T, et al. Canagliflozin reduces epicardial fat in patients with type 2 diabetes mellitus. Diabetes Metab Syndr 2017;9:78.

94. Kusaka H, Koibuchi N, Hasegawa Y, et al. Empagliflozin lessened cardiac injury and reduced visceral adipocyte hypertrophy in prediabetic rats with metabolic syndrome. Cardiovasc Diabetol 2016; 15(1):157.

95. Lin B, Koibuchi N, Hasegawa Y, et al. Glycemic control with empagliflozin, a novel selective SGLT2 inhibitor, ameliorates cardiovascular injury and cognitive dysfunction in obese and type 2 diabetic mice. Cardiovasc Diabetol 2014;13:148.

96. Zinman B, Wanner C, Lachin JM, et al. Empagliflozin, cardiovascular outcomes, and mortality in type 2 diabetes. N Engl J Med 2015;373(22):2117–28.

97. Wiviott SD, Raz I, Bonaca MP, et al. Dapagliflozin and cardiovascular outcomes in type 2 diabetes. N Engl J Med 2018;380(4):347–57.

98. Neal B, Perkovic V, Mahaffey KW, et al. Canagliflozin and cardiovascular and renal events in type 2 diabetes. N Engl J Med 2017;377(7):644–57.

99. Fitchett D, Zinman B, Wanner C, et al. Heart failure outcomes with empagliflozin in patients with type 2

diabetes at high cardiovascular risk: results of the EMPA-REG OUTCOME® trial. Eur Heart J 2016; 37(19):1526–34.

100. Empagliflozin outcome trial in patients with chronic heart failure with preserved ejection fraction (EMPEROR-Preserved). ClinicalTrials.gov Identifier: NCT03057951. Available at: https://clinicaltrials.gov/ct2/show/NCT03057951?term=NCT03057951&draw=2&rank=1. Accessed November 29, 2020.

101. Dapagliflozin evaluation to improve the LIVEs of patients with preserved ejection fraction heart failure. (DELIVER). ClinicalTrials.gov Identifier: NCT03619213. Available at: https://clinicaltrials.gov/ct2/show/NCT03619213. Accessed November 29, 2020.

102. Williams DM, Evans M. Dapagliflozin for heart failure with preserved ejection fraction: will the DELIVER study deliver? Diabetes Ther 2020;11(10):2207–19.

Renal Dysfunction and Heart Failure with Preserved Ejection Fraction

Manjula G. Ananthram, MBBS*, Stephen S. Gottlieb, MD

KEYWORDS

- Renal dysfunction • Heart failure with preserved ejection fraction • Cardiorenal syndrome • CKD
- Renal impairment • HFpEF

KEY POINTS

- Heart failure with preserved ejection fraction (HFpEF) and chronic kidney disease (CKD) constitute a high-risk phenotype with high morbidity and mortality.
- A proinflammatory milieu, endothelial dysfunction, and systemic congestion are pathophysiological drivers of cardiorenal dysfunction in HFpEF and CKD.
- There is a paucity of effective targeted therapies for HFpEF and CKD.

INTRODUCTION

Heart failure with preserved ejection fraction (HFpEF) is a phenotypically heterogeneous syndrome,[1,2] a constellation of symptoms of exercise intolerance, exertional dyspnea, volume overload, and renal dysfunction that are a consequence of abnormal cardiac structure and mechanics resulting in elevated filling pressures. HFpEF comprises about 50%[3] of the cases of acute and chronic heart failure. Multiple comorbidities predispose to HFpEF, and renal dysfunction and HFpEF frequently coexist.[4,5] Chronic kidney disease (CKD) is associated with a worse prognosis, increased mortality, and poor outcomes. Renal dysfunction is associated with increased risk of hospitalizations and increased death in HFpEF.

CHRONIC KIDNEY DISEASE AND WORSENING RENAL FAILURE

CKD is defined as reduced kidney function as evidenced by glomerular filtration rate (GFR) of less than 60 mL/kg/1.73 m^2 or markers of renal damage of at least 3 months duration. Markers of kidney damage include albuminuria, histologic abnormalities, urinary sediment, electrolyte, or other abnormalities owing to tubular disorder, structural abnormalities detected by imaging, and history of kidney transplantation.[6,7]

CKD prevalence is nearly 50% in acute and chronic heart failure.[8,9] Cardiovascular (CV) causes and heart failure are major causes of mortality in CKD.[10–12] CKD, worsening renal function (WRF), and concomitant heart failure are associated with a poor prognosis, increased mortality, and worse outcomes.[8,9,13–15] A multitude of factors contributes to the coexistence of HFpEF in CKD. Shared comorbidities, factors impacting macrovascular and microvascular circulation, contribute to the CKD-HFpEF milieu[16] (**Fig. 1**). WRF is most commonly defined as an absolute increase in creatinine by 0.3 mg/dL[5] or a 25% reduction in eGFR from admission to discharge.[15] Renal dysfunction is associated with increased risk of hospitalizations and increased death in HFpEF.[17]

In a large meta-analysis of more than 1,076,104 patients, Damman and colleagues[8] noted that 32% of patients had CKD at baseline and was associated with an odds ratio (OR) of 2.34 for all-cause mortality.

Both moderate and severe renal dysfunction were associated with reduced survival with a hazard ratio [HR] of 1.59 for moderate CKD, 95% confidence

Department of Internal Medicine, Division of Cardiology, University of Maryland, 110 South Paca Street, 7th Floor, Baltimore, MD 21201, USA
* Corresponding author.
E-mail address: mananthram@som.umaryland.edu

Heart Failure Clin 17 (2021) 357–367
https://doi.org/10.1016/j.hfc.2021.03.005
1551-7136/21/© 2021 Elsevier Inc. All rights reserved.

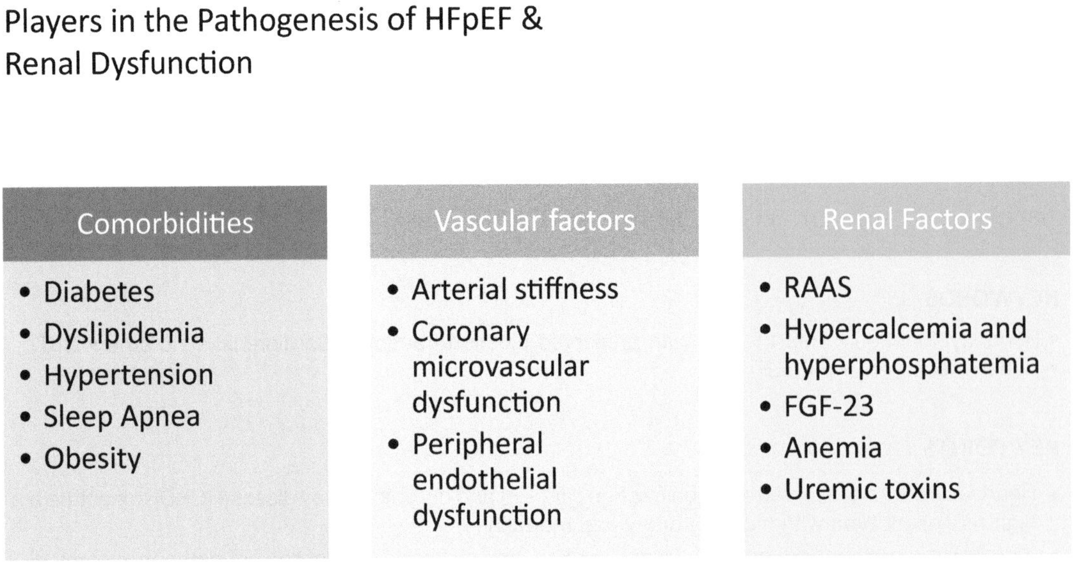

Players in the Pathogenesis of HFpEF & Renal Dysfunction

Comorbidities	Vascular factors	Renal Factors
• Diabetes • Dyslipidemia • Hypertension • Sleep Apnea • Obesity	• Arterial stiffness • Coronary microvascular dysfunction • Peripheral endothelial dysfunction	• RAAS • Hypercalcemia and hyperphosphatemia • FGF-23 • Anemia • Uremic toxins

Fig. 1. Factors involved in the pathogenesis of coexistent HFpEF and renal dysfunction.

interval [CI] 1.49 to 1.69, P<.001, and HR of 2.17 for severe CKD, 95% CI 1.45 to 2.62, P<.001.[8] Of the patients, 23% had WRF and was associated with increased mortality risk with an OR of 1.81, 95% CI 1.55 to 2.12, P<.001. The investigators concluded that CKD and WRF portend unfavorable prognosis and are associated with heightened mortality. Predictors of WRF include baseline CKD, diuretic utilization, presence of comorbidities, such as diabetes and hypertension, and older age.[8] It was found that CKD was a better prognosticator in subjects with HFpEF compared with heart failure with reduced ejection fraction (HFrEF).[8]

CLINICAL FEATURES

Shah and colleagues[1] used machine learning techniques to discern categories of 397 HFpEF patients based on their clinical phenotypes ("phenomapping").[1] They identified 3 phenogroups.

Phenogroup 1 consisted of younger subjects with lower brain natriuretic peptide (BNP) values.[1]

Phenogroup 2 was composed of obese subjects with higher prevalence of diabetes, sleep apnea, and the worst left ventricular (LV) relaxation.[1,18]

Phenogroup 3 comprised of patients that were older, with CKD, evidence of electrical and RV remodeling, RV dysfunction, abnormal ventriculoarterial coupling, highest BNP values and MAGGIC(Meta-analysis Global Group in Chronic Heart Failure)[19] risk scores. These patients comprised phenogroup 3 and had the highest risk of death and hospitalization. among all three phenogroups1 RV dysfunction and enhanced reactive pulmonary hypertension contribute to poor prognosis in this group.[20] Information gleaned from this study can

be used to tailor study design and targeted therapies for HFpEF.

THE HEART'S EFFECT ON THE KIDNEY

The heart-kidney nexus in HFpEF is complex and intriguing and not completely understood. Altered hemodynamics is a pivotal pathophysiological driver of renal dysfunction in heart failure. Conventional thinking supported the concept of decreased cardiac output as the primary cause of decreased renal perfusion in renal dysfunction. However, it is now known that elevated central venous pressure (CVP) and decreased renal perfusion are the most important hemodynamic factors involved in the heart-kidney interplay.[21–23] Elevated CVP is more important than reduced cardiac output in this heart-kidney interplay, and the association between increased CVP and reduced GFR is more robust in preserved cardiac output compared with reduced cardiac output.[5,24] Increased CVP results in decreased renal blood flow and renal perfusion pressure (**Fig. 2**). Decrease in renal perfusion pressure triggers the renin-angiotensin aldosterone and sympathetic (RAAS) nervous systems, resulting in decreased GFR.[5,21] As a consequence of increased CVP, renal venous pressure and renal interstitial pressure increase. When renal interstitial pressure surpasses the intraluminal tubular pressure, tubular collapse occurs and passive filtration ceases because of a reduction in pressure gradient across the glomerulus in the Bowman capsule to inconsequential levels.[21,25] Elevated interstitial pressure engenders tubular interstitial inflammation and fibrosis.[21,26]

Systemic and intrarenal circulation is affected by enhanced sympathetic activity.[27] Heightened

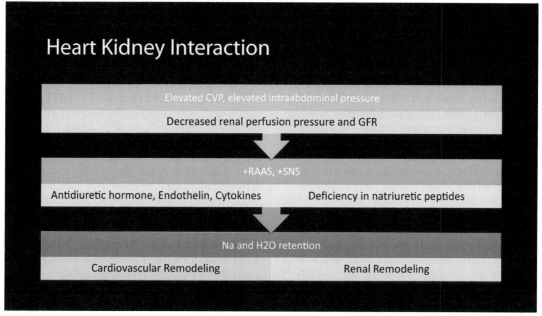

Fig. 2. Proposed mechanism of renal dysfunction in HFpEF. SNS, sympathetic nervous system.

sympathetic system activity results in increased adrenergic tone with a resultant decrease in β-receptor density in the ventricular myocardium with decoupling of the receptors from intracellular signaling mechanisms.[28] This decoupling is associated with altered baroreceptor reflexes, reduced heart rate variability, and susceptibility to arrhythmias.[29] With progression of heart failure, arterial underfilling or systemic venous congestion triggers baroreceptors, leading to renal vasoconstriction and stimulation of renal sympathetic nerves with release of catecholamines and neurohormones. Norepinephrine, arginine vasopressin, angiotensin-II, and endothelin result in efferent arterial vasoconstriction,[30] which leads to increased renal sodium absorption and sodium avidity and fluid retention. In advanced CKD accumulation of uremic toxins, uremia-associated proinflammatory cytokines and advanced glycation end products inhibit endothelial function and increase oxidative stress.

CHRONOTROPIC INCOMPETENCE

One of the important contributors to exercise intolerance in HFpEF is chronotropic incompetence, which was evaluated prospectively in an outpatient HFpEF cohort. Of the patients, 75% was found to have chronotropic incompetence. Reduced GFR, elevated BNP, and increased pulmonary artery systolic pressure correlated with CI. Lower GFR was associated with lower heart rate recovery, worse chronotropic incompetence, and reduced Vo_{2max}. Decreased heart rate reserve

suggests that CKD may be associated with impairment of autonomic function.[31]

ENDOTHELIUM

The endothelium plays a crucial role in maintaining CV homeostasis by modulating cardiac function, vascular tone, and permeability.[32] Undamaged, salubrious endothelium possesses vasoactive, hemostatic, antioxidant, and anti-inflammatory properties.[5] Vascular tone is modulated by the endothelium via the release of NO.[5,33] Stimulation of NADPH oxidase-2 increases myocardial fibrosis via enhanced mesenchymal cell transition, diastolic dysfunction, and inflammation in response to angiotensin-II.[34–36] Proinflammatory cytokines incite endothelial production of reactive oxygen species and cause endothelial dysfunction and oxidative stress[37]; this leads to a decrease in NO bioavailability and reduced cyclic GMP and protein kinase G (PK-G) activity in cardiac myocytes. PK-G is an inhibitor of cardiomyocyte hypertrophy.

Reduced PK-G activity results in cardiac remodeling, impaired relaxation, and myocardial fibrosis.

The endothelium is involved in sodium handling and its transition from the endothelial cell into the extracellular matrix.[5] Elevated plasma sodium or aldosterone levels contribute to a decrease in endothelial pliability and promote stiffening and reduced NO availability, a breach in the endothelial glycocalyx, and vascular endothelial dysfunction,[5,38] which leads to elevated resistance in the microvascular circulation, altered permeability, and extravascular fluid accumulation.[5]

Cardiac as well as peripheral endothelial cell dysfunction plays a role in the pathogenesis of HFpEF.[32,39]

Akiyama and colleagues[39] recruited 373 patients with HFpEF and 173 with no HFpEF and assessed endothelial dysfunction by reactive hyperemia peripheral artery tonometry (RHI). Participants with HFpEF had a lower GFR and higher BNP and high sensitivity C-reactive protein at baseline. Peripheral endothelial dysfunction as measured by RHI correlated with future CV events.[39]

In a postmortem study with an antemortem diagnosis of HFpEF, Mohammed and colleagues[36] studied the cardiac morphologic features of 124 patients and compared it with age-matched controls. HFpEF patients had more hypertrophy, fibrosis, epicardial coronary artery disease, and coronary microvascular rarefaction, which is a reduction in coronary microvascular density.[40] These findings probably play a role in diastolic dysfunction and diminished functional cardiac reserve commonly seen in HFpEF.[40] Microvascular endothelial inflammation possibly triggers microvascular rarefaction and myocardial fibrosis.[41,42]

INFLAMMATION

Paulus and Tschöpe[42] proposed a new paradigm for HFpEF that shifts the focus from LV load to a cascade of events involving inflammation and microvascular dysfunction leading to cardiac remodeling.

CKD is a proinflammatory state.[43,44] A systemic proinflammatory state plays a crucial role in the pathogenesis of HFpeF, and increased levels of inflammatory markers have been demonstrated in several studies.[45] Multiple inflammatory biomarkers, such as vascular cell adhesion molecule (VCAM), E-selectin, interleukin-6 (IL-6) and IL-8, monocyte chemoattractant protein-1, pentraxin-3, suppression of tumorigenicity 2 (ST2), and tumor necrosis factor (TNF)-αreceptor 2, have been identified in HFpEF.[5,46] In patients with HFpEF, enhanced inflammation stimulates accrual of collagen. Migration of inflammatory cells from the endothelium to the myocardium incite cardiac remodeling and diastolic dysfunction.[46]

The microvasculature of the kidneys and its ability to excrete sodium are affected by oxidative stress and systemic inflammation.[20,47]

BIOMARKERS IN RENAL DYSFUNCTION AND HEART FAILURE WITH PRESERVED EJECTION FRACTION

Concomitant HFpEF and CKD foster a deleterious milieu and portend poor prognosis.[33] Biomarkers may be useful in management of renal dysfunction in HFpeF by enhancing the understanding of pathophysiologic processes, identifying patients at risk of developing HFpEF, cardiac remodeling, fibrosis, and predicting outcomes.

In an inpatient cohort of HFpEF and Heart failure with mid-range ejection fraction (HFmrEF) patients with blood urea nitrogen (BUN)/creatinine and N terminal pro BNP (NT pro BNP) below the median admission values, renal impairment was not associated with increased mortality. In participants with both elevated BUN/creatinine ratio and elevated NT-proBNP, those with renal insufficiency had reduced survival when compared with those without renal insufficiency.[48] HFpEF patients with renal impairment with only one of the parameters, either BUN/creatinine ratio or NT-proBNP, elevated, had a significantly higher mortality risk compared with patients without renal insufficiency.[48]

Concomitant use of NT-proBNP values and BUN/creatinine ratio was shown to be useful in risk stratifying HFpEF patients with renal impairment.[48]

Albuminuria is a marker of endothelial dysfunction and is associated with unfavorable outcomes in HFpEF. HFpeF patients with albuminuria may have increased renin angiotensin aldosterone activity when compared with those without albuminuria.[49]

In addition to the above, higher urinary albumin/creatinine ratio was associated with LV/RV remodeling and CKD and was associated with the composite endpoint of CV hospitalization and death in a well-defined HFpEF cohort.[50] Albuminuria in conjunction with eGFR was found to be useful in risk stratification of patients with HFpEF.[49]

Similarly, among HFpEF patients in the PARAMOUNT study, Gori and colleagues[51] found that 62% of the patients had at least 1 parameter of abnormal renal function. Renal dysfunction as assessed by either eGFR or albuminuria (urinary/albumin to creatinine ratio) was associated with cardiac remodeling.

Individuals with microalbuminuria were found to be at increased risk for development of HFpEF in a large community-based cohort.[2,52]

Urinary albumin excretion and cystatin C are risk factors for new-onset HFpEF.[53] Cystatin C is unaffected by muscle mass, age, sex, and race and is a superior and earlier predictor of glomerular function than creatinine.[4,54]

Integrating a plasma multimarker strategy with machine learning to augment risk profiling in HFpEF, Chirinos and colleagues[55] showed that the biomarkers of renal injury, cystatin C and NGAL, clustered with biomarkers of inflammation and remodeling, bringing to light the role of renal dysfunction and systemic inflammation in HFpEF. A biomarker for liver fibrosis YLK-40/CHI3L1 was also found to be tightly clustered with the renal and inflammatory biomarkers, suggesting that the inflammatory process extends beyond the cardiorenal realm. Fibroblast growth factor (FGF) 23 plays a role in phosphate regulation, and FGF-23 levels increase with declining renal function.[56] FGF-23 is a strong predictor of incident heart failure and poor outcomes.[55,57]

In the other direction, a robust association between FGF-23 and elevated risk of CV events was demonstrated in a prospective cohort of 3860 subjects with CKD stage 2 to 4. The association was more pronounced for congestive heart failure (CHF) than atherosclerotic events.[58]

Renocardiovascular biomarkers, such as neutrophil gelatinase associated lipocalin NGAL, cystatin-C, and kidney injury molecule-1 (KIM-1), are useful in risk stratification in acute and chronic renal dysfunction.[56] NGAL is a marker for acute tubular injury.[59] In hospitalized patients with ADHF, predominantly HFrEF elevated NGAL on admission predicts ensuing worsening renal failure.[60]

In a retrospective analysis of the GISSI-HF population, patients with WRF were found to have reduced baseline GFR and elevated levels of NGAL, N-acetyl-beta-glucosamine, and KIM-1. KIM-1 was found to be the strongest predictor of WRF in this study.[61] Investigations regarding these renal biomarkers in the context of HFpEF are warranted to better understand the mechanism and interaction of renal injury and HFpEF.

An association between ST2, diabetes mellitus, renal dysfunction, systemic congestion, right ventricular pressure overload, and dysfunction has been found. Elevated ST2 level may be a marker of the proinflammatory milieu engendered by the comorbidities associated with HFpEF, including renal impairment, and may be of value in risk stratification of HFpEF and renal dysfunction.[62]

Recent studies have revealed abnormal patterns of microRNA in cardiac and renal fibrosis.[63,64]

There are preliminary data regarding microRNA detection to discern preclinical heart failure.[65] Further studies are needed to evaluate microRNAs as a biomarker in renal and myocardial fibrosis especially in the context of HFpeF.

The clinical application of biomarkers in the management of renal dysfunction and HFpEF holds promise but is not well defined, and additional work is needed in this area.

HEMODYNAMIC FACTORS

One of the most important hemodynamic drivers of WRF is elevated CVP.[22,23]

In a retrospective chart review on 2557 patients with a variety of CV disorders who underwent right heart catheterizations, an elevated CVP was associated with impairment of renal function and was an independent predictor of all-cause mortality.[24]

Elevated CVP is more important than reduced cardiac output, and the association between increased CVP and reduced GFR was stronger in preserved cardiac output compared with reduced cardiac output.[5,24]

It is possible that RV dysfunction contributes to renal dysfunction in HFpEF. A small retrospective analysis of hospitalized patients with HFpEF demonstrated that a decreased pulmonary artery pulsatility index was associated with worsening eGFR, whereas an elevated right atrial pressure to pulmonary capillary wedge pressure ratio predicted worse eGFR, but was not statistically signficant.[66] The importance of the RV has been demonstrated in the advanced heart failure and left ventricular assist device population, and further work is needed to determine whether RV dysfunction truly leads to renal dysfunction in HFpEF.

Severity of tricuspid regurgitation was found to be independently associated with GFR reduction in a study of 196 patients with moderate tricuspid regurgitation and heart failure.[67]

When compared with HFrEF patients, HFpEF patients are susceptible to exaggerated blood pressure decrease and attenuated increase in stroke volume and cardiac output with vasodilator therapies.[68] HFpEF patients are susceptible to venodilation and are preload dependent when compared with HFrEF treated with vasodilators.[68] Fixed stroke volume, drop in blood pressure in the setting of lower filling pressures compounded by chronotropic incompetence may contribute to decreased renal perfusion and renal dysfunction. The primary hemodynamic driver of renal dysfunction, however, is elevated CVP, which is a consequence of pulmonary hypertension and RV dysfunction.

RENAL PARAMETERS IN HEART FAILURE WITH PRESERVED EJECTION FRACTION

Renal function is generally estimated by GFR based on serum creatinine. Calculation of eGFR using the Chronic Kidney Disease Epidemiology Collaboration equation rather than the Modification of Diet in Renal Disease equation results in increased estimates of renal impairment in heart failure and provides a better stratification of mortality risk. Renal dysfunction as measured by eGFR is a stronger predictor of all-cause mortality in HFrEF than in HFpEF.[69] Renal Doppler hemodynamics may have incremental value in the assessment of renal function.

Renal arterial resistance index (RI) is a Doppler index of renal blood flow that is reflective of vascular and parenchymal abnormalities.[70] A strong association has been shown between elevated RI and HFpEF.[71] Increased RI prognosticates unfavorable outcomes in HFpEF. Patients with HFpEF display changes in intrarenal vascular hemodynamics, and the severity of these changes correlates with poor outcomes.[71] An RI greater than 75 was associated with heart failure progression and unfavorable prognosis in patients with both normal and impaired renal function. RI is an independent prognostic marker of HF progression, and its prognostic value is additive to that of GFR alone.[70] In a small renal biopsy-based study, an association was demonstrated between RI >0.65 and severe interstitial fibrosis, arteriosclerosis, and deterioration in renal function.[72]

Echo Doppler parameters of diastolic dysfunction correlated with RI in a small study of patients with hypertension without heart failure or renal insufficiency.

This indicates that cardiac and renal involvement occur simultaneously in hypertensive patients.[73]

In conclusion, RI is an independent predictor of outcomes in CHF and may be valuable in clinical practice as a parameter of renal function and aid in risk stratification.

CARDIAC MORPHOLOGY IN RENAL DYSFUNCTION AND HEART FAILURE WITH PRESERVED EJECTION FRACTION

HFpEF, hypertensive heart disease, and left ventricular hypertrophy (LVH) are frequently seen in conjunction with advanced kidney disease.[74] The degree of concentric LVH in chronic uremia is associated with increased risk of heart failure and mortality.[75] Patients with concomitant CKD and HFpEF are likely to have morphologic and echocardiographic features reflective of advanced disease.

A retrospective study found a significant difference between hospitalized HFpEF patients with and without WRF in echocardiographic measures of RV function as evidenced by a decrease in RV fractional area change and adverse remodeling based on increased RV free wall thickness. However, there was no significant difference between RA RV size between the 2 groups.[76]

In a prospective analysis of HFpEF patients with and without CKD, Unger and colleagues[13] assessed routine diastolic indices and novel echocardiographic parameters, such as LA reservoir strain, LV strain, and RV free wall strain. They found that CKD is associated with a greater degree of impaired diastolic dysfunction, impaired systolic LV, and RV dysfunction when compared with those without CKD. CKD was associated

with impaired cardiac remodeling, worse cardiac mechanics, and worse outcomes.[77]

Patel and colleagues[33] evaluated echocardiographic and biomarker indices in the RELAX HFpEF cohort based on the presence or absence of CKD. Echocardiographic parameter of lateral e′ velocity was significantly decreased, and estimated filling pressures (E/e′ average) were elevated in the CKD group. Lower eGFR was associated with elevated biomarkers (aldosterone, uric acid, NT-proBNP, endothelin-1 and galectin-3, NT-procollagen III peptide and C-terminal telopeptide of collagen type 1-CITP). Lower eGFR was associated with lower peak oxygen consumption, and lower hemoglobin was found to be a significant mediator of the association between low eGFR and peak V_{O_2} levels.

RENIN-ANGIOTENSIN-ALDOSTERONE SYSTEM INHIBITION AND RENAL FUNCTION IN HEART FAILURE WITH PRESERVED EJECTION FRACTION

Studies of RAAS inhibition in HFpEF have not shown mortality benefits.[78–80] However, angiotensin converting enzyme inhibitor and angiotensin receptor blockers have been shown to decrease the risk of renal failure and CV events in CKD.[81] The desired approach to reduce proteinuria in CKD is RAAS inhibition. Although RAAS inhibition in HFrEF leads to chronic benefits in renal function, the results in HFpEF are less clear.[81,82] In the Randomized Aldactone Evaluation Study, spironolactone improved survival even in those with WRF.[83] In The Treatment of Preserved Cardiac Function Heart Failure with an Aldosterone Antagonist Trial, there were more deterioration of renal function in the spironolactone arm; however, this did not portend a poorer prognosis.[84]

Furthermore, in the Prospective Comparison of ARNI with ARB Global Outcomes in HFpEF (PARAGON HF) study, a lower rate of reduction in GFR was noted in the sacubitril-valsartan group when compared with the valsartan group.[85,86] The mechanisms and implications of this are not yet certain.

SODIUM GLUCOSE COTRANSPORTER-2 INHIBITORS

Sodium glucose cotransporter 2 inhibitors (SGLT-2i) decrease oxidative stress,[87,88] fibrosis, and intraglomerular hypertension,[89,90] have anti-inflammatory properties,[91,92] and attenuate sympathetic nervous system activity with the potential to mitigate neurohormonal activity in cardiorenal interactions.[93] They have direct cardioprotective and renoprotective effects.[93–96]

In 4 large-scale outcome trials of patients with diabetes mellitus, SGLT-2i have shown significant reduction in composite of sustained worsening of eGFR, end-stage renal disease, or mortality from renal causes.[97] They have robust benefits in reduction of heart failure hospitalizations and progression of renal disease regardless of history of heart failure.[98] A meta-analysis of the 3 large CV outcome trials revealed that patients with worse baseline renal function had greater reduction in heart failure hospitalizations and a lesser effect on progression of renal dysfunction.[98] A decrease in heart failure hospitalizations in patients with HFpEf and HFrEF was observed in one of the trials.[99]

In HFrEF, SGLT-2i have been shown to decrease heart failure hospitalizations and mortality.[97] Empagliflozin has a beneficial effect on cardiac myocyte endothelial cell and cardiac myocyte interaction following exposure of cardiomyocyte to TNF-α via endothelial-derived NO.[100]

Considering the paradigm of inflammation, endothelial dysfunction, fibrosis, coronary microvascular dysfunction, and sympathetic activation in HFpEF, and the aforementioned effects of SGLT-2i, this class of drugs seems promising in HFpEF management.

There are ongoing trials to evaluate the impact of SGLT-2 inhibitors in HFpEF.

Empagliflozin Outcome Trial in Patients With Chronic Heart Failure With Preserved Ejection Fraction (NCT03057951) is a large, double-blind, placebo-controlled trial investigating empagliflozin in HFpEF patients with and without diabetes mellitus. Half of the 5988 patients enrolled in this study have baseline CKD.[101]

Dapagliflozin Evaluation to Improve the Lives of Patients With Preserved Ejection Fraction Heart Failure (NCT03619213) is an international double-blind randomized placebo-controlled study to evaluate the effect of dapagliflozin on reducing CV death or worsening heart failure in patients with HFpEF.[102]

CONNECT AND RECONNECXT

Renal Connection to Microvascular Disease and HFpEF, the next phase (RECONNECXT),[103] is a multicenter consortium created to further research on knowledge gained from Renal Connection to Microvascular Disease and HFpEF (RECONNECT)[5] consortium. Outcomes of RECONNECT highlight that CKD is a significant risk factor in the development, progression, and mortality in HFpEF and plays a pivotal role in the pathogenesis of HFpEF via systemic inflammation and coronary microvascular dysfunction. RECONNECT identified potential targets for therapy in HFpEF.[103] The objectives of RECONNECXT relate to identifying renal drivers for subgroups of HFpEF, to better discern the pathophysiology of the renocardiac nexus, evaluate therapeutic targets, and focus on clinical applications. It is expected that results of this interdisciplinary undertaking will deepen the understanding of mechanistic pathways in HFpEF and pave the way to development of personalized diagnostics and therapeutics.[103]

SUMMARY

HFpEF and CKD constitute a high-risk phenotype with considerable morbidity and mortality and poor outcomes.

Multiple proinflammatory comorbid conditions influence the pathogenesis of HFpEF and CKD. Renal dysfunction in HFpEF is a result of elevated CVP secondary to systemic congestion, pulmonary hypertension, and RV dysfunction. Renal perfusion is compromised by vasodilatation, fixed stroke volume, and chronotropic incompetence. Decreased renal blood flow and reduced sodium excretion promote a proinflammatory state via uremic toxins and fibroblast growth factor, parathyroid hormone, vitamin D deficiency, and erythropoietin. This proinflammatory milieu perpetuates the vicious cycle of cardiac and renal dysfunction in HFpEF.

In contrast to HFrEF, there is a dearth of effective targeted therapies for HFpEF. Tailoring study design toward the different phenotypes and delving into the pathophysiology and biology of these phenotypes may be useful in the development of effective phenotype-specific targeted pharmaceutical therapies for this heterogenous syndrome.

CLINICS CARE POINTS

- Coexistent renal dysfunction and heart failure with preserved ejection fraction present a challenging situation.
- Alleviating symptoms revolves around management of volume status with diuretics and ultrafiltration and mitigating chronotropic incompetence.
- Cautious use or avoidance of vasodilators prevents worsening renal function.
- Comorbid conditions that affect renal dysfunction and HFpEF should be treated.

DISCLOSURE

Dr M.G. Ananthram has nothing to disclose. Dr S.S. Gottlieb reports consulting to Cytokinetics and Eidos.

REFERENCES

1. Shah SJ, Katz DH, Selvaraj S, et al. Phenomapping for novel classification of heart failure with preserved ejection fraction. Circulation 2015;131(3):269–79.
2. Carnes J, Gordon G. Biomarkers in heart failure with preserved ejection fraction: an update on progress and future challenges. Heart Lung Circ 2020;29(1):62–8.
3. Lund LH, Donal E, Oger E, et al. Association between cardiovascular vs. non-cardiovascular comorbidities and outcomes in heart failure with preserved ejection fraction. Eur J Heart Fail 2014; 16(9):992–1001.
4. Lazzeri C, Valente S, Tarquini R, et al. Cardiorenal syndrome caused by heart failure with preserved ejection fraction. Int J Nephrol 2011;2011:634903.
5. Ter Maaten JM, Damman K, Verhaar MC, et al. Connecting heart failure with preserved ejection fraction and renal dysfunction: the role of endothelial dysfunction and inflammation. Eur J Heart Fail 2016;18(6):588–98.
6. Webster AC, Nagler EV, Morton RL, et al. Chronic kidney disease. Lancet 2017;389(10075):1238–52.
7. Evaluation and management of chronic kidney disease: synopsis of the kidney disease: Improving Global Outcomes 2012 Clinical Practice Guideline. Ann Intern Med 2013;158(11):825–30.
8. Damman K, Valente MAE, Voors AA, et al. Renal impairment, worsening renal function, and outcome in patients with heart failure: an updated meta-analysis. Eur Heart J 2014;35(7):455–69.
9. Damman K, Testani JM. The kidney in heart failure: an update. Eur Heart J 2015;36(23):1437–44.
10. Kottgen A, Russell SD, Loehr LR, et al. Reduced kidney function as a risk factor for incident heart failure: the Atherosclerosis Risk in Communities (ARIC) Study. J Am Soc Nephrol 2007;18(4):1307.
11. Bansal N, Katz R, Robinson-Cohen C, et al. Absolute rates of heart failure, coronary heart disease, and stroke in chronic kidney disease: an analysis of 3 community-based cohort studies. JAMA Cardiol 2017;2(3):314–8.
12. Tonelli M, Wiebe N, Culleton B, et al. Chronic kidney disease and mortality risk: a systematic review. J Am Soc Nephrol 2006;17(7):2034–47.
13. Unger ED, Dubin RF, Deo R, et al. Association of chronic kidney disease with abnormal cardiac mechanics and adverse outcomes in patients with heart failure and preserved ejection fraction. Eur J Heart Fail 2016;18(1):103–12.
14. Damman K, Navis G, Voors AA, et al. Worsening renal function and prognosis in heart failure: systematic review and meta-analysis. J Card Fail 2007;13(8):599–608.
15. Rusinaru D, Buiciuc O, Houpe D, et al. Renal function and long-term survival after hospital discharge in heart failure with preserved ejection fraction. Int J Cardiol 2011;147(2):278–82.
16. van de Wouw J, Broekhuizen M, Sorop O, et al. Chronic kidney disease as a risk factor for heart failure with preserved ejection fraction: a focus on microcirculatory factors and therapeutic targets. Front Physiol 2019;10:1108.
17. Georgiopoulou VV, Velayati A, Burkman G, et al. Comorbidities, sociodemographic factors, and hospitalizations in outpatients with heart failure and preserved ejection fraction. Am J Cardiol 2018;121(10):1207–13.
18. Lewis GA, Schelbert EB, Williams SG, et al. Biological phenotypes of heart failure with preserved ejection fraction. J Am Coll Cardiol 2017;70(17):2186–200.
19. Pocock SJ, Ariti CA, McMurray JJV, et al. Predicting survival in heart failure: a risk score based on 39 372 patients from 30 studies. Eur Heart J 2013;34(19):1404–13.
20. Shah SJ, Kitzman DW, Borlaug BA, et al. Phenotype-specific treatment of heart failure with preserved ejection fraction. Circulation 2016;134(1):73–90.
21. Damman K, Voors AA, Navis G, et al. The cardiorenal syndrome in heart failure. Prog Cardiovasc Dis 2011;54(2):144–53. https://doi.org/10.1016/j.pcad.2011.01.003.
22. Mullens W, Abrahams Z, Francis GS, et al. Importance of venous congestion for worsening of renal function in advanced decompensated heart failure. J Am Coll Cardiol 2009;53(7):589–96. https://doi.org/10.1016/j.jacc.2008.05.068.
23. Guyton AC, Jones CE. Central venous pressure: physiological significance and clinical implications. Am Heart J 1973;86(4):431–7. https://doi.org/10.1016/0002-8703(73)90132-4.
24. Damman K, van Deursen VM, Navis G, et al. Increased central venous pressure is associated with impaired renal function and mortality in a broad spectrum of patients with cardiovascular disease. J Am Coll Cardiol 2009;53(7):582–8.
25. Joles JA, Bongartz LG, Gaillard CA, et al. Renal venous congestion and renal function in congestive heart failure. J Am Coll Cardiol 2009;54(17):1632 [author reply: 1632–3].
26. Jin C, Hu C, Polichnowski A, et al. Effects of renal perfusion pressure on renal medullary hydrogen peroxide and nitric oxide production. Hypertension 2009;53(6):1048–53.

27. Boddi M, Sacchi S, Lammel RM, et al. Age-related and vasomotor stimuli-induced changes in renal vascular resistance detected by Doppler ultrasound. Am J Hypertens 1996;9(5):461–6.

28. Bock JS, Gottlieb SS. Cardiorenal syndrome: new perspectives. Circulation 2010;121(23):2592–600.

29. Bongartz LG, Cramer MJ, Doevendans PA, et al. The severe cardiorenal syndrome: "Guyton revisited". Eur Heart J 2005;26(1):11–7.

30. Blankstein R, Bakris GL. Renal hemodynamic changes in heart failure. Heart Fail Clin 2008;4(4):411–23.

31. Klein DA, Katz DH, Beussink-Nelson L, et al. Association of chronic kidney disease with chronotropic incompetence in heart failure with preserved ejection fraction. Am J Cardiol 2015;116(7):1093–100.

32. Lam CSP, Brutsaert DL. Endothelial dysfunction: a pathophysiologic factor in heart failure with preserved ejection fraction. Editorials published in the Journal of the American College of Cardiology reflect the views of the authors and do not necessarily represent the views of JACC or the American College of Cardiology. J Am Coll Cardiol 2012;60(18):1787–9.

33. Patel RB, MEHTA R, REDFIELD MM, et al. Renal dysfunction in heart failure with preserved ejection fraction: insights from the RELAX Trial. J Card Fail 2020;26(3):233–42.

34. Murdoch CE, Chaubey S, Zeng L, et al. Endothelial NADPH oxidase-2 promotes interstitial cardiac fibrosis and diastolic dysfunction through proinflammatory effects and endothelial-mesenchymal transition. J Am Coll Cardiol 2014;63(24):2734–41.

35. Griendling KK, Minieri CA, Ollerenshaw JD, et al. Angiotensin II stimulates NADH and NADPH oxidase activity in cultured vascular smooth muscle cells. Circ Res 1994;74(6):1141–8.

36. Heymes C, Bendall JK, Ratajczak P, et al. Increased myocardial NADPH oxidase activity in human heart failure. J Am Coll Cardiol 2003;41(12):2164–71.

37. Griendling KK, Sorescu D, Ushio-Fukai M. NAD(P)H oxidase: role in cardiovascular biology and disease. Circ Res 2000;86(5):494–501.

38. Oberleithner H, Riethmüller C, Schillers H, et al. Plasma sodium stiffens vascular endothelium and reduces nitric oxide release. Proc Natl Acad Sci U S A 2007;104(41):16281–6.

39. Akiyama E, Sugiyama S, Matsuzawa Y, et al. Incremental prognostic significance of peripheral endothelial dysfunction in patients with heart failure with normal left ventricular ejection fraction. J Am Coll Cardiol 2012;60(18):1778–86.

40. Mohammed SF, Hussain S, Mirzoyev SA, et al. Coronary microvascular rarefaction and myocardial fibrosis in heart failure with preserved ejection fraction. Circulation 2015;131(6):550–9.

41. Gladden JD, Chaanine AH, Redfield MM. Heart failure with preserved ejection fraction. Annu Rev Med 2018;69(1):65–79.

42. Paulus WJ, Tschöpe C. A novel paradigm for heart failure with preserved ejection fraction: comorbidities drive myocardial dysfunction and remodeling through coronary microvascular endothelial inflammation. J Am Coll Cardiol 2013;62(4):263–71.

43. Stenvinkel P, Barany P, Heimbürger O, et al. Mortality, malnutrition, and atherosclerosis in ESRD: what is the role of interleukin-6? Kidney Int 2002;61:S103–8.

44. Herbelin A, Ureña P, Nguyen AT, et al. Elevated circulating levels of interleukin-6 in patients with chronic renal failure. Kidney Int 1991;39(5):954–60.

45. Glezeva N, Baugh JA. Role of inflammation in the pathogenesis of heart failure with preserved ejection fraction and its potential as a therapeutic target. Heart Fail Rev 2014;19(5):681–94.

46. Westermann D, Lindner D, Kasner M, et al. Cardiac inflammation contributes to changes in the extracellular matrix in patients with heart failure and normal ejection fraction. Circ Heart Fail 2011;4(1):44–52.

47. Cowley AWJ, Abe M, Mori T, et al. Reactive oxygen species as important determinants of medullary flow, sodium excretion, and hypertension. Am J Physiol Ren Physiol 2015;308(3):F179–97.

48. Casado J, Sánchez M, Garcés V, et al. Influence of renal dysfunction phenotype on mortality in decompensated heart failure with preserved and midrange ejection fraction. Int J Cardiol 2017;243:332–9.

49. Miura M, Shiba N, Nochioka K, et al. Urinary albumin excretion in heart failure with preserved ejection fraction: an interim analysis of the CHART 2 study. Eur J Heart Fail 2012;14(4):367–76.

50. Katz DH, Burns JA, Aguilar FG, et al. Albuminuria is independently associated with cardiac remodeling, abnormal right and left ventricular function, and worse outcomes in heart failure with preserved ejection fraction. JACC Heart Fail 2014;2(6):586–96.

51. Gori M, Senni M, Gupta DK, et al. Association between renal function and cardiovascular structure and function in heart failure with preserved ejection fraction. Eur Heart J 2014;35(48):3442–51.

52. de Boer RA, Nayor M, deFilippi CR, et al. Association of cardiovascular biomarkers with incident heart failure with preserved and reduced ejection fraction. JAMA Cardiol 2018;3(3):215–24.

53. Brouwers FP, de Boer RA, van der Harst P, et al. Incidence and epidemiology of new onset heart failure with preserved vs. reduced ejection fraction in a community-based cohort: 11-year follow-up of PREVEND. Eur Heart J 2013;34(19):1424–31.

54. Dharnidharka VR, Kwon C, Stevens G. Serum cystatin C is superior to serum creatinine as a marker of kidney function: a meta-analysis. Am J Kidney Dis 2002;40(2):221–6.

55. Chirinos JA, Orlenko A, Zhao L, et al. Multiple plasma biomarkers for risk stratification in patients with heart failure and preserved ejection fraction. J Am Coll Cardiol 2020;75(11):1281–95.

56. Niizuma S, Iwanaga Y, Yahata T, et al. Renocardiovascular biomarkers: from the perspective of managing chronic kidney disease and cardiovascular disease. Front Cardiovasc Med 2017;4:10.

57. Roy C, Lejeune S, Slimani A, et al. Fibroblast growth factor 23: a biomarker of fibrosis and prognosis in heart failure with preserved ejection fraction. ESC Heart Fail 2020;7(5):2494–507.

58. Scialla JJ, Xie H, Rahman M, et al. Fibroblast growth factor-23 and cardiovascular events in CKD. J Am Soc Nephrol JASN 2014;25(2):349–60.

59. Ding H, He Y, Li K, et al. Urinary neutrophil gelatinase-associated lipocalin (NGAL) is an early biomarker for renal tubulointerstitial injury in IgA nephropathy. Clin Immunol 2007;123(2):227–34.

60. Aghel A, Shrestha K, Mullens W, et al. Serum neutrophil gelatinase-associated lipocalin (NGAL) in predicting worsening renal function in acute decompensated heart failure. J Card Fail 2010;16(1):49–54.

61. Damman K, Masson S, Hillege HL, et al. Tubular damage and worsening renal function in chronic heart failure. JACC Heart Fail 2013;1(5):417–24.

62. Abou Ezzeddine OF, McKie PM, Dunlay SM, et al. ST2 in heart failure with preserved ejection fraction. Circulation 2015;132. Available at: https://www.embase.com/search/results?subaction=viewrecord&id=L72180417&from=export.

63. Chung AC-K, Lan HY. MicroRNAs in renal fibrosis. Front Physiol 2015;6:50.

64. Villar AV, García R, Merino D, et al. Myocardial and circulating levels of microRNA-21 reflect left ventricular fibrosis in aortic stenosis patients. Int J Cardiol 2013;167(6):2875–81.

65. D'Alessandra Y, Chiesa M, Carena MC, et al. Differential role of circulating microRNAs to track progression and pre-symptomatic stage of chronic heart failure: a pilot study. Biomedicines 2020;8(12). https://doi.org/10.3390/biomedicines8120597.

66. Lo KB, Mezue K, Ram P, et al. Echocardiographic and hemodynamic parameters associated with diminishing renal filtration among patients with heart failure with preserved ejection fraction. Cardiorenal Med 2019;9(2):83–91.

67. Maeder MT, Holst DP, Kaye DM. Tricuspid regurgitation contributes to renal dysfunction in patients with heart failure. J Card Fail 2008;14(10):824–30.

68. Schwartzenberg S, Redfield MM, From AM, et al. Effects of vasodilation in heart failure with preserved or reduced ejection fraction implications of distinct pathophysiologies on response to therapy. J Am Coll Cardiol 2012;59(5):442–51.

69. McAlister FA, Ezekowitz J, Tarantini L, et al. Renal dysfunction in patients with heart failure with preserved versus reduced ejection fraction impact of the new chronic kidney disease-epidemiology collaboration group formula. Circ Heart Fail 2012;5(3):309–14.

70. Ciccone MM, Iacoviello M, Gesualdo L, et al. The renal arterial resistance index: a marker of renal function with an independent and incremental role in predicting heart failure progression. Eur J Heart Fail 2014;16(2):210–6.

71. Ennezat PV, Maréchaux S, Six-Carpentier M, et al. Renal resistance index and its prognostic significance in patients with heart failure with preserved ejection fraction. Nephrol Dial Transplant 2011;26(12):3908–13.

72. Bigé N, Lévy PP, Callard P, et al. Renal arterial resistive index is associated with severe histological changes and poor renal outcome during chronic kidney disease. BMC Nephrol 2012;13:139.

73. Ogata C, Horio T, Kamide K, et al. Association between left ventricular diastolic dysfunction and renal hemodynamic change in patients with treated essential hypertension. Hypertens Res 2003;26(12):971–8.

74. Levin A, Singer J, Thompson CR, et al. Prevalent left ventricular hypertrophy in the predialysis population: identifying opportunities for intervention. Am J Kidney Dis 1996;27(3):347–54.

75. Parfrey PS, Foley RN, Harnett JD, et al. Outcome and risk factors for left ventricular disorders in chronic uraemia. Nephrol Dial Transplant 1996;11(7):1277–85.

76. Mukherjee M, Sharma K, Madrazo JA, et al. Right-sided cardiac dysfunction in heart failure with preserved ejection fraction and worsening renal function. Am J Cardiol 2017;120(2):274–8.

77. Ter Maaten JM, Voors AA. Renal dysfunction in heart failure with a preserved ejection fraction: cause or consequence? Eur J Heart Fail 2016;18(1):113–4.

78. Massie BM, Carson PE, McMurray JJ, et al. Irbesartan in patients with heart failure and preserved ejection fraction. N Engl J Med 2008;359(23):2456–67.

79. Yusuf S, Pfeffer MA, Swedberg K, et al. Effects of candesartan in patients with chronic heart failure and preserved left-ventricular ejection fraction: the CHARM-Preserved Trial. Lancet Lond Engl 2003;362(9386):777–81.

80. Pitt B, Pfeffer MA, Assmann SF, et al. Spironolactone for heart failure with preserved ejection fraction. N Engl J Med 2014;370(15):1383–92.

81. Beldhuis IE, Streng KW, Ter Maaten JM, et al. Renin-angiotensin system inhibition, worsening renal function, and outcome in heart failure patients with reduced and preserved ejection fraction: a meta-analysis of published study data. Circ Heart Fail 2017;10(2). https://doi.org/10.1161/CIRCHEARTFAILURE.116.003588.

82. Damman K, Perez AC, Anand IS, et al. Worsening renal function and outcome in heart failure patients with preserved ejection fraction and the impact of angiotensin receptor blocker treatment. J Am Coll Cardiol 2014;64(11):1106–13.

83. Vardeny O, Wu DH, Desai A, et al. Influence of baseline and worsening renal function on efficacy of spironolactone in patients with severe heart failure: insights from RALES (Randomized Aldactone Evaluation Study). J Am Coll Cardiol 2012;60(20):2082–9.

84. Bristow MR, Sharma K, Assmann SF, et al. Data and Safety Monitoring Board evaluation and management of a renal adverse event signal in TOP-CAT. Eur J Heart Fail 2017;19(4):457–65.

85. Mc Causland FR, Lefkowitz MP, Claggett B, et al. Angiotensin-neprilysin inhibition and renal outcomes in heart failure with preserved ejection fraction. Circulation 2020;142(13):1236–45.

86. Solomon SD, McMurray JJV, Anand IS, et al. Angiotensin-neprilysin inhibition in heart failure with preserved ejection fraction. N Engl J Med 2019;381(17):1609–20.

87. El-Daly M, Pulakazhi Venu VK, Saifeddine M, et al. Hyperglycaemic impairment of PAR2-mediated vasodilation: prevention by inhibition of aortic endothelial sodium-glucose-co-transporter-2 and minimizing oxidative stress. Vascul Pharmacol 2018;109:56–71.

88. Yaribeygi H, Atkin SL, Butler AE, et al. Sodium-glucose cotransporter inhibitors and oxidative stress: an update. J Cell Physiol 2019;234(4):3231–7.

89. Wanner C. Sodium glucose cotransporter 2 inhibition and the visualization of kidney hemodynamics. Circulation 2019;140(4):316–8.

90. Kidokoro K, Cherney DZI, Bozovic A, et al. Evaluation of glomerular hemodynamic function by empagliflozin in diabetic mice using in vivo imaging. Circulation 2019;140(4):303–15.

91. Ye Y, Bajaj M, Yang H-C, et al. SGLT-2 inhibition with dapagliflozin reduces the activation of the Nlrp3/ASC inflammasome and attenuates the development of diabetic cardiomyopathy in mice with type 2 diabetes. Further augmentation of the effects with saxagliptin, a DPP4 inhibitor. Cardiovasc Drugs Ther 2017;31(2):119–32.

92. Zhang N, Feng B, Ma X, et al. Dapagliflozin improves left ventricular remodeling and aorta sympathetic tone in a pig model of heart failure with preserved ejection fraction. Cardiovasc Diabetol 2019;18(1):107.

93. Zelniker TA, Braunwald E. Mechanisms of cardiorenal effects of sodium-glucose cotransporter 2 inhibitors: JACC state-of-the-art review. J Am Coll Cardiol 2020;75(4):422–34.

94. Mustroph J, Wagemann O, Lücht CM, et al. Empagliflozin reduces Ca/calmodulin-dependent kinase II activity in isolated ventricular cardiomyocytes. ESC Heart Fail 2018;5(4):642–8.

95. Packer M. Reconceptualization of the molecular mechanism by which sodium-glucose cotransporter 2 inhibitors reduce the risk of heart failure events. Circulation 2019;140(6):443–5.

96. Lee YH, Kim SH, Kang JM, et al. Empagliflozin attenuates diabetic tubulopathy by improving mitochondrial fragmentation and autophagy. Am J Physiol Ren Physiol 2019;317(4):F767–80.

97. Zelniker TA, Braunwald E. Clinical benefit of cardiorenal effects of sodium-glucose cotransporter 2 inhibitors: JACC state-of-the-art review. J Am Coll Cardiol 2020;75(4):435–47.

98. Zelniker TA, Wiviott SD, Raz I, et al. SGLT2 inhibitors for primary and secondary prevention of cardiovascular and renal outcomes in type 2 diabetes: a systematic review and meta-analysis of cardiovascular outcome trials. Lancet 2019;393(10166):31–9.

99. Kato ET, Silverman MG, Mosenzon O, et al. Effect of dapagliflozin on heart failure and mortality in type 2 diabetes mellitus. Circulation 2019;139(22):2528–36.

100. Juni RP, Kuster DWD, Goebel M, et al. Cardiac microvascular endothelial enhancement of cardiomyocyte function is impaired by inflammation and restored by empagliflozin. JACC Basic Transl Sci 2019;4(5):575–91.

101. Anker SD, Butler J, Filippatos G, et al. Baseline characteristics of patients with heart failure with preserved ejection fraction in the EMPEROR-Preserved trial. Eur J Heart Fail 2020;22(12):2383–92.

102. AstraZeneca. An international, double-blind, randomised, placebo-controlled phase III study to evaluate the effect of dapagliflozin on reducing CV death or worsening heart failure in patients with heart failure with preserved ejection fraction (HFpEF). clinicaltrials.gov. 2020. Available at: https://clinicaltrials.gov/ct2/show/NCT03619213. Accessed March 4, 2021.

103. About RECONNeXT – RECONNeXT. Available at: https://www.reconnext.eu/about/. Accessed February 28, 2021.

Sleep Disorder and Heart Failure with Preserved Ejection Fraction

Masahiko Kato, MD, PhD[a],*, Kazuhiro Yamamoto, MD, PhD[b]

KEYWORDS

- Sleep disorder • Insomnia • Sleep-disordered breathing • Obstructive sleep apnea
- Central sleep apnea • Heart failure with reduced ejection fraction
- Heart failure with preserved ejection fraction

KEY POINTS

- Almost half of heart failure (HF) patients complain of insomnia, but physicians, health professionals, and patients lack knowledge of this disease in the cardiology clinic.
- Sleep-disordered breathing is highly prevalent in patients with HF. Obstructive sleep apnea may be strongly associated with incident HF with preserved left ventricular ejection fraction (HFpEF).
- Nonpharmacological interventions, such as continuous positive airway pressure and adaptive servo-ventilation, may be effective for improving symptoms, exercise capacity, and left ventricular diastolic function in patients with HFpEF.

INTRODUCTION

Cardiologists aim to identify effective treatments and reduce mortality in patients with heart failure (HF). In the past decade, the importance of multidisciplinary intervention has been demonstrated, not only to cure patients, but also to provide them with better care.[1] One of the most common daily life complaints of patients with HF is poor sleep quality caused by difficulty initiating and maintaining sleep.[2–13] Therefore, physicians and health professionals must evaluate sleep disorders to manage patients with HF. Sleep disorders are grouped into 7 major categories, including insomnia, sleep-related breathing disorders (sleep-disordered breathing [SDB]), central disorders of hypersomnolence, circadian rhythm sleep–wake disorders, parasomnias, sleep-related movement disorders, and other sleep disorders in the third edition of the International Classification of Sleep Disorders (ICSD3).[14] As for the relationship between sleep disorders and HF, both obstructive sleep apnea (OSA) and central sleep apnea (CSA), which belong to SDB, have been well discussed thus far.[10,15] It is generally considered that OSA is a potential cause of HF, and both insomnia and CSA are results of HF. Recently, the number of reports describing the bidirectional relationship between sleep disorder and HF has gradually increased.

Importantly, HF itself is classified into many categories by symptoms and cardiac function, and therapeutic strategies differ depending on left ventricular ejection fraction (EF), such as HF with reduced EF (HFrEF), HF with midrange EF, and HF with preserved EF (HFpEF).[15,16] This article introduces the bidirectional relationship between sleep disorders and HFpEF.

Name of grant: This work was supported by a grant from the Japan Society for the Promotion of Science (JSPS KAKENHI grant number 18K10671).

[a] Division of School of Health Science, Department of Pathobiological Science and Technology, Faculty of Medicine, Tottori University, 86 Nishicho, Yonago, Japan; [b] Department of Cardiovascular Medicine, and Endocrinology and Metabolism, Faculty of Medicine, Tottori University, 36-1 Nishicho, Yonago, Japan
* Corresponding author.
E-mail address: mkato@tottori-u.ac.jp

Heart Failure Clin 17 (2021) 369–376
https://doi.org/10.1016/j.hfc.2021.02.004
1551-7136/21/© 2021 Elsevier Inc. All rights reserved.

Insomnia

Definition of insomnia

Although several previous reports have investigated the association between insomnia and HF,[17,18] there are many variations of diagnostic symptoms and indices of insomnia. The reason that insomnia diagnoses can vary is that insomnia is defined by patients' subjective symptoms, but not by objective indices. Even when patients complain of symptoms of insomnia, objective polysomnographic recordings can appear normal, which is also called sleep misperception.[19] From this, researchers have investigated insomnia in different ways. Therefore, ICSD3 and the Diagnostic and Statistical Manual of Mental Disorders, 5th Edition[20] have defined insomnia as a single disorder: chronic insomnia disorder. The American Academy of Sleep Medicine defines insomnia as a perceived difficulty with sleep initiation, consolidation, duration, or quality, despite an adequate opportunity to sleep and lasting at least 3 months.[21] Javaheri and colleagues highlighted that even the definition of insomnia does not include criteria related to sleep duration measured by objective tools, and the occurrence of short sleep duration with insomnia appears to identify a phenotype with distinct clinical features.[22] Thus, when one interprets data related to sleep disorder, one should be aware that there are many aspects of sleep disorders other than insomnia and SDB.

Insomnia as a symptom of heart failure

Approximately 30% of the general population experience occasional insomnia symptoms, and 10% of those suffer from chronic insomnia.[23,24] As for patients with HF, 23% to 73% complain of poor sleep quality and sleep discontinuity.[7,8] Patients with HF experience a variety of symptoms, such as fatigue, nocturnal dyspnea, depression, anxiety, daytime sleepiness, poor quality of life, and decrements in daily activity. These HF symptoms are associated with its pathophysiological background, such as low cardiac output and fluid congestion, and overlap with insomnia symptoms. The problem in cardiology clinics is that physicians and health professionals tend to underestimate the importance of sleep disorder symptoms, and patients with HF tend not to consult about therapeutic interventions to alleviate these symptoms, except for prescription of hypnotic agents.

Insomnia and incident heart failure

Some large community-based cohort studies have investigated the association between insomnia and incident HF. Ingelsson and colleagues reported that self-reported sleep disturbances imply an increased risk of incident HF in overweight subjects, independent of established risk factors for HF during 3 decades of follow-up in a population-based sample of 2322 middle-aged men.[18] This study demonstrated that the association between sleep disturbance and HF was present only in overweight subjects, indicating that obesity is an important mechanism by which sleep disturbance increases the risk of incident HF. The authors proposed potential mechanisms. First, sleep disturbances cause alterations in growth hormone (GH)/insulin-like growth factor-1 (IGF-1). Previous studies have described that low serum concentrations of IGF-1 are predictive of the risk of incident HF.[25,26] There is an association between obesity and low GH concentrations,[27] which could explain why sleep disturbances only predict HF in overweight participants. Second, sleep disturbances could be related to increased inflammatory activity. Inflammation might be a mechanism by which sleep disturbance leads to HF, as the authors' previous study and other studies demonstrated a close relationship between inflammation and incident HF and poor HF outcomes.[28–30]

OSA is strongly associated with being overweight,[31] and nocturnal hypoxemia or reoxygenation might increase the risk of incident HF. Laugsand and colleagues reported an association between self-reported insomnia symptoms and the risk of incident HF in Norway's Trøndelag Health study, which constituted a large database of clinical, anthropometric, and socioeconomic information collected during a 3-phase population-based health survey in Trøndelag County in Norway.[17] They asked 54,403 participants 3 questions related to insomnia at baseline and followed participants over a mean follow-up period of 11.3 years (standard deviation, 2.9 years). The questions were related to difficulty initiating sleep, difficulty maintaining sleep, and experiencing a feeling of nonrestorative sleep. They found that older participants were more likely to experience symptoms of insomnia compared with younger participants, and symptoms were more frequent in females compared with males. Additionally, the number of insomnia symptoms was positively associated with the risk of HF and overall mortality. They also described potential mechanisms between insomnia and the risk of incident HF. Insomnia is a disorder of hyperarousal that is accompanied by chronic activation of stress responses with increased activity in the hypothalamic–pituitary–adrenal axis and sympathetic nervous system, leading to an increase in the secretion of cortisol and upregulation of the renin–angiotensin–aldosterone system.[32] This stress response is also accompanied by increased heart rate, decreased heart rate variability, increased blood pressure, and secretion of proinflammatory cytokines and catecholamines, which are all risk factors for incident HF.[33] Furthermore, increased sympathetic activation and hypercortisolemia in patients with insomnia have been implicated in the pathophysiology of insulin resistance and metabolic syndrome.[34] Insomnia is associated with an unhealthy lifestyle, including a high prevalence of obesity and physical inactivity.[35] Consequently, patients suffering from insomnia are more likely to have hypertension,[36] dyslipidemia, and glucose intolerance. These may also contribute to endothelial dysfunction, atherosclerosis, renal dysfunction, and progressive left ventricular remodeling. Moreover, Kanno and colleagues reported an association between insomnia and cardiac events in patients with HF.[37] One thousand eleven patients with HF were enrolled and divided into 2 groups according to the presence of insomnia based on symptoms in normal daily life and/or upon hospital discharge. They found that insomnia was an independent predictor of cardiac events in patients with HF after adjusting for multiple known confounding factors. The insomnia group had an activated renin–angiotensin–aldosterone system, impaired renal function, and a lower exercise capacity compared with the noninsomnia group.

Taken together, abnormalities in sympathetic nerve activity, neurohumoral activation, and the inflammatory response may represent a biologically plausible causal link between insomnia and incident HF.

Insomnia and heart failure with preserved left ventricular ejection fraction

No studies have examined the association between insomnia and left ventricular function, except for a study by Strand and colleagues.[38] The study examined the association between insomnia and left ventricular function using echocardiography in 788 patients with HF. Echocardiographic measurements, such as systolic mitral annular excursion, peak velocity of mitral annulus systolic and diastolic motion, and systolic deformation of the left ventricle, were not associated with insomnia symptoms. However, there is insufficient evidence to conclude lack of an association between insomnia and HFpEF. This issue is still open to argument, because the characteristics of patients with insomnia and HFpEF seem to overlap. For example, older age, female sex, excess weight, poor renal function, and impaired exercise capacity are observed in patients with insomnia and in patients with HFpEF. There may be a link between insomnia and HFpEF. More specific studies explaining the association between insomnia and HFpEF are required in the future.

Sleep-Disordered Breathing

Sleep-disordered breathing and incident heart failure

There is a high prevalence of sleep apnea syndrome (SAS) in patients with HF.[10,39] SAS can be classified into OSA and CSA. OSA is characterized by hypopnea (a reduction in breathing coupled with ≥3%–4% desaturation) and apnea (cessation of breathing for at least 10 seconds because of airflow obstruction in the upper pharynx) despite persistent respiratory effort. CSA is characterized by apnea and hypopnea in the absence of a central nervous system signal to breathe, with a cessation in breathing lasting for at least 10 seconds.[14]

Two large community-based, prospective cohort studies on the cardiovascular consequences of OSA were reported from the Sleep Heart Health Study.[40]

Shahar and colleagues examined the association between SDB and self-reported cardiovascular disease in 6424 free-living individuals who underwent overnight, unattended polysomnography at home.[41] They found that SDB was associated more strongly with HF and stroke than coronary heart disease. Gottlieb and colleagues also investigated the association between OSA and incident coronary heart disease and HF.[42] They concluded that OSA predicts incident HF in males but not females. Males with an apnea hypopnea index (AHI) of at least 30 were more likely to develop HF compared with those with an AHI less than 5. These studies suggest the possibility of a bidirectional causal relationship between SDB and incident HF. HF causes instability in ventilatory control, and, through a periodic reduction in neural output to both the diaphragm and pharyngeal dilator muscles, may cause either OSA or CSA. Conversely, the mechanisms by which OSA may cause HF are sympathetic nervous system activation from intermittent hypoxemia and hypercapnia during sleep, as well as hypoxic and oxidative stress resulting from repeated episodes of hypoxemia and reoxygenation.[43] It is hypothesized that these factors cause systemic inflammation, endothelial dysfunction, increased production of vasoactive substances, and insulin resistance, with resultant hypertension, hyperlipidemia, and diabetes mediating the HF consequences of OSA.

Sleep-disordered breathing and heart failure with preserved left ventricular ejection fraction

Because the focus on management of patients with HFpEF is increasing with the aging population, evidence of a relationship between SDB and HFpEF is also increasing.

Bitter and colleagues examined the prevalence of SDB (AHI ≥5) in patients with HR with reduced

EF (HFpEF). SDB was documented in 69.3% of all patients, in 39.8% of patients with OSA, and in 29.5% of patients with CSA.[44] They also evaluated the relative proportions of different types of SDB in patients with different left ventricular in-flow patterns by echocardiography (impaired relaxation, pseudo-normal, and restrictive) in patients with HFpEF. OSA was dominant in patients with a pseudo-normal pattern, and CSA was most common in patients with a restrictive pattern. CSA may be dominant in patients with advanced HF, and OSA may be dominant in patients in the early stages of HF. Herrscher and colleagues evaluated the prevalence of SDB in patients with HFpEF.[45] Patients with HFpEF had nearly the same prevalence of sleep apnea as patients with HFrEF (80% vs 82%, respectively). Patients with HFpEF more frequently had OSA than CSA (62% vs 18%, respectively). Patients with HFpEF and OSA had a higher body mass index and were more likely to have hypertension compared with patients with HFpEF without OSA. Abdullah and colleagues investigated the impact of OSA on hospitalization for HFpEF.[46] They investigated 147,463 patients with a primary diagnosis of HFpEF. The prevalence of OSA in patients with HFpEF was 16.8%, and patients with OSA were older; more likely to be male; and more likely to have hypertension, diabetes mellitus, acute coronary syndrome, a history of coronary artery disease, prior myocardial infarction, chronic kidney disease, atrial fibrillation, and obesity. After adjusting for several confounding factors using multivariate logistic regression and using propensity score matching, OSA was a significant predictor of HFpEF and increased the risk of hospitalization. The authors proposed the clinical hypothesis that patients with OSA experience repeated nocturnal hypoxemia leading to sympathetic activation with a consequent increase in neurohumoral activation and arterial blood pressure, thus predisposing to wall thickening and compromised left ventricular diastolic function. Indeed, the authors previously reported that sympathetic nerve activation, which was evaluated by muscle sympathetic nerve activity, was augmented, and that

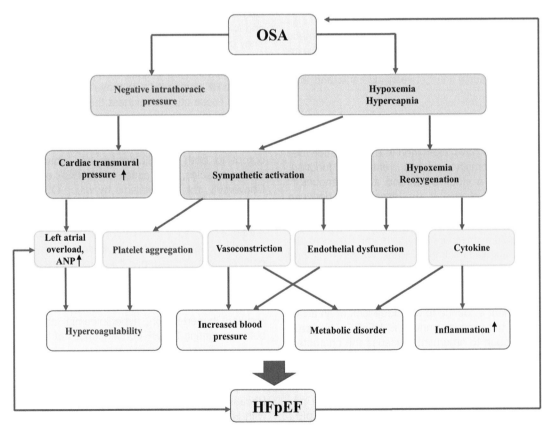

Fig. 1. Mechanisms of the bidirectional relationship between OSA and HFpEF. The pathophysiological status of OSA, such as an increase in the transmural cardiac pressure, sympathetic activation, hypoxemia, and reoxygenation, led to left atrial overload, platelet aggregation, vasoconstriction, endothelial dysfunction, and cytokine induction. This pathophysiological status is plausible to construct the pathophysiology of HFpEF.

endothelial function in resistance vessels was impaired in patients with OSA.[47,48] Moreover, serum C-reactive protein (CRP) was elevated, and continuous positive airway pressure (CPAP) therapy decreased CRP in patients with OSA.[49] The authors' data support the hypothesis that hypoxia and reoxygenation enhance the inflammatory response and sympathetic activity in patients with OSA.

The large-scale studies suggest that OSA may induce a pathophysiological status, such as an increase in transmural cardiac pressure, sympathetic activation, hypoxemia, and reoxygenation, which lead to left atrial overload, platelet aggregation, vasoconstriction, endothelial dysfunction, and cytokine induction.[43] The status is plausible to construct the pathophysiology of HFpEF. Left atrial overload leads to an increase in the secretion of atrial natriuretic peptide and urges urination, which affects the hypercoagulability status. Sympathetic excitation leads to an increase in blood pressure by causing peripheral vasoconstriction and inducing metabolic disorder due to insulin resistance related to vascular insufficiency. Moreover, hypoxia and reoxygenation may lead to cell and vascular damage by activating the inflammatory response (**Fig. 1**). Some reports describe a direct association between OSA and left ventricular diastolic dysfunction, independent of other confounding factors. Usui and colleagues reported that OSA might contribute to left ventricular diastolic dysfunction independent of left ventricular geometry, arterial stiffness, and obesity.[50] Moreover, Shah and colleagues described that both SAS and obesity are associated with left ventricular remodeling, independent of traditional confounding factors in patients with atrial fibrillation and HFpEF.[51] On the other hand, Shim and colleagues reported that improvement of left ventricular diastolic function by 3 months CPAP therapy compared with sham treatment was accompanied by improvements in pulse wave velocity, nighttime diastolic blood pressure, arterial elastance index, and ventricular-vascular coupling index in patients with severe OSA.[52] Kim and colleagues also described that 3 months CPAP therapy improved left ventricular mechanical function assessed by speckle-tracking echocardiography and right ventricular fractional area change assessed by 2-dimensional echocardiography with changing right ventricular size in patients with severe OSA.[53] The direct contribution of OSA to the development of HFpEF is still controversial and requires further detailed studies.

As for the reverse relationship, Yumino and colleagues reported that overnight rostral fluid shift displacement into the neck could contribute to the pathogenesis of OSA in patients with HF.[54]

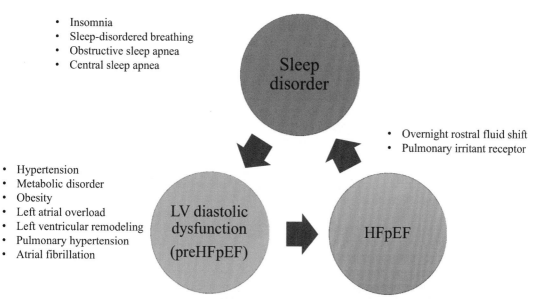

Fig. 2. Bidirectional relationship between sleep disorder and HFpEF. Sleep disorder may contribute to left ventricular diastolic dysfunction by causing hypertension, metabolic disorder, obesity, left atrial overload, left ventricular remodeling, pulmonary hypertension, and atrial fibrillation, which lead to HFpEF. Overnight rostral fluid shift and lung congestion may lead to airway obstruction in the upper pharynx and stimulate pulmonary irritant receptors, which induce hyperventilation and sleep disorder.

Bucca and colleagues reported that diuretic treatment of HFpEF produces a significant decrease in AHI, possibly because of a reduction in fluid retention and pulmonary congestion.[55] Assuming that positive airway pressure therapies, such as CPAP and adaptive servo-ventilation (ASV), improve oxygenation, several previous studies reported that CPAP improved pulmonary congestion and decreased wall stress,[56] atrial overload, right ventricular overload, pulmonary hypertension, and left ventricular hypertrophy[57] in patients with HF. Although an international, multicenter, randomized, parallel-group study did not find the efficacy of ASV on a composite of death from any cause, life-saving cardiovascular intervention, and unplanned hospitalization for worsening chronic HF in patients with HFrEF (SERVE-HF),[58] some studies have shown the beneficial effects of ASV on cardiac function in patients with HFpEF. Bitter and colleagues investigated the effect of ASV on cardiopulmonary exercise capacity, left atrial diameter, and echocardiographic indices of diastolic ventricular performance in 85 patients with HFpEF and Cheyne–Stokes respiration (CSR-CSA).[59] They found that ASV attenuated CSR-CSA events during sleep and improved HF symptoms and diastolic function. Yoshihisa and colleagues reported that ASV improved right cardiac function, pulmonary function, exercise capacity, and cardiac events, such as rehospitalization and cardiac death, in patients with HFpEF and SDB.[60] These studies had small sample sizes; thus, further large-scale randomized controlled trials are required to clarify these observations.

Taken together, sleep disorder may contribute to left ventricular diastolic dysfunction via left atrial overload, left ventricular remodeling, pulmonary hypertension, and atrial fibrillation, which lead to HFpEF. Overnight rostral fluid shift and lung congestion may lead to airflow obstruction in the upper pharynx and stimulate pulmonary irritant receptors, which induce hyperventilation and sleep disorder (**Fig. 2**).

SUMMARY

Sleep disorder is prevalent in patients with HF and is an important factor that may contribute to HF development. Focusing on the association between sleep disorder, particularly OSA, and HFpEF may play a key role in linking many confounding factors to construct a wide variety of HFpEF phenotypes. Although there is insufficient evidence to improve cardiac function and mortality in patients with HFpEF, CPAP and ASV may improve the confounding factors related to HFpEF and prevent HFpEF onset.

CLINICS CARE POINTS

- 23% to 73% of HF patients experience poor sleep quality.
- The abnormalities in sympathetic nerve activity, neurohumoral activation, and the inflammatory response may represent a biologically plausible causal link between insomnia and incident HF.
- OSA may induce the pathophysiology of HFpEF, such as an increase in transmural cardiac pressure, sympathetic activation, hypoxemia, and reoxygenation, which lead to left atrial overload, platelet aggregation, vasoconstriction, endothelial dysfunction, and cytokine induction.
- CPAP and ASV may improve the confounding factors related to HFpEF and prevent HFpEF onset.

DISCLOSURE

K. Yamamoto received a grant from Fukuda Denshi and Teijin Pharma.

ACKNOWLEDGMENTS

The authors thank Emily Woodhouse, PhD, from Edanz Group (https://en-author-services.edanzgroup.com/ac) for editing a draft of this manuscript.

REFERENCES

1. Rich MW, Beckham V, Wittenberg C, et al. A multidisciplinary intervention to prevent the readmission of elderly patients with congestive heart failure. N Engl J Med 1995;333(18):1190–5.
2. Friedman MM, King KB. Correlates of fatigue in older women with heart failure. Heart Lung 1995; 24:512–8.
3. Grady KL, Jalowiec A, Grusk BB, et al. Symptom distress in cardiac transplant candidates. Heart Lung 1992;21:434–9.
4. Jaarsma T, Halfens R, Abu-Saad HH, et al. Quality of life in older patients with systolic and diastolic heart failure. Eur J Heart Fail 1999;1:151–60.
5. Mayou R, Blackwood R, Bryant B, et al. Cardiac failure: symptoms and functional status. J Psychosom Res 1991;35:399–407.
6. Principe-Rodriguez K, Strohl KP, Hadziefendic S, et al. Sleep symptoms and clinical markers of illness

in patients with heart failure. Sleep Breath 2005;9:
127–33.

7. Redeker NS, Stein S. Characteristics of sleep in patients with stable heart failure versus a comparison
group. Heart Lung 2006;35:252–61.

8. Erickson VS, Westlake CA, Dracup KA, et al. Sleep
disturbance symptoms in patients with heart failure.
AACN Clin Iss 2003;14:477–87.

9. Brostrom A, Stromberg A, Dalstrom U, et al. Sleep
difficulties, daytime sleepiness, and health-related
quality of life in patients with chronic heart failure.
J Cardiovasc Nurs 2004;19:234–42.

10. Sin DD, Fitzgerald F, Parker JD, et al. Risk factors for
central and obstructive sleep apnea in 450 men and
women with congestive heart failure. Am J Respir
Crit Care Med 1999;160:1101–6.

11. Ferrier K, Campbell A, Yee B, et al. Sleep-disordered
breathing occurs frequently in stable outpatients
with congestive heart failure. Chest 2005;128:
2116–22.

12. Chan J, Sanderson J, Chan W, et al. Prevalence of
sleep-disordered breathing in diastolic heart failure.
Chest 1997;111:1488–93.

13. Arzt M, Young T, Finn L, et al. Sleepiness and sleep
in patients with both systolic heart failure and
obstructive sleep apnea. Arch Intern Med 2006;
166:1716–22.

14. American Academy of Sleep Medicine. International
classification of sleep disorders. 3rd edition. Darien
(IL): American Academy of Sleep Medicine; 2014.

15. Tsutsui H, Isobe M, Ito H, et al. JCS 2017/JHFS 2017
Guideline on diagnosis and treatment of acute and
chronic heart failure. Circ J 2019;83(10):2084–184.

16. Ponikowski P, Voors AA, Anker SD, et al. 2016 ESC
guidelines for the diagnosis and treatment of acute
and chronic heart failure: the Task Force for the
Diagnosis and Treatment of Acute and Chronic
Heart Failure of the European Society of Cardiology
(ESC) developed with the special contribution of the
Heart Failure Association (HFA) of the ESC. Eur
Heart J 2016;37(27):2129–200.

17. Laugsand LE, Strand LB, Platou C, et al. Insomnia
and the risk of incident heart failure: a population
study. Eur Heart J 2014;35(21):1382–93.

18. Ingelsson E, Lind L, Arnlov J, et al. Sleep disturbances independently predict heart failure in overweight middle-aged men. Eur J Heart Fail 2007;
9(2):184–90.

19. Bastien CH, Ceklic T, St-Hilaire P, et al. Insomnia and
sleep misperception. Pathol Biol (Paris) 2014;62(5):
241–51.

20. American Psychiatric Association. Diagnostic and
Statistical manual of Mental disorders. 5th edition.
Arlington (VA): American Psychiatric Publishing;
2013.

21. Edinger JD, Bonnet MH, Bootzin RR, et al. Derivation
of research diagnostic criteria for insomnia: report of

an American Academy of Sleep Medicine Work
Group. Sleep 2004;27(8):1567–96.

22. Javaheri S, Redline S. Insomnia and Risk of Cardiovascular Disease. Chest 2017;152(2):435–44.

23. Morin CM, LeBlanc M, Daley M, et al. Epidemiology
of insomnia: prevalence, self-help treatments, con-
sultations, and determinant of help-seeking behav-
iors. Sleep Med 2006;7:123–30.

24. Ohayon MM. Epidemiology of insomnia: what we
know and we still need to learn. Sleep Med Rev
2002;6:97–111.

25. Bleumink GS, Rietveld I, Janssen JA, et al. Insulin-
like growth factor-I gene polymorphism and risk of
heart failure (the Rotterdam Study). Am J Cardiol
2004;94(3):384–6.

26. Vasan RS, Sullivan LM, D'Agostino RB, et al. Serum
insulin-like growth factor I and risk for heart failure in
elderly individuals without a previous myocardial
infarction: the Framingham Heart Study. Ann Intern
Med 2003;139(8):642–8.

27. Munzer T, Harman SM, Hees P, et al. Effects of GH
and/or sex steroid administration on abdominal subcutaneous and visceral fat in healthy aged women
and men. J Clin Endocrinol Metab 2001;86(8):
3604–10.

28. Tamaki S, Mano T, Sakata Y, et al. Interleukin-16 promotes cardiac fibrosis and myocardial stiffening in
heart failure with preserved ejection fraction. PLoS
One 2013;8(7):e68893.

29. Kinugasa Y, Kato M, Sugihara S, et al. A simple risk
score to predict in-hospital death of elderly patients
with acute decompensated heart failure–hypoalbu-
minemia as an additional prognostic factor. Circ J
2009;73(12):2276–81.

30. Ingelsson E, Ärnlöv J, Sundström J, et al. Inflammation,
as measured by the erythrocyte sedimentation rate, is
an independent predictor for the development of heart
failure. J Am Coll Cardiol 2005;45(11):1802–6.

31. Young T, Peppard PE, Gottlieb DJ. Epidemiology of
obstructive sleep apnea: a population health
perspective. Am J Respir Crit Care Med 2002;
165(9):1217–39.

32. Basta M, Chrousos GP, Vela-Bueno A, et al. Chronic
insomnia and the stress system. Sleep Med Clin
2007;2:279–91.

33. Speidelhalder K, Scholtes C, Riemann D. The association between insomnia and cardiovascular diseases. Nat Sci Sleep 2010;2:71–8.

34. Mullington JM, Haack M, Toth M, et al. Cardiovascular,
inflammatory, and metabolic consequences of sleep
deprivation. Prog cardiovasc Dis 2009;51:294–302.

35. Janson C, Lindberg E, Gislason T, et al. Insomnia in
men-a 10-year prospective population based study.
Sleep 2001;24:425–30.

36. Kato M, Phillips BG, Sigurdsson G, et al. Effects of
sleep deprivation on neural circulatory control. Hypertension 2000;35(5):1173–5.

37. Kanno Y, Yoshihisa A, Watanabe S, et al. Prognostic significance of insomnia in heart failure. Circ J 2016; 80(7):1571–7.

38. Strand LB, Laugsand LE, Dalen H, et al. Insomnia and left ventricular function - an echocardiography study. Scand Cardiovasc J 2016;50(3):187–92.

39. Javaheri S, Parker TJ, Liming JD, et al. Sleep apnea in 81 ambulatory male patients with stable heart failure. Types and their prevalence, consequences, and presentations. Circulation 1998;97:2154–9.

40. Quan SF, Howard BV, Iber C, et al. The Sleep Heart Health Study: design, rationale, and methods. Sleep 1997;20:1077–85.

41. Shahar E, Whitney CW, Redline S, et al. Sleep-disordered breathing and cardiovascular disease: cross-sectional results of the sleep heart health study. Am J Respir Crit Care Med 2001;163(1):19–25.

42. Gottlieb DJ, Yenokyan G, Newman AB, et al. Prospective study of obstructive sleep apnea and incident coronary heart disease and heart failure: the sleep heart health study. Circulation 2010;122(4): 352–60.

43. Somers VK, White DP, Amin R, et al. Sleep apnea and cardiovascular disease: an American Heart Association/American College of Cardiology Foundation scientific statement. Circulation 2008;118: 1080–111.

44. Bitter T, Faber L, Hering D, et al. Sleep-disordered breathing in heart failure with normal left ventricular ejection fraction. Eur J Heart Fail 2009;11(6):602–8.

45. Herrscher TE, Akre H, Øverland B, et al. High prevalence of sleep apnea in heart failure outpatients: even in patients with preserved systolic function. J Card Fail 2011;17(5):420–5.

46. Abdullah A, Eigbire G, Salama A, et al. Relation of obstructive sleep apnea to risk of hospitalization in patients with heart failure and preserved ejection fraction from the national inpatient sample. Am J Cardiol 2018;122(4):612–5.

47. Narkiewicz K, Kato M, Phillips BG, et al. Nocturnal continuous positive airway pressure decreases daytime sympathetic traffic in obstructive sleep apnea. Circulation 1999;100(23):2332–5.

48. Kato M, Roberts-Thomson P, Phillips BG, et al. Impairment of endothelium-dependent vasodilation of resistance vessels in patients with obstructive sleep apnea. Circulation 2000;102(21):2607–10.

49. Ishida K, Kato M, Kato Y, et al. Appropriate use of nasal continuous positive airway pressure decreases elevated C-reactive protein in patients with obstructive sleep apnea. Chest 2009;136(1):125–9.

50. Usui Y, Takata Y, Inoue Y, et al. Severe obstructive sleep apnea impairs left ventricular diastolic function in non-obese men. Sleep Med 2013;14(2):155–9.

51. Shah RV, Abbasi SA, Heydari B, et al. Obesity and sleep apnea are independently associated with adverse left ventricular remodeling and clinical outcome in patients with atrial fibrillation and preserved ventricular function. Am Heart J 2014; 167(4):620–6.

52. Shim CY, Kim D, Park S, et al. Effects of continuous positive airway pressure therapy on left ventricular diastolic function: a randomised, sham-controlled clinical trial. Eur Respir J 2018;51(2):1701774.

53. Kim D, Shim CY, Cho YJ, et al. Continuous positive airway pressure therapy restores cardiac mechanical function in patients with severe obstructive sleep apnea: a randomized, sham-controlled study. J Am Soc Echocardiogr 2019;32:826–35.

54. Yumino D, Redolfi S, Ruttanaumpawan P, et al. Nocturnal rostral fluid shift: a unifying concept for the pathogenesis of obstructive and central sleep apnea in men with heart failure. Circulation 2010; 121(14):1598–605.

55. Bucca CB, Brussino L, Battisti A, et al. Diuretics in obstructive sleep apnea with diastolic heart failure. Chest 2007;132:440–6.

56. Bellone A, Etteri M, Vettorello M, et al. The effects of continuous positive airway pressure on plasma brain natriuretic peptide concentrations in patients presenting with acute cardiogenic pulmonary edema with preserved left ventricular systolic function. Am J Emerg Med 2010;28:230–4.

57. Colish J, Walker JR, Elmayergi N, et al. Obstructive sleep apnea: effects of continuous positive airway pressure on cardiac remodeling as assessed by cardiac biomarkers, echocardiography, and cardiac MRI. Chest 2012;141:674–81.

58. Cowie MR, Woehrle H, Wegscheider K, et al. Adaptive servo-ventilation for central sleep apnea in systolic heart failure. N Engl J Med 2015;373(12): 1095–105.

59. Bitter T, Westerheide N, Faber L, et al. Adaptive servoventilation in diastolic heart failure and Cheyne-Stokes respiration. Eur Respir J 2010;36(2):385–92.

60. Yoshihisa A, Suzuki S, Yamaki T, et al. Impact of adaptive servo-ventilation on cardiovascular function and prognosis in heart failure patients with preserved left ventricular ejection fraction and sleep-disordered breathing. Eur J Heart Fail 2013;15(5):543–50.

Atrial Fibrillation and Heart Failure with Preserved Ejection Fraction
Two Chronic Troublemakers

In-Cheol Kim, MD, PhD

KEYWORDS

- Atrial fibrillation • Heart failure with preserved ejection fraction • Diagnosis • Management

KEY POINTS

- Heart failure with preserved ejection fraction (HFpEF) and atrial fibrillation (AF) frequently coexist, affecting each other.
- Resting transthoracic echocardiography is the mainstay of the diagnosis in HFpEF to evaluate etiology, systolic function, diastolic function, and intracardiac pressures.
- Noninvasive or invasive exercise tests often are needed to identify the increase in intracardiac pressure during exercise and unmask exercise-induced symptoms.
- There is no single medication proved to increase survival in HFpEF with AF, but symptomatic treatment with management of combined risk factors is important.
- Future phenotype-based patient classification and treatment can improve outcomes by a more specific pathophysiology-based management strategy in HFpEF with AF.

INTRODUCTION

The prevalence of heart failure (HF) with preserved ejection fraction (HFpEF) and atrial fibrillation (AF) is increasing, and they commonly appear together because of the shared pathophysiology and comorbidities. The combination of HFpEF and AF is associated with poor prognoses, such as stroke, hospitalization for HF, and mortality. Diagnosis of HFpEF often is challenging due to its heterogenous clinical presentation and diverse phenotypes. Thus, scoring systems are introduced for improving the diagnostic performance in HFpEF. On the contrary, diagnosis of AF is more straightforward and clear when the electrocardiography is performed adequately. In HFpEF, there is no single medical treatment to show survival benefits. Management of AF based on the current guidelines is focused on anticoagulation, rhythm control, and rate control, according to the risk and symptoms of the patient. Patients with HFpEF and AF need integrated care, including early detection and appropriate treatment of both conditions, with the best management of combined comorbidities. This review focuses on the definition, pathophysiologic interactions, diagnostic modalities, treatments, and future perspectives of HFpEF with AF.

DEFINITIONS OF HEART FAILURE WITH PRESERVED EJECTION FRACTION AND ATRIAL FIBRILLATION

HF is a clinical syndrome characterized by typical symptoms (dyspnea, generalized/lower leg edema, and fatigue) with relevant signs (engorgement of the jugular vein due to elevated venous pressure, lung crackles, and pitting edema) caused by a functional or structural abnormality of the heart. It also is characterized by the decreased cardiac output and increased intracardiac pressures at rest or during stress[1] (**Table 1**).

Division of Cardiology, Department of Internal Medicine, Cardiovascular Center, Keimyung University Dongsan Hospital, Keimyung University School of Medicine, 1035, Dalgubeol-daero, Dalseo-gu, Daegu 42601, Republic of Korea
E-mail address: kimic@dsmc.or.kr

Heart Failure Clin 17 (2021) 377–386
https://doi.org/10.1016/j.hfc.2021.03.001
1551-7136/21/© 2021 Elsevier Inc. All rights reserved.

Table 1
Symptoms and signs of heart failure with preserved ejection fraction and atrial fibrillation

Symptoms of Heart Failure with Preserved Ejection Fraction	Symptoms of Atrial Fibrillation
• Breathlessness • Orthopnea • Paroxysmal nocturnal dyspnea • Reduced exercise tolerance • Fatigue, tiredness, increased time to recover after exercise • Ankle swelling	• Palpitations • Chest tightness • Dizziness • Syncope • Dyspnea • Fatigue • Exercise intolerance
Signs of Heart Failure with Preserved Ejection Fraction	**Signs of Atrial Fibrillation**
• Elevated jugular venous pressure • Hepatojugular reflux • Third heart sound (gallop rhythm) • Laterally displaced apical impulse	• Irregular pulsation • Irregular heart sound

Data from Refs.[1,3]

Although the current definition of HF includes typical symptoms, functional or structural abnormalities, including systolic and/or diastolic dysfunction, precede apparent symptoms.[2] The definition of HFpEF requires echocardiographic evidence of diastolic dysfunction and structural heart disease, including left ventricular (LV) hypertrophy or left atrial (LA) enlargement with preserved ejection fraction (EF) (EF ≥50%). Elevated level of natriuretic peptides (NPs) (B-type NP [BNP] >35 pg/mL or N-terminal-proBNP [NT-proBNP] >125 pg/mL) also is a crucial component (**Table 2**). AF is defined as a supraventricular tachyarrhythmia with uncoordinated atrial electrical activation and consequently ineffective atrial contraction. Electrocardiographic characteristics of AF include irregularly irregular R-R intervals (when atrioventricular conduction is not impaired), absence of distinct repeating P waves, and irregular atrial activations (see **Table 2**).[3] Recent guidelines of the European Society of Cardiology (ESC) distinguished the term, *clinical AF*, from the term, *subclinical AF* (including atrial high-rate episode), depending on the documentation by surface electrocardiography, regardless of the symptoms.[3–5]

MECHANISTIC INTERACTION BETWEEN ATRIAL FIBRILLATION AND HEART FAILURE WITH PRESERVED EJECTION FRACTION

Shared pathophysiologic mechanisms exist between AF and HFpEF. These include up-regulation of the renin-angiotensin-aldosterone system, increased sympathetic tone, and induction of systemic inflammation by common risk factors, including advanced age, smoking, hypertension, diabetes mellitus, anemia, chronic obstructive pulmonary disease, obstructive sleep apnea, renal dysfunction, and obesity (**Fig. 1**).[3,6] Age-related LV diastolic dysfunction and systolic ventricular-vascular uncoupling contribute to HFpEF, which also is linked to the development of AF.[7,8] Systemic inflammation is closely related to endothelial dysfunction, oxidative stress, and microvascular inflammation, leading to end-organ manifestations, such as diastolic dysfunction.[9,10] Elevated inflammatory markers, such as C-reactive protein, interleukin-6, and matrix metalloprotease-2 have been associated with the presence of AF.[3,11,12] Coronary microvascular dysfunction and fibrosis can be induced by endothelial inflammation, which results in both atrial and ventricular myopathy. Epicardial adipose tissue, which is closely located to the myocardium, may augment these inflammatory reactions that influence the electroanatomic dysfunction to develop AF and impairment of LV to develop HFpEF.[13,14] Remodeling of the LA with impairment of the reservoir function and loss of contraction is a mainstay of HFpEF with AF. Elevated LA pressure despite the distension of the chamber causes backward transmission of the pressure resulting in pulmonary hypertension especially during exercise, reflecting the underlying atrial myopathy.[15] Concomitant ventricular myopathy is a hallmark of diastolic dysfunction and elevated LV end-diastolic pressure in HFpEF. Amyloidosis is a protein-misfolding disease characterized by extracellular deposition of a soluble precursor protein that aggregates in the form of insoluble fibrils, causing cell/tissue damage and ultimately organ dysfunction. It appears to play an important role in both HFpEF and AF and in their interaction.[16]

Table 2
Definitions of heart failure with preserved ejection fraction and atrial fibrillation

Definition of Heart Failure with Preserved Ejection Fraction	Definition of Atrial Fibrillation
<ul><li>Symptoms ± signs of HF</li><li>LVEF ≥50%</li><li>1) Elevated levels of NPs (BNP >35 pg/mL, NT-proBNP >125 pg/mL) 2) At least 1 additional criterion - Relevant structural heart disease (LV hypertrophy and/or LA enlargement) - Diastolic dysfunction</li></ul>	<ul><li>A supraventricular tachyarrhythmia with uncoordinated atrial electrical activation and consequently ineffective atrial contraction</li><li>Electrocardiographic characteristics of AF - Irregularly irregular R-R intervals (when AV conduction is not impaired) - Absence of distinct repeating P waves - Irregular atrial activations</li></ul>

Abbreviation: AV, atrioventricular.
Data from Refs.[1,3]

DIAGNOSIS OF HEART FAILURE WITH PRESERVED EJECTION FRACTION IN ATRIAL FIBRILLATION

Unlike HF with reduced EF (HFrEF), diagnosis of HFpEF is challenging because the systolic function is normal. Symptoms of HFpEF often are vague and require meticulous evaluation to differentiate from other comorbidities. Frequently, it shows symptoms only during exertion. Therefore, exercise echocardiography, cardiopulmonary

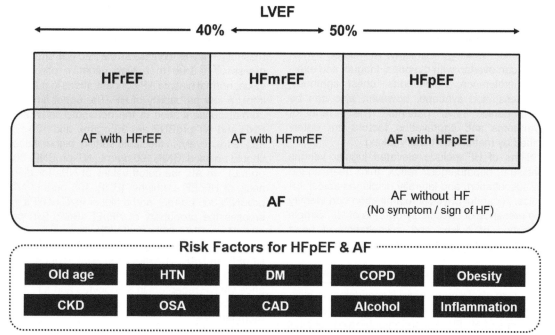

Fig. 1. Schematic image showing classification of HF and its association with AF. Underlying risk factors for both HFpEF and AF also are summarized. HTN, hypertension; DM, diabetes mellitus; COPD, chronic obstructive pulmonary disease; CKD, chronic kidney disease; OSA, obstructive sleep apnea; CAD, coronary artery disease. (*Data from* Refs.[19,20])

exercise test, and right heart catheterization during exercise need to be utilized to increase the sensitivity of the diagnosis.[17–21] The diagnosis of AF is clear with the appropriately performed electrocardiography or 24-hour Holter monitoring. Implantable loop recorder and recently developed wearable devices can aid in accurate diagnosis of AF.[3,22] Diagnosis of combined HFpEF and AF is more complicated. In AF patients, common diastolic parameters are not readily applicable; it usually is accompanied by LA size enlargement, and NP levels are elevated.[1,12,21,23,24] In addition, those with HFpEF and AF might have more advanced HF compared with patients with HFpEF and sinus rhythm. Scoring systems that recently have been suggested can be used to assist the diagnosis of HFpEF irrespective of the presence of AF.[19,20] Proper diagnostic procedures are key to successful treatment and start with detailed history taking and careful physical examination.[24,25] Utilization of appropriate diagnostic modalities, such as electrocardiography, echocardiography, stress tests, and right heart catheterization, as well as interpretation of the result, also is mportant.[12]

History Taking and Physical Examination

A detailed history of typical HF symptoms is important to obtain at the first visit and during follow-ups. Symptoms related to HFpEF include breathlessness, orthopnea, paroxysmal nocturnal dyspnea, reduced exercise tolerance, fatigue, tiredness, increased time to recover after exercise, and ankle swelling.[1] Similarly, AF-related symptoms can overlap with dyspnea, fatigue, and exercise intolerance. Palpitations, chest tightness, dizziness, and syncope, however, also can be accompanied in AF patients.[3] The severity of symptoms and aggravating factors are determined by meticulous history taking.

Signs of HF include elevated jugular venous pressure, hepatojugular reflux, third heart sound by auscultation, and laterally displaced apical impulse. A careful physical examination can identify the presence of specific symptoms of HF. Simple palpation of pulses and auscultation of heart sounds easily can detect the presence of AF.

Electrocardiography and Chest Radiography

A 12-lead electrocardiogram is mandatory to evaluate the evidence of cardiac abnormality and the presence of AF. Electrocardiographic signs of atrial enlargement, ventricular hypertrophy, and ST-T segment abnormality frequently are observed in HFpEF. Chest radiography can detect cardiomegaly, pulmonary congestion, and combined pulmonary diseases of HFpEF. Further pulmonary function test or chest computed tomography might be required for a better understanding of the pulmonary etiology of HFpEF combined with AF.

Echocardiography

Transthoracic echocardiography is the most important diagnostic modality in patients with HFpEF. Abnormal findings of diastolic function parameters with a normal EF are the mainstay for the diagnosis of HFpEF. Increased E/e′ ratio (increased LV filling pressure), elevated pulmonary artery systolic pressure (PASP) derived by tricuspid regurgitation (TR) velocity, LA enlargement, LV hypertrophy, decreased LV early diastolic tissue velocity (e′), decreased global longitudinal strain, right ventricular dysfunction, and dilatation are important findings suggesting diastolic dysfunction.[21,23] Enlargement of LA is a common finding in AF but increased E/e′ ratio and elevated PASP can be observed only in patients with overt HF. In AF patients, it is critical to average several cardiac cycles to measure E/e′. Although velocity measurements from 10 consecutive cycles are recommended for AF, velocities and time intervals averaged from 3 nonconsecutive beats with cycle lengths within 10% to 20% of the average heart rate still can be utilized.[26]

Natriuretic Peptides

The plasma concentration of NPs, NT-proBNP, and BNP are biomarkers to diagnose HF, evaluate the therapeutic response, and predict future prognosis. Plasma NP levels increase as cardiac wall stress increases.[27,28] Due to a high negative predictive value, normal plasma NP concentrations in patients imply a low probability of HF. The upper limits of normal concentration in the nonacute setting for BNP and NT-proBNP are 35 pg/mL and 125 pg/mL, respectively; in the acute setting, higher values should be used (BNP, 100 pg/mL; NT-proBNP, 300 pg/mL).[1] In AF, the cutoff values of NPs for diagnosis of HFpEF are higher (BNP, 105 pg/mL; NT-proBNP, 365 pg/mL), and a higher level of NPs increases the probability of HFpEF (BNP, 240 pg/mL; NT-proBNP, 660 pg/mL) (**Fig. 2**).[20]

Obesity, which is a common comorbidity of HFpEF and AF, is associated with reduced NP levels in plasma. This is due to the increased clearance via NP receptors in adipocytes and a reduction in cardiac chamber distention by pericardial restraint.[12,29]

Invasive and Noninvasive Exercise Testing

Patients with HFpEF commonly show worsening of symptoms during exercise. It is necessary to

		Points	Clinical Variable	Values
H₂FPEF Score	**H₂**	2	Heavy	BMI > 30kg/m²
		1	HTN	≥ 2 antihypertensive drugs
	F	3	AF	Paroxysmal or persistent
	P	1	Pulmonary HTN	PASP > 35 mmHg (by Doppler echocardiography)
	E	1	Elderly	Age > 60 years
	F	1	Filling pressure	Septal E/e' ratio > 9 (by Doppler echocardiography)

		Functional	Morphological	Biomarker (AF)
HFA-PEFF Score	**Major (2 points)**	• Septal e' < 7 cm/s • Lateral e' < 10 cm/s • Average E/e' ratio ≥ 15 • TR velocity > 2.8 m/s (PASP > 35 mmHg)	• LAVI > 40 ml/m² • LVMI ≥ 149/122 g/m² (M/F) and RWT > 0.42	• NT-proBNP > 660 pg/ml • BNP > 240 pg/ml
	Minor (1 points)	• Average E/e' ratio 9–14 • GLS < 16%	• LAVI 34–40 ml/m² • LVMI > 115/95 g/m² (M/F) • RWT > 0.42 • LV wall thickness ≥ 12 mm	• NT-proBNP 365–660 pg/ml • BNP 105–240 pg/ml

HFpEF Probability	Score	0	1	2	3	4	5	6	7	8	9
	H₂FPEF	Low probability		Intermediate probability				High probability			
	HFA-PEFF	Low probability		Intermediate probability		High probability		NA			

Decision Making	Low probability	Search for other cardiac/non-cardiac causes
	Intermediate probability	Need Diastolic stress test (confirm HFpEF when abnormal)
	High probability	Confirm HFpEF

Fig. 2. H₂FPEscore and HFA-PEFF scoring system for diagnosis of HFpEF in AF. BMI, body mass index; HTN, hypertension; GLS, global longitudinal strain; LVMI, left ventricular mass index; RWT, relative wall thickness.

adopt exercise testing to unveil the presence of HFpEF. During rest, measurement of intracardiac pressure by right heart catheterization often shows normal pressures, but remarkably elevated pressures are noted during exercise. Patients with HFpEF display pulmonary capillary wedge pressure greater than or equal to 15 mm Hg at rest and greater than or equal to 25 mm Hg during exercise. Invasive cardiopulmonary exercise testing also is used to assess cardiac output reserve, with the measurement of cardiac output and oxygen consumption.[12,18,24,30]

Exercise echocardiography increasingly has been advocated as an alternative to invasive stress testing.[31] Similar to the invasive test, patients would have normal diastolic echocardiographic parameters at rest, but they may show abnormal results of diastolic echocardiographic parameters (average E/e' ≥15 or TR velocity >3.4 m/s) with an increase in LV filling pressure during exercise, which are hallmarks of the diagnosis of HFpEF.[18,20,31] Doppler echocardiographic parameters, such as the E/e' ratio and TR velocity, correlate well with invasively measured pressures and the correlations were even higher during exercise echocardiography.[24,31]

Application of Scoring Systems

Recently, 2 scoring systems were introduced for the diagnosis of HFpEF. One is the heavy, hypertensive, AF, pulmonary hypertension, elder, and filling pressure (H₂FPEF) score and the other is

Heart Failure Association (HFA)–pretest assessment, echocardiographic and NP score, functional testing in case of uncertainty, and final etiology (PEFF) score, suggested by the HFA of the ESC (see **Fig. 2**).[19,20,24] Patients with AF have a higher prevalence of HFpEF, and the presence of AF has 3 points in the H₂FPEF score. Patient characteristics, such as hypertension (equal or more than 2 antihypertensive drugs use), obesity (body mass index >30 kg/m²), elderly (age >60 years), and increased filling pressure (septal E/e' ratio >9) with pulmonary hypertension (PASP >35 mm Hg) are other components constituting H₂FPEF score. In the HFA-PEFF score, the approach to diagnose HFpEF is focused on a stepwise algorithm. It starts with pretest assessment (step P), which identifies patients with the potential diagnosis of HFpEF, evaluating specific causes for HF-like symptoms. Patients likely to have HFpEF are those with typical demographics (eg, elderly, female, and with comorbidities), a preserved LVEF, and other easily detectable findings, such as elevated NPs and the presence of AF. Alternative causes, such as coronary artery disease, significant valvular disease, pulmonary disease, and anemia, are excluded during the initial work-up. If step P is positive, the is proceeded to next step (step E), which includes a comprehensive echocardiographic evaluation of diastolic parameters, LA volume, and LV wall thickness and measurement of BNP or NT-proBNP, if not already done in step P. Generally, enlarged LA (LA volume index [LAVI] >34 mL/m²) is known to be associated with HF, ischemic stroke, and death even without AF or valvular heart disease.[32] In HFpEF patients with AF, LAVI is larger (approximately 35%) than it is in sinus rhythm regardless of the presence of LV diastolic dysfunction.[23,33] Therefore, a different LAVI cutoff is suggested for AF in the HFA-PEFF score.[20] When the HFA-PEFF score is intermediate, a diastolic stress test needs to be performed (step F1) to confirm the diagnosis of HFpEF. F1 is performed when step E is inconclusive. The last step is designed to identify a specific etiology (step F2) using ergometry, cardiac magnetic resonance imaging, cardiac computed tomography, positron emission tomography, bone scintigraphy, blood test, genetic testing, and endomyocardial biopsy.[16,20]

The probability of HFpEF is determined by the sum of the positive components. HFpEF can be confirmed with high probability when the point is between 6 and 9 by the H_2FPEF score and between 5 and 6 by the HFA-PEFF score. The probability of HFpEF falls in the intermediate class when the point is between 2 and 5 by the H_2FPEF score and between 2 and 4 by the HFA-PEFF score, which would necessitate further diastolic stress test to confirm HFpEF. The low probability of HFpEF by the H_2FPEF score (0–1) does not occur because AF gets 3 points. In the HFA-PEFF score, separate criteria for AF are applied in LA size and NT-proBNP level to avoid over-diagnosis of HFpEF in AF patients.

Except for the anticoagulation treatment, there are no treatments for patients with HFpEF and AF that have been shown to improve prognosis.[1,3] Conventional HFrEF therapies that have been shown to decrease mortality and morbidity, such as angiotensin-converting enzyme inhibitors, angiotensin receptor blockers, angiotensin-neprilysin inhibitor, β-blockers, and mineralocorticoid receptor antagonists, failed to prove similar benefits in HFpEF.[34–44] Combined HF with AF may further diminish the beneficial effects of β-blockers or digoxin.[12,45,46] In patients with AF, anticoagulation treatment is recommended to decrease the risk of thromboembolism or stroke considering the associated clinical risk factors.[3] There is growing evidence of a higher risk of stroke in any form of HF with AF and adequate anticoagulation is highly recommended in patients with AF and HEpEF, especially when congestion symptoms are evident.[47–51] The mainstay of management needs to focus on the best care for combined comorbidities and modifiable risk factors with symptom control. These include volume optimization, blood pressure control, and minimization of ischemia, with the optimal management of obesity, pulmonary disease, anemia, and diabetes.[52] Adequate treatment of comorbidities and risk factors may improve symptom burden, quality of life, and exercise capacity. To date, the AF guidelines recommend the simple Atrial fibrillation Better Care (ABC) holistic pathway (A, anticoagulation/avoid stroke; B, better symptom management; and C, cardiovascular and comorbidity optimization), which emphasizes the integrated care of patients with AF across all health care levels and among different specialties.[3,53] Implementation of the ABC pathway is significantly associated with better outcomes, including a lower risk of all-cause mortality, the composite outcome of stroke/major bleeding/cardiovascular death and first hospitalization, lower rates of cardiovascular events, and lower health-related costs compared with those related to usual care.[3,54–57] In the context of HFpEF with AF, rate control is not expected to improve survival, but it might have some beneficial effect on quality of life, exercise capacity, or cardiac function.[58] Regarding rhythm control, there are challenges, especially in patients with HFpEF. Previous reports have demonstrated a mortality benefit in AF ablation, and it might be considered in selected patients.[3,59,60]

OUTCOMES OF HEART FAILURE WITH PRESERVED EJECTION FRACTION IN ATRIAL FIBRILLATION

In patients with HFpEF, both prevalent and incident AF were associated with increased mortality.[61,62] Likewise, the presence of HF had a poor prognosis in patients with AF.[12,63,64] In addition, the previous data showed the risk of stroke increased in HFpEF patients with AF.[65,66] Women are at higher risk of HFpEF, and they also showed a greater risk of adverse events in the HFpEF trial, implying the need for special attention in female patients.[67] HFrEF patients with sinus rhythm showed worse symptoms, functional capacity, and quality of life than patients with HFpEF with sinus rhythm, whereas in AF patients, there were no differences between HFrEF and HFpEF.[15] The population of AF patients with HFpEF is increasing progressively, and they show similar clinical characteristics, and prognosis as those with HF with midrange EF (HFmrEF) or HFrEF. The risk of death, hospitalization for HF, and stroke or transient ischemic attack in all EF groups were not different in various studies.[3,16,24,65]

FUTURE PERSPECTIVES

Previous trials to identify effective treatment strategies were not successful due to the pathophysiologic diversity within the broader clinical spectrum of HFpEF. Classifying patients with HFpEF into subgroups of clinically or pathophysiologically homogeneous phenotypes is expected to allow more precise and targeted therapies.[68–70] Several strategies have been introduced to classify patients with different characteristics, according to the presence of diverse comorbidities, echocardiographic parameters, invasive hemodynamic results, genetic test results, and plasma biomarker levels.[71] Newer phenotypic approaches might show better classification of HFpEF patients, resulting in superior predictability of therapeutic response and prognosis.[24,69] Further studies using artificial intelligence using big data in HFpEF patients could precisely predict a specific patient group who might benefit from a certain HF medication.

SUMMARY

HFpEF and AF are common diseases that frequently coexist and further affect each other. These also are manifested with similar symptoms, and diagnostic uncertainties exist due to the multiple factors influencing test results. Diverse risk factors should be considered for better diagnostic performance. Resting transthoracic echocardiography is the mainstay of the diagnosis in HFpEF to evaluate etiology, systolic function, diastolic function, and intracardiac pressure. Often, noninvasive or invasive exercise tests are needed to identify increases in intracardiac pressure during exercise and unmask exercise-induced symptoms. The appropriate use of HFpEF diagnostic scores can aid diagnostic procedures and also are useful in patients with AF. Currently, there is no single medication proved to increase survival in patients with HFpEF and AF. Symptomatic treatment with volume optimization and best management of combined risk factors on the basis of lifestyle modification need to be emphasized to improve quality of life. Better survival also can be expected with risk factor management. Future phenotype-based patient classification and treatment can improve outcomes further by more specific pathophysiology-based management strategies.

CLINICS CARE POINTS

- Echocardiographic evidence of enlarged LA volume, LV hypertrophy, diastolic dysfunction, and a high filling pressure increase the probability of HFpEF in AF patients.

- Cutoff value of NT-proBNP (or BNP) is higher in HFpEF patients with AF (2 points: NT-proBNP >660 pg/mL, BNP >240 pg/mL; 1 point: NT-proBNP 365–660 pg/mL, BNP 105–240 pg/mL).

- Management of underlying comorbidities and appropriate use of diuretics to control symptoms are required to treat HFpEF, and anticoagulation therapy as per indication with adequate rate and rhythm control is recommended to treat AF.

ACKNOWLEDGMENTS

This research was supported by the Bisa Research Grant of Keimyung University in 2017.

REFERENCE

1. Ponikowski P, Voors AA, Anker SD, et al. 2016 ESC Guidelines for the diagnosis and treatment of acute and chronic heart failure: The Task Force for the diagnosis and treatment of acute and chronic heart failure of the European Society of Cardiology (ESC) Developed with the special contribution of the Heart Failure Association (HFA) of the ESC. Eur Heart J 2016;37(27):2129–200.

2. Wang TJ, Evans JC, Benjamin EJ, et al. Natural history of asymptomatic left ventricular systolic dysfunction in the community. Circulation 2003; 108(8):977–82.

3. Hindricks G, Potpara T, Dagres N, et al. 2020 ESC Guidelines for the diagnosis and management of atrial fibrillation developed in collaboration with the European Association for Cardio-Thoracic Surgery (EACTS): The Task Force for the diagnosis and management of atrial fibrillation of the European Society of Cardiology (ESC) Developed with the special contribution of the European Heart Rhythm Association (EHRA) of the ESC. Eur Heart J 2020. https://doi.org/10.1093/eurheartj/ehaa612.

4. Calkins H, Hindricks G, Cappato R, et al. 2017 HRS/EHRA/ECAS/APHRS/SOLAECE expert consensus statement on catheter and surgical ablation of atrial fibrillation: Executive summary. Europace 2018; 20(1):157–208.

5. Charitos EI, Stierle U, Ziegler PD, et al. A comprehensive evaluation of rhythm monitoring strategies for the detection of atrial fibrillation recurrence: insights from 647 continuously monitored patients and implications for monitoring after therapeutic interventions. Circulation 2012;126(7):806–14.

6. Mentz RJ, Kelly JP, von Lueder TG, et al. Noncardiac comorbidities in heart failure with reduced versus preserved ejection fraction. J Am Coll Cardiol 2014;64(21):2281–93.

7. Lam CS, Roger VL, Rodeheffer RJ, et al. Cardiac structure and ventricular-vascular function in persons with heart failure and preserved ejection fraction from Olmsted County, Minnesota. Circulation 2007;115(15):1982–90.

8. Kawaguchi M, Hay I, Fetics B, et al. Combined ventricular systolic and arterial stiffening in patients with heart failure and preserved ejection fraction: implications for systolic and diastolic reserve limitations. Circulation 2003;107(5):714–20.

9. Paulus WJ, Tschöpe C. A novel paradigm for heart failure with preserved ejection fraction: comorbidities drive myocardial dysfunction and remodeling through coronary microvascular endothelial inflammation. J Am Coll Cardiol 2013;62(4):263–71.

10. Frustaci A, Chimenti C, Bellocci F, et al. Histological substrate of atrial biopsies in patients with lone atrial fibrillation. Circulation 1997;96(4):1180–4.

11. Sasaki N, Okumura Y, Watanabe I, et al. Increased levels of inflammatory and extracellular matrix turnover biomarkers persist despite reverse atrial structural remodeling during the first year after atrial fibrillation ablation. J Interv Card Electrophysiol 2014;39(3):241–9.

12. Kotecha D, Lam CS, Van Veldhuisen DJ, et al. Heart failure with preserved ejection fraction and atrial fibrillation: vicious twins. J Am Coll Cardiol 2016; 68(20):2217–28.

13. Packer M, Lam CSP, Lund LH, et al. Interdependence of atrial fibrillation and heart failure with a preserved ejection fraction reflects a common underlying atrial and ventricular myopathy. Circulation 2020;141(1):4–6.

14. Kim I-C, Han S. Epicardial adipose tissue: fuel for COVID-19-induced cardiac injury? Eur Heart J 2020. https://doi.org/10.1093/eurheartj/ehaa474.

15. Patel RB, Shah SJ. Therapeutic Targeting of Left Atrial Myopathy in Atrial Fibrillation and Heart Failure With Preserved Ejection Fraction. JAMA Cardiol 2020;5(5):497–9.

16. van den Berg MP, Mulder BA, Klaassen SHC, et al. Heart failure with preserved ejection fraction, atrial fibrillation, and the role of senile amyloidosis. Eur Heart J 2019;40(16):1287–93.

17. Borlaug BA, Nishimura RA, Sorajja P, et al. Exercise hemodynamics enhance diagnosis of early heart failure with preserved ejection fraction. Circ Heart Fail 2010;3(5):588–95.

18. Obokata M, Kane GC, Reddy YN, et al. Role of Diastolic Stress Testing in the Evaluation for Heart Failure With Preserved Ejection Fraction: A Simultaneous Invasive-Echocardiographic Study. Circulation 2017; 135(9):825–38.

19. Reddy YNV, Carter RE, Obokata M, et al. A simple, evidence-based approach to help guide diagnosis of heart failure with preserved ejection fraction. Circulation 2018;138(9):861–70.

20. Pieske B, Tschöpe C, de Boer RA, et al. How to diagnose heart failure with preserved ejection fraction: the HFA-PEFF diagnostic algorithm: a consensus recommendation from the Heart Failure Association (HFA) of the European Society of Cardiology (ESC). Eur Heart J 2019;40(40):3297–317.

21. Obokata M, Reddy YNV, Borlaug BA. Diastolic dysfunction and heart failure with preserved ejection fraction: understanding mechanisms by using noninvasive methods. JACC Cardiovasc Imaging 2020;13(1 Pt 2):245–57.

22. Ding EY, Marcus GM, McManus DD. Emerging technologies for identifying atrial fibrillation. Circ Res 2020;127(1):128–42.

23. Nagueh SF, Smiseth OA, Appleton CP, et al. Recommendations for the Evaluation of Left Ventricular Diastolic Function by Echocardiography: An Update from the American Society of Echocardiography and the European Association of Cardiovascular Imaging. J Am Soc Echocardiogr 2016;29(4):277–314.

24. Borlaug BA. Evaluation and management of heart failure with preserved ejection fraction. Nat Rev Cardiol 2020;17(9):559–73.

25. Patel RB, Vaduganathan M, Shah SJ, et al. Atrial fibrillation in heart failure with preserved ejection fraction: Insights into mechanisms and therapeutics. Pharmacol Ther 2017;176:32–9.

26. Nagueh SF, Kopelen HA, Quiñones MA. Assessment of left ventricular filling pressures by Doppler in the presence of atrial fibrillation. Circulation 1996; 94(9):2138–45.

27. Wong CM, Hawkins NM, Jhund PS, et al. Clinical characteristics and outcomes of young and very young adults with heart failure: The CHARM programme (Candesartan in Heart Failure Assessment of Reduction in Mortality and Morbidity). J Am Coll Cardiol 2013;62(20):1845–54.

28. Wong CM, Hawkins NM, Petrie MC, et al. Heart failure in younger patients: the Meta-analysis Global Group in Chronic Heart Failure (MAGGIC). Eur Heart J 2014;35(39):2714–21.

29. McKie PM, Schirger JA, Costello-Boerrigter LC, et al. Impaired natriuretic and renal endocrine response to acute volume expansion in pre-clinical systolic and diastolic dysfunction. J Am Coll Cardiol 2011;58(20):2095–103.

30. Henning RJ. Diagnosis and treatment of heart failure with preserved left ventricular ejection fraction. World J Cardiol 2020;12(1):7–25.

31. Ha JW, Andersen OS, Smiseth OA. Diastolic stress test: invasive and noninvasive testing. JACC Cardiovasc Imaging 2020;13(1 Pt 2):272–82.

32. Abhayaratna WP, Seward JB, Appleton CP, et al. Left atrial size: physiologic determinants and

clinical applications. J Am Coll Cardiol 2006;47(12): 2357–63.

33. Lam CS, Rienstra M, Tay WT, et al. Atrial fibrillation in heart failure with preserved ejection fraction: association with exercise capacity, left ventricular filling pressures, natriuretic peptides, and left atrial volume. JACC Heart Fail 2017;5(2):92–8.

34. Hollenberg SM, Warner Stevenson L, Ahmad T, et al. 2019 ACC Expert Consensus Decision Pathway on Risk Assessment, Management, and Clinical Trajectory of Patients Hospitalized With Heart Failure: A Report of the American College of Cardiology Solution Set Oversight Committee. J Am Coll Cardiol 2019;74(15):1966–2011.

35. Kim K-J, Cho H-J, Kim M-S, et al. Focused Update of 2016 Korean Society of Heart Failure guidelines for the management of chronic heart failure. Int J Heart Fail 2019;1(1):4–24.

36. Seferovic PM, Ponikowski P, Anker SD, et al. Clinical practice update on heart failure 2019: pharmacotherapy, procedures, devices and patient management. An expert consensus meeting report of the Heart Failure Association of the European Society of Cardiology. Eur J Heart Fail 2019;21(10): 1169–86.

37. Velazquez EJ, Morrow DA, DeVore AD, et al. Angiotensin-Neprilysin Inhibition in Acute Decompensated Heart Failure. N Engl J Med 2019;380(6): 539–48.

38. Cleland JG, Tendera M, Adamus J, et al. The perindopril in elderly people with chronic heart failure (PEP-CHF) study. Eur Heart J 2006;27(19):2338–45.

39. Massie BM, Carson PE, McMurray JJ, et al. Irbesartan in Patients with Heart Failure and Preserved Ejection Fraction. N Engl J Med 2008;359(23): 2456–67.

40. Yusuf S, Pfeffer MA, Swedberg K, et al. Effects of candesartan in patients with chronic heart failure and preserved left-ventricular ejection fraction: the CHARM-Preserved Trial. Lancet 2003;362(9386): 777–81.

41. Solomon SD, McMurray JJV, Anand IS, et al. Angiotensin–Neprilysin Inhibition in Heart Failure with Preserved Ejection Fraction. N Engl J Med 2019; 381(17):1609–20.

42. Pitt B, Pfeffer MA, Assmann SF, et al. Spironolactone for Heart Failure with Preserved Ejection Fraction. N Engl J Med 2014;370(15):1383–92.

43. Yamamoto K, Origasa H, Hori M. Effects of carvedilol on heart failure with preserved ejection fraction: the Japanese Diastolic Heart Failure Study (J-DHF). Eur J Heart Fail 2013;15(1):110–8.

44. Conraads VM, Metra M, Kamp O, et al. Effects of the long-term administration of nebivolol on the clinical symptoms, exercise capacity, and left ventricular function of patients with diastolic dysfunction: results of the ELANDD study. Eur J Heart Fail 2012;14(2): 219–25.

45. Ziff OJ, Lane DA, Samra M, et al. Safety and efficacy of digoxin: systematic review and meta-analysis of observational and controlled trial data. BMJ 2015; 351:h4451.

46. Kotecha D, Holmes J, Krum H, et al. Efficacy of β blockers in patients with heart failure plus atrial fibrillation: an individual-patient data meta-analysis. Lancet 2014;384(9961):2235–43.

47. Zannad F, Anker SD, Byra WM, et al. Rivaroxaban in patients with heart failure, sinus rhythm, and coronary disease. N Engl J Med 2018;379(14):1332–42.

48. Greenberg B, Neaton JD, Anker SD, et al. Association of Rivaroxaban With Thromboembolic Events in Patients With Heart Failure, Coronary Disease, and Sinus Rhythm: A Post Hoc Analysis of the COMMANDER HF Trial. JAMA Cardiol 2019;4(6):515–23.

49. Kotecha D, Chudasama R, Lane DA, et al. Atrial fibrillation and heart failure due to reduced versus preserved ejection fraction: A systematic review and meta-analysis of death and adverse outcomes. Int J Cardiol 2016;203:660–6.

50. Kotecha D, Banerjee A, Lip GY. Increased stroke risk in atrial fibrillation patients with heart failure: does ejection fraction matter? Stroke 2015;46(3): 608–9.

51. Sandhu RK, Hohnloser SH, Pfeffer MA, et al. Relationship between degree of left ventricular dysfunction, symptom status, and risk of embolic events in patients with atrial fibrillation and heart failure. Stroke 2015;46(3):667–72.

52. Kotecha D, Piccini JP. Atrial fibrillation in heart failure: what should we do? Eur Heart J 2015;36(46): 3250–7.

53. Lip GYH. The ABC pathway: an integrated approach to improve AF management. Nat Rev Cardiol 2017; 14(11):627–8.

54. Proietti M, Romiti GF, Olshansky B, et al. Improved Outcomes by Integrated Care of Anticoagulated Patients with Atrial Fibrillation Using the Simple ABC (Atrial Fibrillation Better Care) Pathway. Am J Med 2018;131(11):1359–66.e6.

55. Yoon M, Yang PS, Jang E, et al. Improved Population-Based Clinical Outcomes of Patients with Atrial Fibrillation by Compliance with the Simple ABC (Atrial Fibrillation Better Care) Pathway for Integrated Care Management: A Nationwide Cohort Study. Thromb Haemost 2019;119(10):1695–703.

56. Pastori D, Pignatelli P, Menichelli D, et al. Integrated Care Management of Patients With Atrial Fibrillation and Risk of Cardiovascular Events: The ABC (Atrial fibrillation Better Care) Pathway in the ATHERO-AF Study Cohort. Mayo Clin Proc 2019;94(7):1261–7.

57. Pastori D, Farcomeni A, Pignatelli P, et al. ABC (Atrial fibrillation Better Care) Pathway and Healthcare

Costs in Atrial Fibrillation: The ATHERO-AF Study. Am J Med 2019;132(7):856–61.

58. Kotecha D, Calvert M, Deeks JJ, et al. A review of rate control in atrial fibrillation, and the rationale and protocol for the RATE-AF trial. BMJ Open 2017;7(7):e015099.

59. Packer DL, Mark DB, Robb RA, et al. Effect of Catheter Ablation vs Antiarrhythmic Drug Therapy on Mortality, Stroke, Bleeding, and Cardiac Arrest Among Patients With Atrial Fibrillation: The CABANA Randomized Clinical Trial. JAMA 2019;321(13):1261–74.

60. Marrouche NF, Brachmann J, Andresen D, et al. Catheter Ablation for Atrial Fibrillation with Heart Failure. N Engl J Med 2018;378(5):417–27.

61. Zakeri R, Chamberlain AM, Roger VL, et al. Temporal relationship and prognostic significance of atrial fibrillation in heart failure patients with preserved ejection fraction: a community-based study. Circulation 2013;128(10):1085–93.

62. Owan TE, Hodge DO, Herges RM, et al. Trends in prevalence and outcome of heart failure with preserved ejection fraction. N Engl J Med 2006;355(3):251–9.

63. Santhanakrishnan R, Wang N, Larson MG, et al. Atrial Fibrillation Begets Heart Failure and Vice Versa: Temporal Associations and Differences in Preserved Versus Reduced Ejection Fraction. Circulation 2016;133(5):484–92.

64. Olsson LG, Swedberg K, Ducharme A, et al. Atrial fibrillation and risk of clinical events in chronic heart failure with and without left ventricular systolic dysfunction: results from the Candesartan in Heart failure-Assessment of Reduction in Mortality and morbidity (CHARM) program. J Am Coll Cardiol 2006;47(10):1997–2004.

65. Son MK, Park JJ, Lim NK, et al. Impact of atrial fibrillation in patients with heart failure and reduced, mid-range or preserved ejection fraction. Heart 2020;106(15):1160–8.

66. Oluleye OW, Rector TS, Win S, et al. History of atrial fibrillation as a risk factor in patients with heart failure and preserved ejection fraction. Circ Heart Fail 2014;7(6):960–6.

67. Lam CS, Carson PE, Anand IS, et al. Sex differences in clinical characteristics and outcomes in elderly patients with heart failure and preserved ejection fraction: the Irbesartan in Heart Failure with Preserved Ejection Fraction (I-PRESERVE) trial. Circ Heart Fail 2012;5(5):571–8.

68. Tromp J, Westenbrink BD, Ouwerkerk W, et al. Identifying Pathophysiological Mechanisms in Heart Failure With Reduced Versus Preserved Ejection Fraction. J Am Coll Cardiol 2018;72(10):1081–90.

69. Tromp J, Ouwerkerk W, Demissei BG, et al. Novel endotypes in heart failure: effects on guideline-directed medical therapy. Eur Heart J 2018;39(48):4269–76.

70. Tromp J, Khan MA, Klip IT, et al. Biomarker Profiles in Heart Failure Patients With Preserved and Reduced Ejection Fraction. J Am Heart Assoc 2017;6(4). https://doi.org/10.1161/jaha.116.003989.

71. Borlaug BA, Obokata M. Is it time to recognize a new phenotype? Heart failure with preserved ejection fraction with pulmonary vascular disease. Eur Heart J 2017;38(38):2874–8.

Valvular Disease and Heart Failure with Preserved Ejection Fraction

Yiting Fan, PhD[a], Alex Pui-Wai Lee, MBChB, MD, FRCP, FESC[b,c],*

KEYWORDS

- Valvular heart disease • Heart failure with preserved ejection fraction • Primary HFpEF
- Secondary HFpEF

KEY POINTS

- Half of patients with heart failure (HF) have preserved left ventricular ejection fraction (EF).
- Heart failure with preserved ejection fraction (HFpEF) is classified into primary and secondary, according to the cause.
- Valvular heart disease (VHD) is commonly seen in patients with HFpEF and can be the primary cause of HFpEF or secondary to HFpEF.
- In general, primary VHD with secondary HFpEF is amenable to surgery or transcatheter intervention.
- There is an increasing recognition of the existence of secondary VHD complicating primary HFpEF. The mechanisms and best management approach remain to be defined.

INTRODUCTION

Heart failure (HF) with preserved ejection fraction (HFpEF), referring to HF in the presence of left ventricular (LV) ejection fraction (EF) greater than 50%, is an emerging global health problem. HFpEF has a prognosis similar to HF with reduced ejection fraction (HFrEF) and accounts for approximately half of all patients with HF.[1,2] The understanding of the pathophysiology of HFpEF has grown in recent years but is still limited in certain aspects, including its relationship with valvular heart diseases (VHD).

There are two forms of HFpEF in relation to VHD: primary and secondary HFpEF (**Fig. 1**). Primary HFpEF, as a clinical entity, is often diagnosed in cases where there is a primary diastolic dysfunction leading to HF symptoms and signs. Multiple risk factors, including hypertension, aging, systemic inflammatory status, and metabolic disorders, may contribute to the development of HFpEF, but often there is no single specific underlying cause identified. Currently, there are no definitive medical or surgical therapies for primary HFpEF.[3] Patients with primary HFpEF may develop secondary/functional valvular diseases in association with atrial fibrillation or ventricular/atrial dysfunction, among which functional mitral regurgitation (MR) and functional tricuspid regurgitation (TR) are most commonly observed.

Secondary HFpEF refers to a condition where HF symptoms and signs are relevant to certain identifiable causes, such as primary VHD. Generally, secondary HFpEF runs a clinical trajectory that is specific to the underlying VHD, such as mitral/aortic stenosis (AS)/regurgitation; its

The authors have nothing to disclose.
[a] Department of Cardiology, Shanghai Chest Hospital, Shanghai Jiao Tong University, 241 West Huaihai Road, Xu Hui District, Shanghai, China; [b] Laboratory of Cardiac Imaging and 3D Printing, Li Ka Shing Institute of Health Science, The Chinese University of Hong Kong, Hong Kong SAR, China; [c] Division of Cardiology, Department of Medicine and Therapeutics, The Chinese University of Hong Kong, Hong Kong SAR, China
* Corresponding author. Prince of Wales Hospital, Room 114037, 9/F, Lui Che Woo Clinical Sciences Building, Shatin, N.T., Hong Kong SAR, China.
E-mail address: alexpwlee@cuhk.edu.hk

Heart Failure Clin 17 (2021) 387–395
https://doi.org/10.1016/j.hfc.2021.02.005
1551-7136/21/© 2021 Elsevier Inc. All rights reserved.

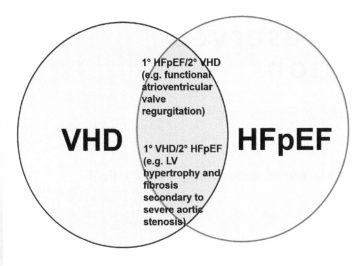

Fig. 1. Venn diagram showing relationships between VHD and HFpEF. 1° HFpEF/2° VHD denotes HFpEF caused by primary LV diastolic dysfunction leading to secondary VHD (mainly atrioventricular valve regurgitation) through mechanisms including alterations of the atrial/ventricular/valvular geometry and hemodynamic burdens secondary to elevated left ventricular filling pressures. 1° VHD/2° HFpEF denotes VHD as a primary cause of HFpEF (mainly stenosis and/or regurgitation of the left heart valves) with secondary atrial/ventricular remodeling secondary to the valve lesions, contributing to the HFpEF hemodynamic burdens. A typical example is LV hypertrophy and fibrosis with resultant diastolic dysfunction secondary to aortic stenosis.

prognosis is generally good if intervention/surgery to the underlying primary VHD is performed in a timely manner but may progress if the diagnosis is established late or if the patient is denied surgery/intervention because of severe comorbidities. Early referral for surgery and the availability of emerging catheter-based valve interventions in inoperable/high-risk surgical candidates can prevent HF development and prolong survival. However, there are still long-term issues, such as the risk of recurrent HF with prosthetic valve malfunction and the need for redo-surgery/interventions.

We herein review the prevalence, clinical features, diagnostic approach, management, and prognosis of HFpEF in structural heart disease in a primary and secondary form.

PRIMARY HEART FAILURE WITH PRESERVED EJECTION FRACTION AND SECONDARY VALVULAR HEART DISEASE

In primary HFpEF, secondary (or functional) VHD may develop in the absence of intrinsic structural valve disease. In particular, secondary (or functional) atrioventricular (ie, mitral and/or tricuspid) valve regurgitation is frequently observed in patients with primary HFpEF, without obvious primary leaflet lesions, such as prolapse, flail, rheumatic changes, or endocarditis, or severe calcification.

Primary Heart Failure with Preserved Ejection Fraction and Secondary Mitral Regurgitation

Secondary MR may occur in patients with HFpEF without apparent intrinsic mitral valve pathologies.[4] However, unlike secondary MR in patients with HFrEF, the clinical picture of secondary MR in HFpEF is less well defined; limited data exist

regarding the prevalence of valve disease in general, and MR specifically, in HFpEF. Most clinical trials, observational studies, and clinical diagnostic algorithms of HFpEF exclude patients with significant mitral or aortic valve disease.[5–7] However, mild to moderate degree of MR and TR is frequently observed in HFpEF and is often considered as "bystanders" rather than the cause of HF symptoms. Most HFpEF registries/clinical trials/observational studies reported the prevalence for any MR in HFpEF patients to be approximately 60% and approximately 10% to 15% for moderate-to-severe or greater MR. The Treatment of Preserved Cardiac Function Heart Failure with an Aldosterone Antagonist (TOPCAT) trial enrolled 3445 patients with HFpEF to determine whether treatment with spironolactone would reduce mortality and morbidity.[5] Baseline echocardiographic data of the TOPCAT trial showed that MR was found in 61% of patients, with moderate or more regurgitation present in 12% of the overall patient population.[8] Prior surgical replacement of the mitral and/or aortic valve was noted in 3% of the TOPCAT population. In the New York Heart Failure Registry, MR was present in more than 60% of the 619 patients with HFpEF studied, with moderate-to-severe or greater degrees of MR evident in approximately 10%.[9] The prevalence was higher in women than men. Consistently, in the Northwestern HFpEF Registry, moderate MR was noted in approximately 14% of patients[7]; however, these registries excluded patients with more than moderate MR, hence they may be underestimating the true prevalence of secondary MR in HFpEF. Of note, even a mild degree of MR may have an important hemodynamic burden in patients with HFpEF. In a smaller study of 70 patients with HFpEF, 30% of patients had secondary

MR, which is linked to more significant pulmonary hypertension compared with patients with HFpEF without MR even though the mean regurgitant volume in these patients was only 15 mL.[10] The reported prevalence of secondary MR in HFpEF may also depend on the timing of echocardiographic assessment because the occurrence and severity of MR alters significantly with the hemodynamic status of the patients. In a study of patients hospitalized for acute HFpEF, 32 of the 37 (86%) patients with HFpEF had MR on admission as opposed to none of the non-HFpEF patients had MR.[11] The prevalence and degree of acute MR often improve after diuretics therapy and tend to become mild if assessed during the compensated state of HFpEF.

Scarce data exist regarding the prognostic significance of secondary MR in HFpEF. In a retrospective study of 54 hospitalized patients with HFpEF, residual MR at discharge was predictive of future cardiac death and/or HF readmission, with 2.4 times increase risk per one grade MR increase over 20 months postdischarge.[12] Another study showed that the HF readmission rate of patients with HFpEF/atrial fibrillation who had moderate/severe MR was even higher than that of patients with HFrEF with no/mild MR.[13] Consistently in another study of 298 patients with atrial fibrillation and LVEF greater than or equal to 50% (11% had prior HF admission), patients with significant functional MR had poorer prognosis, with an event-free (death, HF hospitalization, or valve surgery) rate of 39% versus 94% in patients without significant functional MR at a mean follow-up of 24 months.[14]

Compared with HFrEF, the pathophysiology of HFpEF is more heterogeneous.[15–18] It is therefore not surprising that the mechanism of secondary MR in HFpEF is less well defined than secondary in HFrEF. Just like the heterogeneous nature of the pathophysiology of HFpEF, the mechanism of secondary MR in HFpEF may also be heterogeneous. Because concentric hypertrophy is the primary pattern of LV remodeling in HFpEF, subvalvular leaflet tethering is, therefore, unlike HFrEF, a major mechanism of MR in HFpEF. The exception is a phenotypic subgroup of HFpEF in which local/eccentric LV remodeling may contribute to MR.[19] More commonly, MR in HFpEF in the absence of intrinsic leaflet pathologies is normal leaflet motion MR (Carpentier type I) associated with left atrial (LA) dilatation, an important feature of HFpEF.[20] A primary mechanism of functional MR in preserved LVEF is mitral annulus dilatation and dysfunction.[21] In HFpEF, LA dilatation secondary to chronically elevated LA pressure and/or atrial fibrillation, which is common in HFpEF, causes mitral annular dilatation independent of LV remodeling.[22] Atrial myopathy has been suggested because MR/atrial dysfunction in HFpEF can occur without atrial fibrillation.[22] The loss of atrial contraction in atrial fibrillation predisposes to MR occurrence as a result of the loss of late diastolic mitral annular contraction that normally serves to bring the mitral leaflets to approximation at end-diastole.[23] More recently, our group demonstrated that longitudinal LV deformation may be important in the pathogenesis of atrial functional MR (which may therefore be a misnomer).[21] Intriguingly, the notion of atrial functional MR has recently been associated with hypertensive older female patients with atrial fibrillation, a similar group of patients affected by HFpEF, who develop normal-EF-normal-leaflet-motion MR.[24,25] There seems to be a significant overlap in clinical manifestation and pathogenic mechanisms for atrial functional MR and HFpEF/MR. The longitudinal descend of the posterior portion of mitral annulus along with the contraction of the longitudinal LV fibers normally has the function to fold the annulus into a deeper saddle shape, which helps to bring the two mitral leaflets close to each other during systole. Loss of the systolic annular saddle-shape is evident in patients with atrial functional MR.[21] Although mitral tenting is caused by a reduced leaflet closing force from the impaired LV in HFrEF, mitral tenting in HFpEF can be caused by an excessive pushing force from an elevated LA pressure that prevents leaflet closure. A high E/e', a surrogate of elevated LA pressure, has been shown to be a primary determinant of functional MR in HFpEF.[19] Moreover, severe atrial dilatation can tether the posterior mitral leaflet from the atrial side and produce restricted systolic leaflet motion MR (Carpentier type IIIa).[26]

Similar to HFrEF, a closer look of the mitral valve leaflets often shows that their structures are not completely normal. Nodular thickening of the leaflets, especially over the line of coaptation where stress is maximal, is frequently observed in elderly patients.[27] Associated with aging, mitral annular calcifications are a common occurrence in HFpEF, further distorting annular function and leaflet motions.[28] Mitral leaflet remodeling in adaptation to mitral annular enlargement may occur in patients with preserved LVEF, but the adaptive mechanism can eventually fail to compensate for progressive annular dilatation resulting in MR.[29]

Primary Heart Failure with Preserved Ejection Fraction and Secondary Tricuspid Regurgitation

The reported prevalence of moderate/severe TR in patients with HFpEF ranges from approximately 9% to 51%.[30–32] This variability in reported prevalence is probably related to the varying definitions/stages of HFpEF among studies. In an older study of 576 patients with HF, of the 44% of patients who had LVEF greater than 35%, the prevalence of semiquantitatively defined moderate/severe TR was approximately 9%.[30] Similarly, in a study of 2014 patients with stage B/C HFpEF, moderate/severe TR, defined visually, was prevalent in 11% of patients.[31] However, in a recent study enrolling patients with apparently more advanced HFpEF, as evident by a higher N-terminal pro–B-type natriuretic peptide level than previous studies, a much higher prevalence of moderate/severe TR of 51% was reported.[32] The presence of moderate/severe TR carries important prognostic implications in HFpEF, predictive of a worse outcome, with a higher risk of death,[30,31] HF hospitalization,[31] heart transplant,[30] and LV-assist device implantation.[30] The risk-stratifying power of TR is even stronger in HFpEF than in HFrEF.[30]

The mechanisms of secondary TR in HFpEF most likely involve dilatation of the right atrium and right ventricle with dilation of the tricuspid annulus and subvalvular tethering of the tricuspid valve leaflets.[33] Alterations in ventricular geometry can lead to TR by altering tricuspid annulus size and papillary muscle position.[34] Right ventricular dilatation, tricuspid annular dilatation, and tricuspid leaflet tethering may result from any underlying causes of HFpEF that also directly involves the right ventricle (eg, cardiomyopathy, ischemia) or causes an elevation in right ventricular systolic pressure with pulmonary hypertension secondary to elevated LA pressure/MR associated with HFpEF. Significant secondary TR is also associated with atrial fibrillation, which commonly occurs in HFpEF, but whether the TR is the cause of right atrial dilatation and thus predisposes to atrial fibrillation or whether chronic atrial fibrillation causes tricuspid annular dilatation and causes TR is not known.[35,36]

PRIMARY VALVULAR HEART DISEASE AND SECONDARY HEART FAILURE WITH PRESERVED EJECTION FRACTION

Secondary HFpEF, also known as HFpEF mimics, has an identifiable cause. Such conditions have distinctive clinical manifestations and courses and may respond to treatments targeting the underlying causes. Among secondary forms of HFpEF, VHD is most commonly seen. Stenosis/regurgitation of the left heart valves (mitral/aortic) creates acute/chronic loading burden to the LV/LA, leading eventually to HF signs and symptoms often indistinguishable from primary HFpEF. The prompt identification and early detection of valve

disease rely on a comprehensive history, physical examination, electrocardiogram, and imaging, including cardiac computed tomography, cardiac MRI, and, especially, echocardiography. Tailored treatments, according to their specific pathophysiology, may improve the HF symptoms and the prognosis.

Aortic Stenosis and Secondary Heart Failure with Preserved Ejection Fraction

AS is more than just a valvular disease but also a myocardial disease caused by chronic afterload increase on the LV, which leads to remodeling in form of hypertrophy. Diffuse myocardial fibrosis associated with AS is detectable on cardiac MRI and worsens LV diastolic dysfunction and dyspnea and HFpEF outcomes.[37] There are four gradient patterns in severe AS with HFpEF, including normal flow/normal gradient AS, low flow/low gradient AS, normal flow/low gradient (NF-LG) AS, and low flow/low gradient (LF-LG) AS.[38] The latter two patterns are classified as paradoxic low-gradient AS, which deserve special attention because they are believed to present with a syndrome akin to HFpEF.[39] Paradoxic low-gradient AS predominates in older patients and has a higher prevalence of coronary artery disease, diabetes, hypertension, and a tendency to female predisposition, which are all characteristics of HFpEF.[40] A meta-analysis revealed that 30% to 50% of the AS population with HFpEF are LF-LG AS, and 25% to 50% are NF-LG AS. Most of the studies found that LF-LG AS had worse symptomatic status and an increased risk of mortality compared with other subtypes of AS, including moderate AS, NF-LG AS, and high gradient AS.[38,41–50] However, some studies found a similar prognosis for patients with LF-LG AS versus those with other AS subtypes.[51–53] The discrepancies can possibly be explained by the differences in patients' baseline characteristics, variability in the echocardiographic measurements of stroke volume, aortic valve area and/or gradient, and the definition of LF-LG AS among these studies. The outcomes of patients with NF-LG AS are similar to those with high-gradient AS and better than patients with LF-LG AS.

Surgical or transcatheter aortic valve replacement is recommended for symptomatic patients with LF-LG severe AS (class IIa recommendation). It is confirmed to be associated with a major survival benefit. Although patients with NF-LG AS represent an important proportion of the AS population with HFpEF, the current guidelines do not draw a clear recommendation for this group of patients. For asymptomatic patients with severe AS and preserved LVEF, the optimal timing of intervention remains controversial. To date, early surgery is recommended in asymptomatic patients with high-gradient severe AS and preserved EF.[54]

Aortic Regurgitation Secondary Heart Failure with Preserved Ejection Fraction

AR causes a chronic volume and pressure overload on LV, which leads to progressive LV enlargement and LV dysfunction.[55,56] The current guidelines[57,58] recommend surgery for symptomatic patients with severe AR with preserved or reduced EF. For asymptomatic patients with severe AR, surgery should be considered when LV end-systolic diameter greater than 55 mm (25 mm/m^2) or LVEF decreases to less than 50%.[59] The optimal timing of cardiac surgery for patients not meeting these criteria remains controversial, with the development of LV systolic dysfunction often preceding symptom onset in more than one-fourth of patients.[60] Once LV starts to fail and LVEF drops in severe AR, HF symptoms develop, and a dramatic decrease in survival without surgery is expected.[61–63] Several studies suggested early surgery in asymptomatic patients with severe AR and preserved EF, proposing a lower threshold of LV dimensions for surgical referral.[64,65] In addition, new echocardiographic markers of early LV systolic dysfunction, including a decrease in the mitral annular plane excursion, systolic mitral annular velocity (s') measured by tissue Doppler,[66–68] and global LV longitudinal strain measured by speckle tracking,[69–72] may be helpful for detection of early LV dysfunction when EF is preserved.

Little attention has been paid to nonsevere (mild or moderate) AR, which was thought to have little impact on the outcome. However, a recent study[73] found that in a group of patients with HF hospitalized for acute HF (n = 505), mild/moderate AR was associated with increased all-cause mortality in the subgroup of patients presenting with acute HFpEF. A possible explanation of the detrimental effect of nonsevere AR in patients with acute HFpEF is the small LV cavity and increased LV wall stiffness in these patients, that even a small amount of AR can cause a disproportionately elevated end-diastolic pressure.

Mitral Stenosis and Secondary Heart Failure with Preserved Ejection Fraction

MS is characterized by a chronic elevation in LA pressure and underfilling of LV leading to pulmonary hypertension and HF symptoms. Although LVEF is "preserved" in patients with MS caused by a low preload, up to 84.2% of patients with severe MS were found to have impaired global longitudinal strain.[74] The cause of myocardial dysfunction in MS may be related to the underlying rheumatic inflammatory process, tethering effect by the rigid mitral apparatus,[75] or lack of LV vortex formation.[76] Mitral valve surgery or percutaneous transcatheter mitral commissurotomy are strongly recommended in symptomatic patients with severe MS, irrespective of LVEF. An MS patient with reduced EF was reported to have higher in-hospital postoperative HF. Besides, those patients had higher HF deaths and admissions during the 9-year follow-up. However, no difference of overall mortality was found compared with control subjects.[77]

Mitral Regurgitation and Secondary Heart Failure with Preserved Ejection Fraction

HFpEF secondary to primary MR (eg, mitral valve prolapse) is called secondary HFpEF.[78] Patients with severe primary MR presents with symptoms and signs of HF with preserved EF. In fact, in the acute phase and early compensatory phase of severe primary MR, LVEF is typically hypernormal (>70%). Unlike severe aortic valve disease in which LV concentric hypertrophy occurs consequentially to chronic afterload increase, LV remodeling is typically eccentric in the compensatory phase of chronic severe primary MR with progressive dilatation of LV but the preservation of LVEF. Because of LV afterload reduction in chronic severe MR, an LVEF less than 60% (rather than <50%) is already considered as "reduced" EF and is an indication for mitral valve intervention.[78] Treatment of HFpEF secondary to primary degenerative MR is surgical repair or replacement; for patients with prohibitive risk for surgery, transcatheter approach to mitral valve repair is an alternative treatment strategy.[79]

SUMMARY

Although VHD occurs less frequently than coronary artery disease or hypertension, it has drawn increasing clinical attention recently because it represents a major health problem globally with an increasing prevalence in the aging population and even more so among the HFpEF patient population. Future studies will better define the complex interactions in the pathophysiology and pathogenic mechanisms of primary/secondary HFpEF with various forms of VHD. Understanding their mechanisms is of paramount importance for developing optimal diagnostic and therapeutic strategies for these complex yet interesting HFpEF/VHD syndromes.

CLINICS CARE POINTS

- To date, there is no single gold standard diagnostic test for HFpEF; the incidence and prevalence in its primary and secondary forms are not fully understood. Current guidelines recommend a multiparametric approach to diagnose HFpEF, with emphasis on the use of natriuretic peptide tests and echocardiography.

- When accessing a patient with suspected HFpEF, it is important to distinguish between primary and secondary HFpEF because secondary causes (eg, VHD or pericardial disease) are often treatable, and current guidelines recommend early intervention in symptomatic patients.

- The optimal approach to VHD (eg, functional mitral and tricuspid regurgitation, secondary to primary HFpEF), however, is controversial. The success of valvular interventions has been reported for this group of patients, but their long-term benefit has not been established by randomized controlled trials.

ACKNOWLEDGMENTS

This work was funded by the Hong Kong Special Administrative Region Government Health and Medical Research Fund (05160976).

REFERENCES

1. Owan TE, Hodge DO, Herges RM, et al. Trends in prevalence and outcome of heart failure with preserved ejection fraction. N Engl J Med 2006; 355(3):251–9.
2. Tribouilloy C, Rusinaru D, Mahjoub H, et al. Prognosis of heart failure with preserved ejection fraction: a 5 year prospective population-based study. Eur Heart J 2008;29(3):339–47.
3. Pfeffer MA, Shah AM, Borlaug BA. Heart failure with preserved ejection fraction in perspective. Circ Res 2019;124(11):1598–617.
4. Marechaux S, Pibarot P, Ennezat PV. Insights into functional mitral regurgitation despite preserved LVEF. Arch Cardiovasc Dis 2011;104(2):131–3.
5. Desai AS, Lewis EF, Li R, et al. Rationale and design of the treatment of preserved cardiac function heart failure with an aldosterone antagonist trial: a randomized, controlled study of spironolactone in patients with symptomatic heart failure and preserved ejection fraction. Am Heart J 2011;162(6):966–72. e10.
6. Solomon SD, McMurray JJV, Anand IS, et al. Angiotensin-neprilysin inhibition in heart failure with preserved ejection fraction. N Engl J Med 2019; 381(17):1609–20.
7. Katz DH, Beussink L, Sauer AJ, et al. Prevalence, clinical characteristics, and outcomes associated with eccentric versus concentric left ventricular hypertrophy in heart failure with preserved ejection fraction. Am J Cardiol 2013;112(8):1158–64.
8. Shah AM, Shah SJ, Anand IS, et al. Cardiac structure and function in heart failure with preserved ejection fraction: baseline findings from the echocardiographic study of the treatment of preserved cardiac function heart failure with an aldosterone antagonist trial. Circ Heart Fail 2014;7(1):104–15.
9. Klapholz M, Maurer M, Lowe AM, et al. Hospitalization for heart failure in the presence of a normal left ventricular ejection fraction: results of the New York Heart Failure Registry. J Am Coll Cardiol 2004; 43(8):1432–8.
10. Marechaux S, Neicu DV, Braun S, et al. Functional mitral regurgitation: a link to pulmonary hypertension in heart failure with preserved ejection fraction. J Card Fail 2011;17(10):806–12.
11. Ennezat PV, Marechaux S, Bouabdallaoui N, et al. Dynamic nature of pulmonary artery systolic pressure in decompensated heart failure with preserved ejection fraction: role of functional mitral regurgitation. J Card Fail 2013;19(11):746–52.
12. Ito K, Abe Y, Watanabe H, et al. Prognostic significance of residual functional mitral regurgitation in hospitalized heart failure patients with chronic atrial fibrillation and preserved ejection fraction after medical therapies. J Echocardiogr 2019;17(4): 197–205.
13. Saito C, Minami Y, Arai K, et al. Prevalence, clinical characteristics, and outcome of atrial functional mitral regurgitation in hospitalized heart failure patients with atrial fibrillation. J Cardiol 2018;72(4): 292–9.
14. Abe Y, Akamatsu K, Ito K, et al. Prevalence and prognostic significance of functional mitral and tricuspid regurgitation despite preserved left ventricular ejection fraction in atrial fibrillation patients. Circ J 2018;82(5):1451–8.
15. Sanderson JE. HFNEF, HFpEF, HF-PEF, or DHF: what is in an acronym? JACC Heart Fail 2014;2(1):93–4.
16. Kawaguchi M, Hay I, Fetics B, et al. Combined ventricular systolic and arterial stiffening in patients with heart failure and preserved ejection fraction: implications for systolic and diastolic reserve limitations. Circulation 2003;107(5):714–20.
17. Wang J, Fang F, Yip GW, et al. Importance of chronotropic response and left ventricular long-axis function for exercise performance in patients with heart failure and preserved ejection fraction. Int J Cardiol 2016;202:339–43.

18. Wang J, Fang F, Wai-Kwok Yip G, et al. Left ventricular long-axis performance during exercise is an important prognosticator in patients with heart failure and preserved ejection fraction. Int J Cardiol 2015; 178:131–5.

19. Marechaux S, Pincon C, Poueymidanette M, et al. Elevated left atrial pressure estimated by Doppler echocardiography is a key determinant of mitral valve tenting in functional mitral regurgitation. Heart 2010;96(4):289–97.

20. Ennezat PV, Marechaux S, Pibarot P, et al. Secondary mitral regurgitation in heart failure with reduced or preserved left ventricular ejection fraction. Cardiology 2013;125(2):110–7.

21. Tang Z, Fan YT, Wang Y, et al. Mitral annular and left ventricular dynamics in atrial functional mitral regurgitation: a three-dimensional and speckle-tracking echocardiographic study. J Am Soc Echocardiogr 2019;32(4):503–13.

22. Tamargo M, Obokata M, Reddy YNV, et al. Functional mitral regurgitation and left atrial myopathy in heart failure with preserved ejection fraction. Eur J Heart Fail 2020;22(3):489–98.

23. Lee AP, Jin CN, Fan Y, et al. Functional implication of mitral annular disjunction in mitral valve prolapse: a quantitative dynamic 3D echocardiographic study. JACC Cardiovasc Imaging 2017; 10(12):1424–33.

24. Gertz ZM, Raina A, Saghy L, et al. Evidence of atrial functional mitral regurgitation due to atrial fibrillation: reversal with arrhythmia control. J Am Coll Cardiol 2011;58(14):1474–81.

25. Fan Y, Wan S, Wong RH, et al. Atrial functional mitral regurgitation: mechanisms and surgical implications. Asian Cardiovasc Thorac Ann 2020;28(7): 421–6.

26. Abe Y, Takahashi Y, Shibata T. Functional mitral regurgitation, updated: ventricular or atrial? J Echocardiogr 2020;18(1):1–8.

27. Gumpangseth T, Mahakkanukrauh P, Das S. Gross age-related changes and diseases in human heart valves. Anat Cell Biol 2019;52(1):25–33.

28. Barasch E, Gottdiener JS, Larsen EK, et al. Clinical significance of calcification of the fibrous skeleton of the heart and aortosclerosis in community dwelling elderly. The Cardiovascular Health Study (CHS). Am Heart J 2006;151(1):39–47.

29. Kim DH, Heo R, Handschumacher MD, et al. Mitral valve adaptation to isolated annular dilation: insights into the mechanism of atrial functional mitral regurgitation. JACC Cardiovasc Imaging 2019;12(4): 665–77.

30. Neuhold S, Huelsmann M, Pernicka E, et al. Impact of tricuspid regurgitation on survival in patients with chronic heart failure: unexpected findings of a long-term observational study. Eur Heart J 2013;34(11): 844–52.

31. Ren QW, Li XL, Fang J, et al. The prevalence, predictors, and prognosis of tricuspid regurgitation in stage B and C heart failure with preserved ejection fraction. ESC Heart Fail 2020;7(6):4051–60.

32. Mascherbauer J, Kammerlander AA, Zotter-Tufaro C, et al. Presence of isolated tricuspid regurgitation should prompt the suspicion of heart failure with preserved ejection fraction. PLoS One 2017; 12(2):e0171542.

33. Sagie A, Schwammenthal E, Padial LR, et al. Determinants of functional tricuspid regurgitation in incomplete tricuspid valve closure: Doppler color flow study of 109 patients. J Am Coll Cardiol 1994; 24(2):446–53.

34. Spinner EM, Lerakis S, Higginson J, et al. Correlates of tricuspid regurgitation as determined by 3D echocardiography: pulmonary arterial pressure, ventricle geometry, annular dilatation, and papillary muscle displacement. Circ Cardiovasc Imaging 2012;5(1): 43–50.

35. Mutlak D, Aronson D, Lessick J, et al. Functional tricuspid regurgitation in patients with pulmonary hypertension: is pulmonary artery pressure the only determinant of regurgitation severity? Chest 2009; 135(1):115–21.

36. Yamasaki N, Kondo F, Kubo T, et al. Severe tricuspid regurgitation in the aged: atrial remodeling associated with long-standing atrial fibrillation. J Cardiol 2006;48(6):315–23.

37. Lee H-J, Lee H, Kim SM, et al. Diffuse myocardial fibrosis and diastolic function in aortic stenosis. JACC Cardiovasc Imaging 2020;13(12):2561–72.

38. Hachicha Z, Dumesnil JG, Bogaty P, et al. Paradoxical low-flow, low-gradient severe aortic stenosis despite preserved ejection fraction is associated with higher afterload and reduced survival. Circulation 2007;115(22):2856–64.

39. Chin CWL, Ding ZP, Lam CSP, et al. Paradoxical low-gradient aortic stenosis: the HFpEF of aortic stenosis. J Am Coll Cardiol 2016;67(20):2447–8.

40. Dayan V, Vignolo G, Magne J, et al. Outcome and impact of aortic valve replacement in patients with preserved LVEF and low-gradient aortic stenosis. J Am Coll Cardiol 2015;66(23):2594–603.

41. Clavel MA, Dumesnil JG, Capoulade R, et al. Outcome of patients with aortic stenosis, small valve area, and low-flow, low-gradient despite preserved left ventricular ejection fraction. J Am Coll Cardiol 2012;60(14):1259–67.

42. Mehrotra P, Jansen K, Flynn AW, et al. Differential left ventricular remodelling and longitudinal function distinguishes low flow from normal-flow preserved ejection fraction low-gradient severe aortic stenosis. Eur Heart J 2013;34(25):1906–14.

43. Barasch E, Fan D, Chukwu EO, et al. Severe isolated aortic stenosis with normal left ventricular systolic function and low transvalvular gradients:

pathophysiologic and prognostic insights. J Heart Valve Dis 2008;17(1):81–8.

44. Pai RG, Varadarajan P, Razzouk A. Survival benefit of aortic valve replacement in patients with severe aortic stenosis with low ejection fraction and low gradient with normal ejection fraction. Ann Thorac Surg 2008;86(6):1781–9.

45. Belkin RN, Khalique O, Aronow WS, et al. Outcomes and survival with aortic valve replacement compared with medical therapy in patients with low-, moderate-, and severe-gradient severe aortic stenosis and normal left ventricular ejection fraction. Echocardiography 2011;28(4):378–87.

46. Tarantini G, Covolo E, Razzolini R, et al. Valve replacement for severe aortic stenosis with low transvalvular gradient and left ventricular ejection fraction exceeding 0.50. Ann Thorac Surg 2011; 91(6):1808–15.

47. Lancellotti P, Magne J, Donal E, et al. Clinical outcome in asymptomatic severe aortic stenosis: insights from the new proposed aortic stenosis grading classification. J Am Coll Cardiol 2012; 59(3):235–43.

48. Mohty D, Magne J, Deltreuil M, et al. Outcome and impact of surgery in paradoxical low-flow, low-gradient severe aortic stenosis and preserved left ventricular ejection fraction: a cardiac catheterization study. Circulation 2013;128(11 Suppl 1): S235–42.

49. Eleid MF, Sorajja P, Michelena HI, et al. Flow-gradient patterns in severe aortic stenosis with preserved ejection fraction: clinical characteristics and predictors of survival. Circulation 2013;128(16): 1781–9.

50. Eleid MF, Sorajja P, Michelena HI, et al. Survival by stroke volume index in patients with low-gradient normal EF severe aortic stenosis. Heart 2015; 101(1):23–9.

51. Maes F, Boulif J, Pierard S, et al. Natural history of paradoxical low-gradient severe aortic stenosis. Circ Cardiovasc Imaging 2014;7(4):714–22.

52. Tribouilloy C, Rusinaru D, Marechaux S, et al. Low-gradient, low-flow severe aortic stenosis with preserved left ventricular ejection fraction: characteristics, outcome, and implications for surgery. J Am Coll Cardiol 2015;65(1):55–66.

53. Jander N, Minners J, Holme I, et al. Outcome of patients with low-gradient "severe" aortic stenosis and preserved ejection fraction. Circulation 2011; 123(8):887–95.

54. Bohbot Y, Pasquet A, Rusinaru D, et al. Asymptomatic severe aortic stenosis with preserved ejection fraction: early surgery versus conservative management. J Am Coll Cardiol 2018;72(23 Pt A):2938–9.

55. Wisenbaugh T, Spann JF, Carabello BA. Differences in myocardial performance and load between patients with similar amounts of chronic aortic versus chronic mitral regurgitation. J Am Coll Cardiol 1984;3(4):916–23.

56. Carabello BA. Aortic regurgitation. A lesion with similarities to both aortic stenosis and mitral regurgitation. Circulation 1990;82(3):1051–3.

57. Nishimura RA, Otto CM, Bonow RO, et al. 2014 AHA/ACC guideline for the management of patients with valvular heart disease: a report of the American College of Cardiology/American Heart Association Task Force on Practice Guidelines. J Am Coll Cardiol 2014;63(22):e57–185.

58. Nishimura RA, Otto CM, Bonow RO, et al. 2017 AHA/ACC focused update of the 2014 AHA/ACC guideline for the management of patients with valvular heart disease: a report of the American College of Cardiology/American Heart Association Task Force on Clinical Practice Guidelines. J Am Coll Cardiol 2017;70(2):252–89.

59. Baumgartner H, Falk V, Bax JJ, et al. 2017 ESC/EACTS guidelines for the management of valvular heart disease. Rev Esp Cardiol (Engl Ed) 2018; 71(2):110.

60. Bonow RO, Lakatos E, Maron BJ, et al. Serial long-term assessment of the natural history of asymptomatic patients with chronic aortic regurgitation and normal left ventricular systolic function. Circulation 1991;84(4):1625–35.

61. Klodas E, Enriquez-Sarano M, Tajik AJ, et al. Optimizing timing of surgical correction in patients with severe aortic regurgitation: role of symptoms. J Am Coll Cardiol 1997;30(3):746–52.

62. Dujardin KS, Enriquez-Sarano M, Schaff HV, et al. Mortality and morbidity of aortic regurgitation in clinical practice. A long-term follow-up study. Circulation 1999;99(14):1851–7.

63. Greves J, Rahimtoola SH, McAnulty JH, et al. Preoperative criteria predictive of late survival following valve replacement for severe aortic regurgitation. Am Heart J 1981;101(3):300–8.

64. Park HW, Song JM, Choo SJ, et al. Effect of preoperative ejection fraction, left ventricular systolic dimension and hemoglobin level on survival after aortic valve surgery in patients with severe chronic aortic regurgitation. Am J Cardiol 2012;109(12): 1782–6.

65. Mentias A, Feng K, Alashi A, et al. Long-term outcomes in patients with aortic regurgitation and preserved left ventricular ejection fraction. J Am Coll Cardiol 2016;68(20):2144–53.

66. Paraskevaidis IA, Kyrzopoulos S, Farmakis D, et al. Ventricular long-axis contraction as an earlier predictor of outcome in asymptomatic aortic regurgitation. Am J Cardiol 2007;100(11): 1677–82.

67. Vinereanu D, Ionescu AA, Fraser AG. Assessment of left ventricular long axis contraction can detect early myocardial dysfunction in asymptomatic patients

with severe aortic regurgitation. Heart 2001;85(1):30–6.

68. Paraskevaidis IA, Tsiapras D, Kyrzopoulos S, et al. The role of left ventricular long-axis contraction in patients with asymptomatic aortic regurgitation. J Am Soc Echocardiogr 2006;19(3):249–54.

69. Olsen NT, Sogaard P, Larsson HB, et al. Speckle-tracking echocardiography for predicting outcome in chronic aortic regurgitation during conservative management and after surgery. JACC Cardiovasc Imaging 2011;4(3):223–30.

70. Smedsrud MK, Pettersen E, Gjesdal O, et al. Detection of left ventricular dysfunction by global longitudinal systolic strain in patients with chronic aortic regurgitation. J Am Soc Echocardiogr 2011;24(11):1253–9.

71. Kusunose K, Agarwal S, Marwick TH, et al. Decision making in asymptomatic aortic regurgitation in the era of guidelines: incremental values of resting and exercise cardiac dysfunction. Circ Cardiovasc Imaging 2014;7(2):352–62.

72. Mizariene V, Grybauskiene R, Vaskelyte J, et al. Strain value in the assessment of left ventricular function and prediction of heart failure markers in aortic regurgitation. Echocardiography 2011;28(9):983–92.

73. Abdurashidova T, Monney P, Tzimas G, et al. Non-severe aortic regurgitation increases short-term mortality in acute heart failure with preserved ejection fraction. ESC Heart Fail 2020;7(6):3901–9.

74. Sengupta SP, Amaki M, Bansal M, et al. Effects of percutaneous balloon mitral valvuloplasty on left ventricular deformation in patients with isolated severe mitral stenosis: a speckle-tracking strain echocardiographic study. J Am Soc Echocardiogr 2014;27(6):639–47.

75. Bolen JL, Lopes MG, Harrison DC, et al. Analysis of left ventricular function in response to afterload changes in patients with mitral stenosis. Circulation 1975;52(5):894–900.

76. Sengupta PP, Pedrizzetti G, Kilner PJ, et al. Emerging trends in CV flow visualization. JACC Cardiovasc Imaging 2012;5(3):305–16.

77. Mangoni AA, Koelling TM, Meyer GS, et al. Outcome following mitral valve replacement in patients with mitral stenosis and moderately reduced left ventricular ejection fraction. Eur J Cardiothorac Surg 2002;22(1):90–4.

78. Enriquez-Sarano M, Akins CW, Vahanian A. Mitral regurgitation. Lancet 2009;373(9672):1382–94.

79. Feldman T, Foster E, Glower DD, et al. Percutaneous repair or surgery for mitral regurgitation. N Engl J Med 2011;364(15):1395–406.

Exercise Intolerance in Heart Failure with Preserved Ejection Fraction

Andrea Salzano, MD, PhD, MRCP(London)[a,*], Mariarosaria De Luca, MD[b],
Muhammad Zubair Israr, PhD[c], Giulia Crisci, MD[b],
Mohamed Eltayeb, MRCP(UK)[c], Radek Debiec, MRCP(UK)[c],
Brigida Ranieri, PhD[a], Roberta D'Assante, PhD[b], Salvatore Rega[b],
Anna D'Agostino, PhD[a], Ciro Mauro, MD[d], Iain B. Squire, MD, FRCP[c],
Toru Suzuki, MD, PhD, FRCP[c], Eduardo Bossone, MD, PhD, FCCP, FESC, FACC[d],
Marco Guazzi, MD, PhD[e], Alberto M. Marra, MD, PhD[b]

KEYWORDS

- Heart failure with preserved ejection fraction • Exercise tolerance • Exercise training
- Aerobic capacity • Cardiac function • Skeletal muscle function

KEY POINTS

- Exercise intolerance (EI) is defined as the impaired ability to perform physical activity in the presence of symptoms, such as dyspnea and/or fatigue. Associated with a poor quality of life, frequent hospitalizations, and increased all-cause mortality, EI represents a typical feature of HFpEF.
- Distinct systems contribute to EI in patients with HF, influencing their treatment and prognosis. Factors contributing to reduced exercise and functional capacity are classified into two main groups: cardiac and extracardiac.
- Numerous objective methods have been proposed to quantify the severity of EI (eg, 6-minute-walk test [6MWT], graded exercise testing with electrocardiography [ECG]); among them, cardiopulmonary exercise testing (CPET) is the best suited for detecting the main mechanism responsible for the exercise limitation.
- Exercise training programs have shown to improve exercise tolerance in HFpEF, with improvement in cardiopulmonary performance, as testified by the improvement of Vo$_2$ peak, ventilatory threshold, and 6MWT distance. Further studies are needed to identify the most appropriate type of ET.

INTRODUCTION

Heart failure (HF) with preserved ejection fraction (HFpEF) is defined as a complex clinical syndrome caused by structural and or functional impairment of ventricular filling or ejection, characterized by left ventricular ejection fraction greater than or equal to 50% and typical signs and symptoms.[1–4] It represents a growing epidemiologic issue representing about half of all patients with HF, predominantly in the elderly and patients with multiple comorbidities, such as hypertension, coronary

A. Salzano and M. De Luca equally contributed.

[a] IRCCS SDN Nuclear and Diagnostic Research Institute, Naples, Italy; [b] Department of Translational Medical Sciences, Federico II University, Naples, Italy; [c] Department of Cardiovascular Sciences, University of Leicester, NIHR Biomedical Research Centre, Glenfield Hospital, Leicester, UK; [d] AORN A Cardarelli, Cardiac Rehabilitation Unit, Naples, Italy; [e] Heart Failure Unit, Cardiopulmonary Laboratory, University Cardiology Department, IRCCS Policlinico San Donato University Hospital, Milan, Italy
* Corresponding author. IRCCS SDN Nuclear and Diagnostic Research Institute, Via E Gianturco 113, Naples 80143, Italy.
E-mail address: andrea.salzano@leicester.ac.uk

Heart Failure Clin 17 (2021) 397–413
https://doi.org/10.1016/j.hfc.2021.03.004
1551-7136/21/© 2021 Elsevier Inc. All rights reserved.

artery disease, kidney failure, and diabetes.[5] The clinical presentation of HFpEF is heterogeneous, ranging from nonspecific symptoms to severe cardiac manifestations, making early recognition and diagnosis a particular challenging.[1] Recently, the European Society of Cardiology suggested a new score for the diagnosis of HFpEF: the Heart Failure Association-Pre-Test Assessment, Echocardiography & Natriuretic Peptide, Functional Testing, and Final Etiology score, which is a stepwise approach that includes the detection of elevated levels of natriuretic peptides and echocardiographic diastolic dysfunction parameters.[4] HFpEF should be suspected in all patients with different degrees of exercise intolerance (EI), manifesting as dyspnea and fatigue, both of which are hallmark symptoms of the disease and are associated with worse health-related quality of life and increased morbidity and mortality.

Exercise tolerance describes the ability to endure exercise and to achieve the predicted age-related level or exercise duration.[6] EI is defined as the impaired ability to perform physical activity in the presence of symptoms, such as dyspnea and/or fatigue.[6] Associated with a poor quality of life, frequent hospitalizations, and increased all-cause mortality, EI represents a typical feature of HFpEF. The decline in exercise capacity results from several factors; together with the physiologic aging processes, multiple alterations that involve cardiac and extracardiac systems are observed, including reduced lung reserve and dysfunction of peripheral skeletal muscles.

Distinct systems contribute to EI in patients with HF, influencing their treatment and prognosis. Numerous objective methods have been proposed to quantify the severity of EI (eg, 6-minute-walk test [6MWT], graded exercise testing with electrocardiography [ECG]); among them, cardiopulmonary exercise testing (CPET) is the best suited for detecting the main mechanism responsible for the exercise limitation.

This review discusses the pathophysiology of exercise limitation in HFpEF, describes methods of determining exercise tolerance class, and evaluates prognostic implications and potential therapeutic strategies.

EXERCISE INTOLERANCE IN HEART FAILURE WITH PRESERVED EJECTION FRACTION
Pathophysiology of Exercise Intolerance in Heart Failure with Preserved Ejection Fraction

EI is a key feature of HFpEF. It is determined by several multiorgan system disorders. Factors contributing to reduced exercise and functional capacity are classified into two main groups:

cardiac and extracardiac. Extracardiac are mainly related to pulmonary and muscle impairment or comorbidities (**Fig. 1**).

The main cardiac contributors to EI are chronotropic incompetence, reduction in left heart reserve capacity, elevated filling pressures, and the right ventricle pulmonary vascular dysfunction.[7] Chronotropic incompetence, defined as the inability to increase heart rate (HR) proportionally to the degree of metabolic demands, is commonly observed in patients with HFpEF and constrains cardiac output augmentation during physical exertion. Furthermore, left ventricular stiffness, a consequence of extensive fibrosis, titin hypophosphorylation, and myocyte rigidity, prevents left ventricular diastolic volume increase and venous return, impairing Frank-Starling mechanism.[8] During exercise, pulmonary wedge pressure progressively increases, but this phenomenon is not accompanied by an increase in end-diastolic volume. Consequently, diastolic pressures rise, and unsustainable sensation of dyspnea appears in the absence of overt systolic dysfunction.[9] Decreased cardiac output results in skeletal muscle hypoperfusion, the activation of anaerobic metabolism, and the synthesis of muscle lactates and other metabolites, with consequent peripheral and central fatigue.[9]

Chief among cardiovascular contributors to exercise tolerance (and consequently dyspnea) is the capability of the right ventricle to adapt to the increased workload imposed by exercise,[6] a mechanism also known as "exercise right ventricle to pulmonary circulation uncoupling." Indeed, right ventricle dysfunction is likely to become manifest during the effort, although it might appear as preserved at rest.[10] Hallmarks of right ventricle dysfunction differ between HF with reduced ejection fraction (HFrEF) and HFpEF, the latter being characterized by the early occurrence of diastolic dysfunction and reduced ventricular compliance before dilatation and systolic dysfunction occur.[11] Furthermore, according to a recently published study performed by Bandera and coworkers,[12] functional mitral regurgitation during exercise is particularly common in HFpEF and associated with ventilatory inefficiency, right ventricle to pulmonary circulation uncoupling, increased chronotropic response, and peripheral O_2 extraction.

With regard to extracardiac contributors, the reduced pulmonary reserve is frequently observed in patients with HFpEF.[9] Multiple pulmonary comorbidities often coexist, such as chronic obstructive pulmonary disease, reported in about 20% of patients with HF when self-reported or up to 50% when function tests were used to evaluate airflow obstruction,[13–15] and sleep-disordered

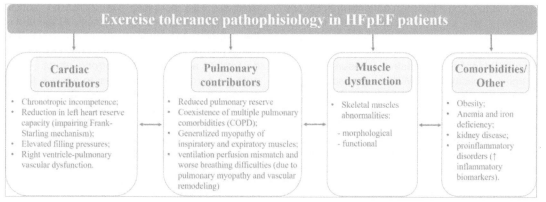

Fig. 1. Pathophysiology of patients with HFpEF. COPD, chronic obstructive pulmonary disease.

breathing.[16] Moreover, a generalized myopathy of inspiratory and expiratory muscles has been described and related to aging, systemic inflammation, and oxidative stress.[17,18] Pulmonary arterial hypertension–related myopathy[19] and vascular remodeling can result in ventilation-perfusion mismatch and exacerbate breathing difficulties. Finally, pulmonary hypertension often complicates HF, dramatically impacting exercise capacity, quality of life, and prognosis, resulting in atrial function impairment, inflammation, and vasoconstriction.[20–22] EI is exacerbated by structural and functional abnormalities of skeletal muscles.[23,24] The main causes are a shift in muscle fiber distribution, with fewer type I fibers and a reduced capillary-to-fiber ratio.[25–27] In addition, defects in oxygen pathways (oxygen-carrying blood capacity, distribution, and extraction by peripheral tissue) are involved. Finally, increased inflammatory response,[28] impaired anabolic signaling,[29–32] hypoxemia, and abnormalities of mitochondrial function[23,24] are involved in the pathophysiology of this process.

Exercise tolerance is often worsened by several comorbid conditions frequently associated with HFpEF, such as obesity,[33] metabolic syndrome,[34] anemia,[35] kidney disease,[36] and proinflammatory disorders that increase plasma levels of inflammatory biomarkers.[28] Obese patients typically present with simultaneous high left- and right-sided filling pressures, elevated circulating plasma volume, metabolically active fatty tissue deposits that promote inflammation, hypertension, insulin resistance, and dyslipidemia, leading to a reduction in functional capacity.[33,37,38] The high prevalence of anemia and iron deficiency reduces oxygen refueling capacity. Furthermore, iron is an essential coenzyme in mitochondrial respiration, and its deficiency negatively regulates cell metabolism.[35] Kidney diseases contribute to myopathy and skeletal muscle mass wasting

through the defective protein metabolism, promoting the development of chronic proinflammatory states, anemia, increased plasma volume, and vascular dysfunction.[6,36]

In summary, a single mechanism underlying EI in patients with HFpEF cannot be identified, because of the complexity of the syndrome. Several studies have attempted to clarify the determinants of EI in HFpEF to obtain new therapeutic strategies that improve exercise and functional capacity, quality of life, and prognosis. However, EI pathophysiology in HFpEF is still poorly understood. Some authors have speculated that different phenotypes are included in the HFpEF category.[27,39] Identifying a specific phenotype with peculiar clinical presentation and the preponderant pathophysiologic mechanism would make it possible to target the main conditions responsible for physical effort intolerance and identify novel therapeutic targets. With this regard, Houstis and colleagues,[40] investigating the mechanism of EI in 134 patients with HFpEF, demonstrated that most patients held defects at multiple steps of the oxygen pathway, with an important entity of disease heterogeneity. As a result, this finding suggests that to identify the specific altered step (often related to comorbidities) would lead to a more tailored and successful treatment; notably, exercise training (ET) is able to correct multiple of these defects at once.[40]

Evaluation of Exercise Intolerance in Heart Failure with Preserved Ejection Fraction

Current modalities to assess EI in patients affected with HFpEF are classified into three categories: (1) subjective assessment tools, (2) noninvasive objective methods, and (3) invasive procedures.

The first group includes methods that depend on the subjective impression of the degree of functional compromise. New York Heart Association classification is the most commonly applied tool to assess functional status in patients with HF and provides an initial evaluation of exercise limitation.[6]

The second includes noninvasive methods that express objective quantitative measurements of exercise capacity: the 6MWT,[41] graded exercise testing with ECG, and CPET.[6] CPET, the gold standard technique to assess exercise capacity, is usually performed using a cycle ergometer or a treadmill protocol and involves the integrative measurements of pulmonary, cardiovascular, hematopoietic, neurologic, and skeletal muscle systems parameters at rest, during exercise, and during recovery.[42] CPET analyzes gas exchange measuring breath-by-breath oxygen uptake (VO_2), carbon dioxide output (VCO_2), and ventilation (VE), in addition to conventional exercise testing parameters (blood pressure, ECG findings, HR, and symptoms). The sum of these measurements provides a comprehensive assessment of exercise tolerance and response and recognizes the predominant mechanism of exercise limitation. Considering its importance, CPET is discussed next.

The third group is formed of invasive methods: CPET is integrated with cardiac imaging or invasive hemodynamics, but these additional techniques are available and applied only in highly specialized tertiary referral centers.[43]

Clinical Relevance of Cardiopulmonary Exercise Testing in Heart Failure with Preserved Ejection Fraction

EI is assessed by CPET through the gas exchange analysis during exercise[44]; in particular, EI is identified and quantified by a reduction in the maximal oxygen consumption (VO_2) peak (VO_2 peak).[45] VO_2 peak is a function of peak cardiac output (Q peak) and arteriovenous oxygen difference (A-V O_2) peak, conforming to the Fick principle (VO_2 peak = Q peak × A-V O_2 peak).[45] Therefore, measuring age, sex, and weight-corrected peak VO_2 is the gold standard to assess EI in patients with HF.[46,47] Alterations in these parameters are directly related to the pathophysiology of HFpEF. Indeed, oxygen delivery disorders (ie, O_2 or CO_2 arterial content, peripheral vascular function) and consumption (ie, diffusion and extraction) can modify peak oxygen consumption. During physical activity, the skeletal muscle pump promotes venous return, the intra-abdominal pressure increases, and the chest wall expands. Venous return increases cardiac output without an untoward elevation in cardiac filling pressures. This effect is achieved through chronotropic, inotropic, and lusitropic mechanisms.[6] During

exercise, HR increases via increased activity of the sympathetic nervous system. At the end of the exercise, the sympathetic effect diminishes, the action of parasympathetic tone prevails and determines a negative chronotropic effect.[6] Chronotropic competence is crucial to achieve the increase in cardiac output and the ability to perform sustained aerobic exercise.

Parameters derived from CPET should be integrated and combined into clinical practice with demographics, medical history, laboratory data, and ongoing treatments to provide valuable information about a diagnosis, prognosis, and therapeutic response in patients with HFpEF.

Peak VO_2 evaluation has a potential diagnostic role in identifying patients with dyspnea of predominantly cardiac versus noncardiac cause. However, no guidelines recommend using peak VO_2 in the assessment of possible HFpEF; indeed, until now, guideline recommendations are focused on HFrEF, without clear recommendations on HFpEF. However, Reddy and colleagues demonstrated that very low peak VO_2 values (<14 mL/kg/min) discriminated HFpEF patients from patients with noncardiac dyspnea with high specificity (91%) but poor sensitivity (50%).[48] Conversely, preserved peak VO_2 (>20 mL/kg/min) excluded HFpEF with high sensitivity (90%) and low specificity (49%). Intermediate peak VO_2 cutoff points need additional invasive tests.[48]

When a diagnosis of HFpEF has already been established, CPET measurements (eg, the VE/VCO_2 slope and peak VO_2) could be used to assess the evolution of exercise tolerance in response to therapeutic lifestyle, pharmacologic, and surgical interventions.[49,50]

Several studies investigated the prognostic role of CPET variables in patients with HFpEF. In the Henry Ford HospITal CardioPulmonary EXercise Testing (FIT-CPX) project, a retrospective cohort of 173 patients with HFpEF, peak VO_2 and percent predicted maximum oxygen uptake (ppMVO$_2$) showed a significant association with the composite outcome of all-cause mortality or cardiac transplant after adjusting for confounders.[51] In contrast, Guazzi and colleagues[44,52] described a strong correlation between VE/VCO_2 slope, but not peak VO_2, hospitalization, cardiovascular events, and all-cause mortality even if multivariable adjustment clinical risk factors was not performed. Finally, Nadruz and colleagues[53] showed that peak VO_2 and VE/VCO_2 slope provided incremental prognostic value for the composite of all-cause death, left ventricular assist device implantation, or heart transplant, and for incident HF hospitalization in a large cohort of patients with HF regardless of ejection fraction;

notably, in this study CPET variables provided greater risk discrimination in patients with HFpEF than with HFrEF. Based on these data, the Heart Failure Association of the European Society of Cardiology recommended a flowchart for the interpretation of CPET results and confirmed the important prognostic power of percent predicted peak V_{O_2}, calculated using the Wasserman equation[54]: a peak V_{O_2} cutoff of 50% has been established to allow risk stratification for poor outcome in patients with HFpEF.[55]

In summary, CPET parameters are impaired in HFpEF; this group of patients shows abnormal ventilatory and hemodynamic responses to exercise.[6] The main alteration is the depression of peak V_{O_2}, as described in several studies.[45,56] Peak V_{O_2} reduction correlates with the severity of impairment in peak cardiac output and stroke volume, reduced peak HR, and A-V O_2.[55] When compared with HFrEF, patients with HFpEF displayed milder or similar impairment in peak V_{O_2} and VE/VCO_2 slope.[55]

EFFECTS OF EXERCISE TRAINING IN HEART FAILURE WITH PRESERVED EJECTION FRACTION

In contrast to well-established treatment pathways for HFrEF, there is no evidence-based treatment of patients with HFpEF.[1] A few pharmacologic interventions have shown to be a benefit on exercise tolerance in patients with HFpEF (**Table 1**). Indeed, in the Perindopril in Elderly People With Chronic HF (PEP-CHF) study, perindopril, despite showing no effects on hard outcomes (ie, composite of all-cause mortality or unplanned HF-related hospitalization using a time-to-first-event analysis) but HF hospitalization, significantly improved symptoms (expressed as an improvement of New York Heart Association functional class) and exercise capacity (ie, a mean of 14 m in difference in change in 6MWT) compared with placebo.[57] In a randomized controlled trial (RCT) including 150 patients with HFpEF, after a 6 months therapy with spironolactone, the active group showed an increment in peak V_{O_2} (2.9 mL/min/kg) and improvement in anaerobic threshold (2.0 mL/min/kg) and O_2 uptake efficiency (0.19), with a reduction in exercise-induced increase in E/e' (−3.0) when compared with placebo (respectively, 0.3 mL/min/kg, −0.9 mL/min/kg, −0.07, and 0.5).[58] However, other RCTs (eg, the Aldo-DHF, the CHARM-preserved, the I-Preserve, the TOPCAT, and the PARAGON-HF) investigating several molecules (eg, β-blockers, irbesartan, candesartan, sacubitril/valsartan) showed inconsistent results.[59] However, in February 2021, the US Food and Drug

Administration has expanded the indication for sacubitril/valsartan "to reduce the risk of cardiovascular death and hospitalization for heart failure in adult patients with chronic heart failure," whereas in the previous version it was for "or heart failure in patients with chronic heart failure and reduced ejection fraction."

The lack of evidence regarding pharmacologic interventions in HFpEF perhaps emphasizes the potential role of ET in the management of HFpEF. Several studies demonstrated that ET improves cardiorespiratory fitness and reduced mortality risk in HFrEF and HFpEF.[17,60] A recent systematic review identified nine studies on 348 patients with HFpEF who performed ET two to three sessions weekly.[61] Overall, ET produces positive effects on exercise tolerance in terms of peak oxygen uptake, 6MWT distance, and ventilatory threshold[61–64]; furthermore, positive effects on quality of life have been demonstrated.[65,66] With regard to the possible mechanisms underpinning the utility of ET in HFpEF, Edelmann and colleagues reported ET to be associated with improved V_{O_2} peak after 3 months of ET, associated with positive effects on cardiac structure and diastolic function (decrease in left atrial volume index and E/e' ratio)[67,68]; Fu and colleagues[69] reported similar findings, whereas Murad and colleagues[70] reported improvement in HR variability.

However, other investigators did not find any improvement in cardiovascular stiffness or function in patients who performed ET, as assessed by echocardiography, flow-mediated dilation, or right heart catheterization.[71–73] Additionally, 6 weeks of ET improved peak V_{O_2} without demonstrable effects on endothelial function or arterial stiffness in a randomized controlled trial conducted in elderly patients with HFpEF.[74] Based on this evidence, some authors suggested that the improvement in V_{O_2} peak observed with structured ET program in HFpEF is primarily the result of peripheral adaptation mechanisms and the consequent increase in oxygen extraction by skeletal muscle.[74,75] After 4 months of ET, a higher peak V_{O_2} was associated with higher estimated peak A-V O_2 and peak HR, but not with peak end-diastolic volume, stroke volume, or cardiac output. Exercise-induced improvement in V_{O_2} peak was primarily driven by increased estimated peak exercise A-V O_2 in a population of HFpEF who performed aerobic interval training.[69] However, the molecular mechanisms remain unclear, and more studies are needed to fully understand the underlying physiopathology.

Concerning the type of exercise, several studies compared moderate continuous training (MCT) with high-intensity interval training (HIIT), with

Table 1
Comparison between main characteristics of HFpEF and HFrEF subjects

Characteristics	HFpEF	HFrEF
LVEF	Normal LVEF ($\geq$50%)	Reduced LVEF (<40%)
Age	Older	Younger
Gender	Females > males	Males > females
Dysfunction	LV diastolic dysfunction	LV systolic dysfunction
Cardiac hypertrophy	Concentric	Eccentric
Risk factors/comorbidities	Obesity, hypertension, diabetes, kidney disease	
	COPD, age, anemia, inflammation, liver disease, sleep apnea, gout, cancer	Volume overload, myocarditis, myocardial infarction
Pulmonary capillary wedge pressures	Normal or less impaired	Increased (at rest and under stress)
Compensative cardiac mechanisms	Unable to use the Frank-Starling mechanism to increase stroke volume during exercise, despite normal contractile function and markedly increased LV filling pressure	LV stroke volume is reduced in HFrEF because of the systolic contractile dysfunction per se, even if LV filling pressure increases the use of the Frank-Starling mechanism
Preponderant determinant mechanisms	Greater role of the peripheral impairments	Greater role of the central impairments
C(A-V) O_2	The primary cause of impaired exercise capacity in 40% of patients with HFpEF Lower in HFpEF	Cause of impaired exercise capacity in only 2% of patients with HFrEF
Regular ET	Safe and improve Vo_2 peak	Safe and improve Vo_2 peak
Endothelial dysfunction	Early stage symptom $\downarrow\downarrow$ NO bioavailability	Late-stage symptom < $\downarrow$ NO bioavailability
Therapies	Reversal of LV dilation = no effective	Reversal of LV dilation = improve outcome
Cardiomyocyte cell death	Absent	Present

Abbreviations: COPD, chronic obstructive pulmonary disease; LV, left ventricle LVEF, left ventricle ejection fraction; VO_2, oxygen uptake.

inconsistent results. In a small pilot study involving 15 patients, Angadi and colleagues[76] suggested that HIIT may provide a more robust stimulus than moderate-intensity aerobic continuous training; in a more recent RCT enrolling 38 patients with HFpEF, Donelli da Silveira and colleagues demonstrated that MCT and HIIT are equally effective in improving ventilatory efficiency and other CPET parameters, quality of life score, and diastolic function after 3 months of training, with the latter showing superiority in improving peak Vo_2.[77,78] However, a more recent RCT, in which 180 chronic stable patients with HFpEF have been randomly assigned to HIIT, MCT, or guideline-based physical activity advice, showed no statistically significant difference in change in

peak VO_2 between those assigned to HIIT versus MCT, with a better patient-reported quality of life in the latter group.[79] As a result, it has been suggested that MCT may be the preferred ET approach in older patients with HFpEF.[80]

Table 2 summarized the key studies investigating the role of ET in HFpEF.

EXERCISE TOLERANCE DIFFERENCES BETWEEN HEART FAILURE WITH PRESERVED EJECTION FRACTION AND HEART FAILURE WITH REDUCED EJECTION FRACTION

The different pathophysiologic mechanisms responsible for the decreased peak Vo_2 in clinically stable patients with HFrEF and HFpEF are

Table 2
Key studies investigating the role of exercise training in heart failure with preserved ejection fraction

First Author, Year of Publication (Ref.)	Study Design; Duration; Type of Exercise	Patients; Age; Women (%)	Principal Outcomes Investigated	Major Findings
Kitzman et al,[72] 2010	Randomized, prospective, attention-controlled, single-blind study 16 wk 1 h ET (warm-up, stimulus, and cool-down phases), 3 times/wk	n = 26 ET 70 ± 6 y 83% n = 27 UC 69 ± 5 y 91%	CPET functional parameters Echocardiographic parameters 6MWT distance Natriuretic peptides QoL scores	Peak VO₂, power output, and exercise time were significantly increased in the ET Peak respiratory exchange ratio was not different between the groups Peak heart rate, heart rate reserve, and oxygen pulse were increased in ET No significant differences were observed in any resting Doppler echocardiography measures 6MWT distance was significantly increased in ET No significant differences in BNP ET group had a significantly lower (improved) physical score
Edelmann et al,[67] 2011	Prospective, randomized 2:1 controlled trial 12 wk Endurance/resistance training	n = 44 64 ± 8 y 55% n = 20 UC 65 ± 6 y 60%	CPET functional parameters Echocardiographic parameters 6MWT distance QoL scores	Peak VO₂ increased with ET and remained unchanged with UC E/e' and left atrial volume index decreased with ET and remained unchanged with UC Increase in the 6MWT distance in the training group by 24 m The physical functioning score improved with ET and remained unchanged with UC

(continued on next page)

Table 2
(continued)

First Author, Year of Publication (Ref.)	Study Design; Duration; Type of Exercise	Patients; Age; Women (%)	Principal Outcomes Investigated	Major Findings
Smart et al,[62] 2012	Randomized, controlled trial 16 wk Cycle ergometer exercise training at 60 rpm	n = 12 ET 67 ± 5.8 y 42% n = 13 UC 61.9 ± 6.9 y 53%	CPET functional parameters Echocardiographic parameters QoL scores QoL	Peak VO_2 in ET increased and was unchanged in UC, although this was not significant between groups VE/VCO_2 slope was reduced in ET but was unchanged in UC No significant changes in diastolic or systolic function were noted in either group QoL and depression scores were unchanged with ET
Murad et al,[70] 2012	Randomized, controlled, single-blinded design 16 wk 1 h ET (warm-up, stimulus, and cool-down phases), 3 times/wk	n = 35 ET 70.1 ± 5.6 63% n = 31 UC 68.0 ± 4.8 64.5%	SDNN RMSSD	ET group had a significantly greater increase in SDNN ET group had a significantly greater increase in RMSSD
Alves et al,[68] 2012	Randomized controlled trial 24 wk Interval training	n = 20 ET; n = 11 UC 63 ± 11 29%	Echocardiographic parameters Exercise tolerance (MET)	LVEF increased after ET Diastolic function improved after ET LV dimensions were not altered by ET ET improved exercise tolerance (MET)

(continued on next page)

Table 2
(continued)

First Author, Year of Publication (Ref.)	Study Design; Duration; Type of Exercise	Patients; Age; Women (%)	Principal Outcomes Investigated	Major Findings
Kitzman et al,[74] 2013	Randomized, controlled, single-blind trial 16 wk Walking, arm, and leg ergometry	n = 32 ET 70 ± 7 y 72% n = 31 UC 70 ± 7 y 80%	Peak VO_2 Echocardiographic parameters Brachial artery FMD Carotid artery distensibility QoL scores	ET significantly improves VO_2 peak without altering brachial FMD or carotid arterial stiffness No significant differences for resting LV volumes, ejection fraction, Doppler LV filling, or pulse pressure/ stroke volume ratio ET did not alter brachial FMD ET did not alter carotid arterial stiffness The emotional and physical Short Form-36 scores were higher in ET than UC, but the MLWHFQ scores were not significantly different
Angadi et al,[76] 2015	Randomized comparison trial/pilot study 4 wk HIIT vs MI-ACT	n = 9 HIIT 69.0 ± 6.1 y 11% n = 6: MCT 71.5 ± 11.7 y 33%	CPET functional parameters Diastolic function FMD	VO_2 peak increased after HIIT but was unchanged after MCT Ventilation threshold, VE/ VCO_2 slope, peak HR, respiratory exchange ratio, VE/ VCO_2, and rate-pressure product were not changed in either group Diastolic dysfunction grade was reduced after HIIT No significant echocardiographic changes were observed after MCT Brachial artery FMD did not change in either group

(continued on next page)

Table 2
(continued)

First Author, Year of Publication (Ref.)	Study Design; Duration; Type of Exercise	Patients; Age; Women (%)	Principal Outcomes Investigated	Major Findings
Nolte et al,[65] 2015	Prospective, randomized, controlled trial 12 wk Endurance/resistance training	n = 44 supervised endurance/resistance training; n = 20 UC 65 ± 7 y 56%	QoL scores	The MLWHFQ total scale and the MLWHFQ physical limitation scale improved with ET
Kitzman et al,[73] 2016	Randomized, attention-controlled, 2 × 2 factorial trail 20 wk Walking exercise 3 times/wk	n = 26 ET n = 24 diet group n = 25 ET + diet group n = 25 UC 67 ± 5 y 81%	Peak VO_2 QoL scores	Peak VO_2 was increased significantly by exercise and diet The combination of exercise + diet was additive for peak VO_2 The change in peak VO_2 was positively correlated with the change in percent lean body mass and the change in thigh muscle No statistically significant change in MLHF total score with exercise and with diet
Fu et al,[69] 2016	Randomized, controlled trial 12 wk Aerobic interval training	n = 30 ET 60.5 ± 2.7 33% n = 30 UC 63.1 ± 2.6 40%	CPET functional parameters Echocardiographic diastolic function QoL scores	ET heightened VO_2 peak in HFpEF and HFrEF groups and lowered the VE/VCO_2 slope ET improved diastolic function with reduction of the E/E' ratio ET improved the Short Form-36 physical/mental component scores and decreased the MLWHFQ score

(continued on next page)

Table 2
(continued)

First Author, Year of Publication (Ref.)	Study Design; Duration; Type of Exercise	Patients; Age; Women (%)	Principal Outcomes Investigated	Major Findings
Maldonado-Martin et al,[63] 2017	Prospective, randomized, single-blinded trial 16 wk Cycling and walking at 50% to 70% of VO_2 peak intensity	n = 23 ET; n = 24 UC $\geq$ 65 y 87%	VO_2 peak, VT 6MWT distance	VO_2 peak and VT values increased in the ET group but decreased in the UC group 6MWT distance was higher than at the baseline in both the groups The change in 6MWT distance and VT was not significantly correlated in both groups The change in VO_2 peak vs 6MWT distance after training was not significantly correlated in both groups
Lang et al,[66] 2018	Randomized controlled trial 12 wk Home-based comprehensive self-management rehabilitation program	n = 25 ET 71.8 $\pm$ 9.9 y 64% n = 25 UC 76 $\pm$ 6.6 y 44%	QoL scores	Improvement in MLWHFQ total score
Palau et al,[64] 2019	Investigator-initiated, open-label, randomized controlled study 12 wk IMT vs FES vs IMT + FES vs UC	n = 15 IMT 75 $\pm$ 10 y 53% n = 15 FES 72 $\pm$ 9 y 60% n = 15 IMT + FES 73 $\pm$ 10 y 50% n = 16 UC 75 $\pm$ 9 y 69%	CPET functional parameter Echocardiographic data Natriuretic peptides QoL scores	IMT, FES, or IMT + FES intervention was associated with significant improvement in exercise capacity Decrease in the D-E/E0 ratio in all intervention groups; D-left atrial volume index showed no significant differences for any of the active treatment groups compared with UC No significant differences for NT-proBNP Significant increases in QoL scores

(continued on next page)

Table 2
(continued)

First Author, Year of Publication (Ref.)	Study Design; Duration; Type of Exercise	Patients; Age; Women (%)	Principal Outcomes Investigated	Major Findings
Donelli da Silveira et al,[77] 2020	Single-blinded, parallel randomized clinical trial 3 d per wk 12 wk HIIT vs MCT	n = 10 HIIT 60 ± 10 y 70% n = 9 MCT 60 ± 9 y 56%	CPET functional parameter Echocardiographic data Natriuretic peptides QoL scores	Peak VO_2 was higher in HIIT compared with MCT Peak RER was not different between groups Anaerobic threshold increased similarly in both groups Respiratory compensation point had a greater improvement with HIIT Echocardiographic resting diameters, ejection fraction, indexed volumes, and LV mass were not significantly different pre-exercise and postexercise training and between groups NT-proBNP decreased over time in both groups QoL improved after training in both groups
Mueller et al,[79] 2021	Randomized controlled trial 3 mo supervised followed by 9 mo of telemedical monitored home-based training HIIT vs MCT vs UC	n = 58 HIIT 70 ± 7 y 71% n = 58 MCT 70 ± 8 y 60% n = 60 UC 69 ± 10 y 68%	CPET functional parameters Diastolic function Natriuretic peptides QoL	No differences in peak VO_2 between patients assigned to HIIT vs MCT No significant changes in diastolic function No significant differences in natriuretic peptides Better in MCT after 12 mo

Abbreviations: BNP, B-type natriuretic peptide; FES, functional electrical stimulation group; FMD, flow-mediated dilation; IMT, inspiratory muscle training; LV, left ventricle; LVEF, left ventricular ejection fraction; MET, metabolic equivalent task; MI-ACT, moderate-intensity aerobic continuous training; MLWHFQ, Minnesota living with heart failure questionnaire; NT-proBNP, N-terminal pro–B-type natriuretic peptide; QoL, quality of life; RER, respiratory exchange ratio; RMSSD, root mean square of successive differences in normal RR intervals; SDNN, standard deviation of all normal RR intervals; UC, usual care; VO_2, oxygen uptake; VT, ventilatory threshold.

multifactorial.[1,6,52] In addition, exercise-related cardiac compensatory mechanisms are different in the two groups. Compared with HFpEF, patients with HFrEF also have higher mean pulmonary capillary wedge pressures at rest and under stress.[81] In HFrEF, as a manifestation of systolic dysfunction per se, left ventricular stroke volume is reduced, even as left ventricular filling pressure increases via the Frank-Starling mechanism. In contrast, despite normal contractile function and markedly increased left ventricle filling pressure, patients with HFpEF are unable to use the Frank-Starling mechanism to increase stroke volume during exercise.[81]

Although the mechanisms involved are similar (**Table 2**), the contribution to EI of central and peripheral determinants seems to be different in the two main phenotypes of HF, with a greater role of the peripheral impairments in HFpEF when compared with patients with HFrEF. Dhakal and colleagues[82] measured peripheral O_2 extraction directly throughout exercise in HFpEF, HFrEF, and healthy control subjects, using invasive CPET. They found that the peak exercise arterio-mixed venous O_2 content difference (C[a-v] O_2) was lower in HFpEF compared with HFrEF (11.5 mL/dL vs 13.5 mL/dL), representing the primary cause of impaired exercise capacity in 40% of patients with HFpEF and in only 2% of patients with HFrEF.[82] Similarly, regular ET is safe and effective in improving Vo_2 peak in HFpEF and HFrEF. In the latter group, results from a meta-analysis including 13 studies showed that ET (particularly high insensitivity interval training) ameliorated cardiac, vascular, and skeletal muscle function with an effect on attenuation of left ventricular remodeling.[50]

CLINICAL IMPLICATIONS AND FUTURE PERSPECTIVES

Exercise tolerance is often severely reduced in patients with HFpEF, the degree of limitation correlating with the degree of reduction in quality of life and prognosis.[49] As a result of the pathophysiologic mechanisms determining EI in HFpEF, a reduction is observed in the reserve capacity required to deliver and consume O_2 in exercising muscle.[25] Exercise limitation, which is an early symptom and a therapeutic end point, should be evaluated by physicians at every disease stage. Understanding the causes of exercise limitations and targeting physiologic abnormalities could be useful in establishing a tailored therapy based on the dominant HFpEF syndrome phenotype. Even if there is not certain evidence of mechanisms responsible for exercise-mediated improvements

in Vo_2 peak in patients with HFpEF, ET programs have shown to improve exercise tolerance in HFpEF, with improvement in cardiopulmonary performance, as testified by the improvement of Vo_2 peak, ventilatory threshold, and 6MWT distance.[17,61] Finally, further studies are needed to identify the most appropriate type of ET.

SUMMARY

HFpEF represents a major and growing health care issue for which there are no evidence-based pharmacologic or mechanical interventions. EI is the central key feature of HFpEF, limiting patients' quality of life and predicting poor outcome. It is appropriate that research should focus on the identification of the causes of EI in what is a complex condition with multiple potential etiologies and for which there may be numerous contributors in an individual patient. The underlying pathophysiologic mechanism remains not fully understood because of the complex interplay of several determinants. CPET is nowadays considered the gold standard to assess the grade of EI impairment and to guide therapeutic interventions directly related to prognostic implications. Thus, a multidisciplinary clinical approach should consider not only the direct HF-related conditions but also the optimal management of comorbidities, involving different members of the health care team (eg, physicians, dieticians, trainers, psychologists, nurses, pharmacists) and individualized patient management.

DISCLOSURE

Dr A.M. Marra was supported by an institutional grant from Italian Healthcare Ministry (Ricerca Finalizzata for young researchers) project GR-2016-02364727.

CLINICS CARE POINTS

- Exercise intolerance (EI) is defined as the impaired ability to perform physical activity in the presence of symptoms, such as dyspnea and/or fatigue. Associated with a poor quality of life, frequent hospitalizations, and increased all-cause mortality, EI represents a typical feature of HFpEF.

- Distinct systems contribute to EI in patients with HF, influencing their treatment and prognosis. Factors contributing to reduced exercise and functional capacity can be classified into two main groups: cardiac and extracardiac.

- Numerous objective methods have been proposed to quantify the severity of EI (eg, 6-minute walk test [6MWT], graded exercise testing with electrocardiography [ECG]); among them, cardiopulmonary exercise testing (CPET) is the best suited for detecting the main mechanism responsible for the exercise limitation.

- Exercise training programs have shown to improve exercise tolerance in HFpEF, with improvement in cardiopulmonary performance, as testified by the improvement of Vo_2 peak, ventilatory threshold, and 6MWT distance. Further studies are needed to identify the most appropriate type of ET.

REFERENCES

1. Ponikowski P, Voors AA, Anker SD, et al. 2016 ESC Guidelines for the diagnosis and treatment of acute and chronic heart failure: the task force for the diagnosis and treatment of acute and chronic heart failure of the European Society of Cardiology (ESC). Developed with the special contribution of the Heart Failure Association (HFA) of the ESC. Eur J Heart Fail 2016;18(8):891–975.

2. Yancy CW, Jessup M, Bozkurt B, et al. 2017 ACC/AHA/HFSA Focused Update of the 2013 ACCF/AHA Guideline for the Management of Heart Failure: a Report of the American College of Cardiology/American Heart Association Task Force on Clinical Practice Guidelines and the Heart Failure Society of America. J Am Coll Cardiol 2017;70(6):776–803.

3. Yancy CW, Jessup M, Bozkurt B, et al. 2013 ACCF/AHA guideline for the management of heart failure: a report of the American College of Cardiology Foundation/American Heart Association Task Force on Practice Guidelines. J Am Coll Cardiol 2013; 62(16):e147–239.

4. Pieske B, Tschöpe C, de Boer RA, et al. How to diagnose heart failure with preserved ejection fraction: the HFA-PEFF diagnostic algorithm: a consensus recommendation from the Heart Failure Association (HFA) of the European Society of Cardiology (ESC). Eur Heart J 2019;40(40):3297–317.

5. Oktay AA, Rich JD, Shah SJ. The emerging epidemic of heart failure with preserved ejection fraction. Curr Heart Fail Rep 2013;10(4):401–10.

6. Del Buono MG, Arena R, Borlaug BA, et al. Exercise intolerance in patients with heart failure. J Am Coll Cardiol 2019;73(17):2209–25.

7. Borlaug BA, Kane GC, Melenovsky V, et al. Abnormal right ventricular-pulmonary artery coupling with exercise in heart failure with preserved ejection fraction. Eur Heart J 2016;37(43):3294–302.

8. Borlaug BA, Melenovsky V, Russell SD, et al. Impaired chronotropic and vasodilator reserves limit exercise capacity in patients with heart failure and a preserved ejection fraction. Circulation 2006; 114(20):2138–47.

9. Obokata M, Olson TP, Reddy YNV, et al. Haemodynamics, dyspnoea, and pulmonary reserve in heart failure with preserved ejection fraction. Eur Heart J 2018;39(30):2810–21.

10. Guazzi M, Villani S, Generati G, et al. Right ventricular contractile reserve and pulmonary circulation uncoupling during exercise challenge in heart failure: pathophysiology and clinical phenotypes. JACC Heart Fail 2016;4(8):625–35.

11. Obokata M, Reddy YNV, Melenovsky V, et al. Deterioration in right ventricular structure and function over time in patients with heart failure and preserved ejection fraction. Eur Heart J 2019;40(8):689–97.

12. Bandera F, Barletta M, Fontana M, et al. Exercise-induced mitral regurgitation and right ventricle to pulmonary circulation uncoupling across the heart failure phenotypes. Am J Physiol Heart Circ Physiol 2021;320(2):H642–53.

13. Pellicori P, Cleland JGF, Clark AL. Chronic obstructive pulmonary disease and heart failure: a breathless conspiracy. Heart Fail Clin 2020;16(1):33–44.

14. Gulea C, Zakeri R, Quint JK. Impact of chronic obstructive pulmonary disease on readmission after hospitalization for acute heart failure: a nationally representative US cohort study. Int J Cardiol 2019; 290:113–8.

15. Andrea R, Lopez-Giraldo A, Falces C, et al. Lung function abnormalities are highly frequent in patients with heart failure and preserved ejection fraction. Heart Lung Circ 2014;23(3):273–9.

16. Coniglio AC, Mentz RJ. Sleep breathing disorders in heart failure. Heart Fail Clin 2020;16(1):45–51.

17. Pandey A, Parashar A, Kumbhani DJ, et al. Exercise training in patients with heart failure and preserved ejection fraction meta-analysis of randomized control trials. Circulation-Heart Fail 2015;8(1):33–U73.

18. Tromp J, Shen L, Jhund PS, et al. Age-related characteristics and outcomes of patients with heart failure with preserved ejection fraction. J Am Coll Cardiol 2019;74(5):601–12.

19. Marra AM, Arcopinto M, Bossone E, et al. Pulmonary arterial hypertension-related myopathy: an overview of current data and future perspectives. Nutr Metab Cardiovasc Dis 2015;25(2):131–9.

20. Marra AM, Benjamin N, Cittadini A, et al. When pulmonary hypertension complicates heart failure. Heart Fail Clin 2020;16(1):53–60.

21. Marra AM, Bossone E, Salzano A, et al. Biomarkers in pulmonary hypertension. Heart Fail Clin 2018; 14(3):393–402.

22. Marra AM, Benjamin N, Eichstaedt C, et al. Gender-related differences in pulmonary arterial hypertension targeted drugs administration. Pharmacol Res 2016;114:103–9.

23. Saccà F, Puorro G, Marsili A, et al. Long-term effect of epoetin alfa on clinical and biochemical markers in Friedreich ataxia. Mov Disord 2016;31(5):734–41.

24. Pane C, Salzano A, Trinchillo A, et al. Safety and feasibility of upper limb cardiopulmonary exercise test in Friedreich ataxia. Full research article. Eur J Prev Cardiol 2020. https://doi.org/10.1093/eurjpc/zwaa134.

25. Haykowsky MJ, Tomczak CR, Scott JM, et al. Determinants of exercise intolerance in patients with heart failure and reduced or preserved ejection fraction. J Appl Physiol 2015;119(6):739–44.

26. Kitzman DW, Nicklas B, Kraus WE, et al. Skeletal muscle abnormalities and exercise intolerance in older patients with heart failure and preserved ejection fraction. Am J Physiology-Heart Circulatory Physiol 2014;306(9):H1364–70.

27. Cohen JB, Schrauben SJ, Zhao L, et al. Clinical phenogroups in heart failure with preserved ejection fraction detailed phenotypes, prognosis, and response to spironolactone. JACC Heart Fail 2020; 8(3):172–84.

28. Marra AM, Arcopinto M, Salzano A, et al. Detectable interleukin-9 plasma levels are associated with impaired cardiopulmonary functional capacity and all-cause mortality in patients with chronic heart failure. Int J Cardiol 2016;209:114–7.

29. Arcopinto M, Salzano A, Giallauria F, et al. Growth hormone deficiency is associated with worse cardiac function, physical performance, and outcome in chronic heart failure: insights from the T.O.S.CA. GHD Study. PLoS One 2017;12(1):e0170058.

30. Bossone E, Arcopinto M, Iacoviello M, et al. Multiple hormonal and metabolic deficiency syndrome in chronic heart failure: rationale, design, and demographic characteristics of the T.O.S.CA. Registry. Intern Emerg Med 2018;13(5):661–71.

31. Cittadini A, Salzano A, Iacoviello M, et al. Multiple hormonal and metabolic deficiency syndrome predicts outcome in heart failure: the T.O.S.CA. Registry. Full research paper. Eur J Prev Cardiol 2021. https://doi.org/10.1093/eurjpc/zwab020.

32. Salzano A, Marra AM, Ferrara F, et al. Multiple hormone deficiency syndrome in heart failure with preserved ejection fraction. Int J Cardiol 2016;225:1–3.

33. Carbone S, Lavie CJ, Elagizi A, et al. The impact of obesity in heart failure. Heart Fail Clin 2020;16(1): 71–80.

34. Arcopinto M, Schiavo A, Salzano A, et al. Metabolic syndrome in heart failure: friend or foe? Heart Fail Clin 2019;15(3):349–58.

35. Magrì D, De Martino F, Moscucci F, et al. Anemia and iron deficiency in heart failure: clinical and prognostic role. Heart Fail Clin 2019;15(3):359–69.

36. Costanzo MR. The cardiorenal syndrome in heart failure. Heart Fail Clin 2020;16(1):81–97.

37. Jamaly S, Carlsson L, Peltonen M, et al. Heart failure development in obesity: underlying risk factors and mechanistic pathways. ESC Heart Fail 2020. https://doi.org/10.1002/ehf2.13081.

38. Oh A, Okazaki R, Sam F, et al. Heart failure with preserved ejection fraction and adipose tissue: a story of two tales. Front Cardiovasc Med 2019;6110. https://doi.org/10.3389/fcvm.2019.00110.

39. Shah SJ, Kitzman DW, Borlaug BA, et al. Phenotype-specific treatment of heart failure with preserved ejection fraction a multiorgan roadmap. Circulation 2016;134(1):73–+.

40. Houstis NE, Eisman AS, Pappagianopoulos PP, et al. Exercise intolerance in heart failure with preserved ejection fraction: diagnosing and ranking its causes using personalized O2 pathway analysis. Circulation 2018;137(2):148–61.

41. Giannitsi S, Bougiakli M, Bechlioulis A, et al. 6-minute walking test: a useful tool in the management of heart failure patients. Ther Adv Cardiovasc Dis 2019;13. 1753944719870084.

42. Guazzi M, Arena R, Halle M, et al. 2016 Focused update: clinical recommendations for cardiopulmonary exercise testing data assessment in specific patient populations. Circulation 2016;133(24):E694–711.

43. Jain CC, Borlaug BA. Performance and interpretation of invasive hemodynamic exercise testing. Chest 2020;158(5):2119–29.

44. Guazzi M, Myers J, Arena R. Cardiopulmonary exercise testing in the clinical and prognostic assessment of diastolic heart failure. J Am Coll Cardiol 2005;46(10):1883–90.

45. Abudiab MM, Redfield MM, Melenovsky V, et al. Cardiac output response to exercise in relation to metabolic demand in heart failure with preserved ejection fraction. Eur J Heart Fail 2013;15(7):776–85.

46. Guazzi M, Adams V, Conraads V, et al. Clinical recommendations for cardiopulmonary exercise testing data assessment in specific patient populations. Circulation 2012;126(18):2261–74.

47. Corra U, Piepoli MF, Adamopoulos S, et al. Cardiopulmonary exercise testing in systolic heart failure in 2014: the evolving prognostic role: a position paper from the Committee on Exercise Physiology and Training of the Heart Failure Association of the ESC. Eur J Heart Fail 2014;16(9):929–41.

48. Reddy YNV, Olson TP, Obokata M, et al. Hemodynamic correlates and diagnostic role of cardiopulmonary exercise testing in heart failure with preserved ejection fraction. JACC Heart Fail 2018; 6(8):665–75.

49. Abbate A, Van Tassell BW, Canada JM, et al. Pharmacologic and surgical interventions to improve functional capacity in heart failure. Heart Fail Clin 2015;11(1):117–+.

50. Neto MC, Duraes AR, Conceicao LSR, et al. High intensity interval training versus moderate intensity continuous training on exercise capacity and quality of life in patients with heart failure with reduced

ejection fraction: a systematic review and meta-analysis. Int J Cardiol 2018;261:134–41.

51. Shafiq A, Brawner CA, Aldred HA, et al. Prognostic value of cardiopulmonary exercise testing in heart failure with preserved ejection fraction. The Henry Ford HosplTal CardioPulmonary EXercise Testing (FIT-CPX) project. Am Heart J 2016;174:167–72.

52. Guazzi M, Myers J, Peberdy MA, et al. Exercise oscillatory breathing in diastolic heart failure: prevalence and prognostic insights. Eur Heart J 2008;29(22):2751–9.

53. Nadruz W, West E, Sengelov M, et al. Prognostic value of cardiopulmonary exercise testing in heart failure with reduced, midrange, and preserved ejection fraction. J Am Heart Assoc 2017;6(11):e006000.

54. Sietsema KE, Sue DY, Stringer WW, et al. Wasserman & Whipp's Principles of Exercise Testing and Interpretation: Including Pathophysiology and Clinical Applications – sixth edition. Publisher: Wolters Kluwer Health. ISBN-10: 1975136438. ISBDN-13: 978-1975136437.

55. Corra U, Agostoni PG, Anker SD, et al. Role of cardiopulmonary exercise testing in clinical stratification in heart failure. A position paper from the Committee on Exercise Physiology and Training of the Heart Failure Association of the European Society of Cardiology. Eur J Heart Fail 2018;20(1):3–15.

56. Obokata M, Kane GC, Reddy YNV, et al. Role of diastolic stress testing in the evaluation for heart failure with preserved ejection fraction: a simultaneous invasive-echocardiographic study. Circulation 2017;135(9):825–38.

57. Cleland JGF, Tendera M, Adamus J, et al. The Perindopril in Elderly People With Chronic Heart Failure (PEP-CHF) study. Eur Heart J 2006;27(19):2338–45.

58. Kosmala W, Rojek A, Przewlocka-Kosmala M, et al. Effect of aldosterone antagonism on exercise tolerance in heart failure with preserved ejection fraction. J Am Coll Cardiol 2016;68(17):1823–34.

59. Kuno T, Ueyama H, Fujisaki T, et al. Meta-analysis evaluating the effects of renin-angiotensin-aldosterone system blockade on outcomes of heart failure with preserved ejection fraction. Am J Cardiol 2020;125(8):1187–93.

60. Ross R, Blair SN, Arena R, et al. Importance of assessing cardiorespiratory fitness in clinical practice: a case for fitness as a clinical vital sign a scientific statement from the American Heart Association. Circulation 2016;134(24):E653–99.

61. Leggio M, Fusco A, Loreti C, et al. Effects of exercise training in heart failure with preserved ejection fraction: an updated systematic literature review. Heart Fail Rev 2020;25(5):703–11.

62. Smart NA, Haluska B, Jeffriess L, et al. Exercise training in heart failure with preserved systolic function: a randomized controlled trial of the effects on cardiac function and functional capacity. Congest Heart Fail 2012;18(6):295–301.

63. Maldonado-Martín S, Brubaker PH, Eggebeen J, et al. Association between 6-minute walk test distance and objective variables of functional capacity after exercise training in elderly heart failure patients with preserved ejection fraction: a randomized exercise trial. Arch Phys Med Rehabil 2017; 98(3):600–3.

64. Palau P, Domínguez E, López L, et al. Inspiratory muscle training and functional electrical stimulation for treatment of heart failure with preserved ejection fraction: the TRAINING-HF Trial. Rev Esp Cardiol (Engl Ed 2019;72(4):288–97.

65. Nolte K, Herrmann-Lingen C, Wachter R, et al. Effects of exercise training on different quality of life dimensions in heart failure with preserved ejection fraction: the Ex-DHF-P trial. Eur J Prev Cardiol 2015;22(5):582–93.

66. Lang CC, Smith K, Wingham J, et al. A randomised controlled trial of a facilitated home-based rehabilitation intervention in patients with heart failure with preserved ejection fraction and their caregivers: the REACH-HFpEF Pilot Study. BMJ Open 2018; 8(4):e019649.

67. Edelmann F, Gelbrich G, Düngen HD, et al. Exercise training improves exercise capacity and diastolic function in patients with heart failure with preserved ejection fraction: results of the Ex-DHF (Exercise training in Diastolic Heart Failure) pilot study. J Am Coll Cardiol 2011;58(17):1780–91.

68. Alves AJ, Ribeiro F, Goldhammer E, et al. Exercise training improves diastolic function in heart failure patients. Med Sci Sports Exerc 2012;44(5):776–85.

69. Fu TC, Yang NI, Wang CH, et al. Aerobic interval training elicits different hemodynamic adaptations between heart failure patients with preserved and reduced ejection fraction. Am J Phys Med Rehabil 2016;95(1):15–27.

70. Murad K, Brubaker PH, Fitzgerald DM, et al. Exercise training improves heart rate variability in older patients with heart failure: a randomized, controlled, single-blinded trial. Congest Heart Fail 2012;18(4):192–7.

71. Fujimoto N, Prasad A, Hastings JL, et al. Cardiovascular effects of 1 year of progressive endurance exercise training in patients with heart failure with preserved ejection fraction. Am Heart J 2012; 164(6):869–77.

72. Kitzman DW, Brubaker PH, Morgan TM, et al. Exercise training in older patients with heart failure and preserved ejection fraction: a randomized, controlled, single-blind trial. Circulation-Heart Fail 2010;3(6):659–67.

73. Kitzman DW, Brubaker P, Morgan T, et al. Effect of caloric restriction or aerobic exercise training on peak oxygen consumption and quality of life in obese older patients with heart failure with preserved ejection fraction: a randomized clinical trial. JAMA 2016;315(1):36–46.

74. Kitzman DW, Brubaker PH, Herrington DM, et al. Effect of endurance exercise training on endothelial function and arterial stiffness in older patients with heart failure and preserved ejection fraction: a randomized, controlled, single-blind trial. J Am Coll Cardiol 2013;62(7):584–92.

75. Tucker WJ, Lijauco CC, Hearon CM, et al. Mechanisms of the improvement in peak VO2 with exercise training in heart failure with reduced or preserved ejection fraction. Heart Lung Circ 2018;27(1):9–21.

76. Angadi SS, Mookadam F, Lee CD, et al. High-intensity interval training vs. moderate-intensity continuous exercise training in heart failure with preserved ejection fraction: a pilot study. J Appl Physiol (1985) 2015;119(6):753–8.

77. Donelli da Silveira A, Beust de Lima J, da Silva Piardi D, et al. High-intensity interval training is effective and superior to moderate continuous training in patients with heart failure with preserved ejection fraction: a randomized clinical trial. Eur J Prev Cardiol 2020;27(16):1733–43.

78. Beckers PJ, Gevaert AB. High intensity interval training for heart failure with preserved ejection fraction: high hopes for intense exercise. Eur J Prev Cardiol 2020;27(16):1730–2.

79. Mueller S, Winzer EB, Duvinage A, et al. Effect of high-intensity interval training, moderate continuous training, or guideline-based physical activity advice on peak oxygen consumption in patients with heart failure with preserved ejection fraction: a randomized clinical trial. JAMA 2021;325(6):542–51.

80. Pandey A, Kitzman DW. Searching for the optimal exercise training regimen in heart failure with preserved ejection fraction. JAMA 2021;325(6):537–9.

81. Kitzman DW, Groban L. Exercise intolerance. Cardiol Clin 2011;29(3):461–77.

82. Dhakal BP, Malhotra R, Murphy RM, et al. Mechanisms of exercise intolerance in heart failure with preserved ejection fraction the role of abnormal peripheral oxygen extraction. Circ Heart Fail 2015;8(2):286–94.

Invasive Hemodynamics in Heart Failure with Preserved Ejection Fraction

Importance of Detecting Pulmonary Vascular Remodeling and Right Heart Function

Nandini Nair, MD, PhD

KEYWORDS

- Diastolic pulmonary gradient • Transpulmonary gradient • Pulmonary arterial compliance
- Pulmonary vascular resistance • Pulmonary arterial pulsatility index

KEY POINTS

- Arterial remodeling and failure impact prognosis.
- Right ventricular dysfunction and pulmonary hypertension are important prognostic factors.
- Pulmonary arterial compliance is an independent predictor of mortality.

INTRODUCTION

The prevalence of heart failure (HF) in the United States is approximately 6.5 million. HF causes significant morbidity, mortality, and astronomical rises in health care costs to the tune of billions of dollars. Grossly 50% of the patients with HF have HF with preserved Ejection Fraction (HFpEF).[1] HFpEF has a similar morbidity and mortality profile as HF with reduced EF (HFrEF). HFpEF diagnosis presents challenges because of the multiple etiologies that underlie its pathophysiology. Hence various approaches have been used to diagnose HFpEF including epidemiologic criteria (Framingham, Gothenburg, Boston, and the European Society of Cardiology).[2–5] Phenomapping and applying artificial intelligence/machine learning algorithms to large databases may be beneficial in delineating homogenous groups and subgroups in this population.[6,7]

Invasive hemodynamics have shown varied results in HFpEF patients, possibly because of the heterogenous etiology of this condition or due to study populations with patients in different stages of HFpEF. Patients in the early stages of HFpEF do not manifest a high pulmonary capillary wedge pressure (PCWP) as do those in later stages of HFpEF. PCWP increases secondary to increasing chamber stiffness, impaired diastolic suction effect, and abnormal relaxation.[8–12] Chronic elevation of PCWP may precede pulmonary vascular remodeling with consequent increases in pulmonary vascular resistance (PVR) and decreases in pulmonary artery compliance (PAC). This article attempts to summarize the importance of detecting pulmonary vascular modeling in HFpEF using invasive hemodynamics.

HEMODYNAMICS USING LEFT HEART CATHETERIZATION

Left ventricular (LV) hemodynamic assessment yields several important parameters depicting the alterations in end diastolic/systolic volumes with changes in ventricular pressure. The parameters of relevance in HFpEF patients are LV diastolic pressure (LVEDP), end systolic pressures (ESPs), arterial elastance (EA), and LV end systolic elastance (Ees) measured using pressure volume loops. **Fig. 1** shows the upward and leftward shift

Department of Medicine, Texas Tech University Health Sciences Center, 3601, 4th Street, Lubbock, TX 79430, USA
E-mail address: nandini.nair@gmail.com

Heart Failure Clin 17 (2021) 415–422
https://doi.org/10.1016/j.hfc.2021.03.003

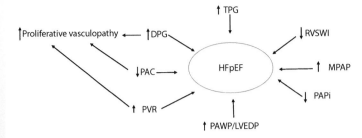

Fig. 1. Pressure volume loops in normal and HFpEF.

of the pressure volume loop in HFpEF. Existing literature shows that Ees and EA are both elevated in addition to LVEDP in HFpEF patients. Another important measure of LV diastolic reserve is the measurement of relaxation, which is prolonged in HFpEF at baseline, with inadequate shortening of tau, the relaxation constant on exercise, and LV filling driven by increased left atrial pressure and increased LVEDP.[13] These measurements done by the pressure volume loop analysis can be useful in the diagnosis of HFpEF in patients with unexplained dyspnea.[14] Patients in early stages of HFpEF may not experience dyspnea at rest and require provocative measures such as exercise or pacer-induced tachycardia to show symptoms and corresponding PCWP increases in invasive hemodynamic testing.[15] The provocation of symptoms with exercise is because of the increase in PCWP. Increase in PCWP is secondary to impaired diastolic function and results from poor suction effect due to inefficient relaxation/increased chamber stiffness. Additionally, a component of systolic dysfunction exists in HFpEF patients, which is a predictor for poorer outcomes in this population. Such systolic dysfunction gets accentuated on exercise, unmasking the exercise-induced findings in HFpEF. Increases in ventricular stiffness are coupled to increases in arterial stiffness, wherein pressure changes with load are more pronounced. Higher filling pressures in HFpEF are a consequence of higher chamber stiffness rather than preload.[10,16–22]

ROLE OF ATRIAL REMODELING AND FAILURE

The structural impairment and functional impairment of left and right atria result in adverse hemodynamics and prognosis. Both interatrial and intra-atrial dyssynchrony can lead to late atrial activation, delayed contraction, shortened emptying, reduced compliance, and increased filling pressures. Such abnormalities can lead to atrial fibrillation, which confers a worse prognosis on HFpEF patients. Pathophysiological mechanisms underlying atrial remodeling include a myopathy and microvascular endothelial activation. Severe dilation of atria can cause annular

dilatation and atrial functional mitral regurgitation. Atrial functional mitral regurgitation exists in about 53% of HFpEF patients. This leads to malcoaptation of leaflets and a decrease in closing force because of increased LA pressure and decreased annular contraction.[23] The right atrium (RA) drives right ventricular (RV) filling and magnitude of central venous pressure (CVP). Structural/functional remodeling of the RA contributes to worsening clinical status in HFpEF patients. Mechanism of RA modeling is unclear at this time but could be caused by pulmonary hypertension, increased RV filling pressure, tricuspid regurgitation, atrial fibrillation, and neurohormonal activation. RA remodeling and dilation are associated with a congestive hepatopathy picture consisting of increased serum hepatobiliary enzymes. Hemodynamic abnormalities if uncorrected contributing to RA remodeling have been noted.[23,24] In a recent study by Ikoma and colleagues,[24] the event-free survival was significantly worse in patients with RA dilation with or without concurrent atrial fibrillation. However, RA dilation and reservoir dysfunction worsened in the population with atrial fibrillation. The effects of atrial fibrillation on bi-atrial remodeling are pronounced when both atria are enlarged. The HFpEF patients with RA dilation had worse outcomes compared to those with normal LA size.[24] RA dilation was associated with increased LA volume/index, higher RV systolic pressures, higher prevalence of tricuspid regurgitation and worse RA reservoir function.[24] Therefore, emphasizing the fact that assessment of PCWP and RAP to drive diuretic management in addition to other measures such as restoring sinus rhythm and structural intervention to reduce annular size should be strongly considered.[23–25]

RIGHT VENTRICULAR HEMODYNAMICS

RV dysfunction and pulmonary hypertension (PH) are important prognostic factors in the HFpEF population. Many comorbidities that influence RV function include diabetes, hypertension, chronic obstructive pulmonary disease (COPD), and obesity. Atrial fibrillation occurs usually secondary to atrial structural and functional remodeling and further contributes to RV dysfunction. Hemodynamics derived from right heart catheterization as shown in **Table 1** provide adequate information about the RA, right ventricle, and the pulmonary artery. PVR, PCWP, pulmonary arterial compliance (PAC), diastolic pulmonary gradient (DPG), transpulmonary gradient (TPG), pulmonary arterial pulsatility index (PAPi), right atrial pressure (RAP), and RV stroke work index (RVSWI) provide extensive characterization of right atrial and ventricular function in HFpEF.

Pulmonary arterial hypertension (PAH), Group 1 PH by World Health Organization (WHO) classification, is rare, with 2 to 5 cases per million in the adult population.[26] Endothelial dysfunction, smooth muscle cell proliferation, pro-inflammatory processes, and vasoconstriction lead to diffuse remodeling of the pulmonary arterial system and finally cause precapillary PH.[27] However, PH secondary to left heart disease (WHO Group 2 PH) is the most common type of PH globally, amounting to 50% of all PH. HFpEF has been noted as a prominent etiology of PH, with the increasing prevalence of aging, obesity, diabetes

mellitus, and systemic hypertension.[28–30] The right ventricle adapts to PH by balancing RV contractility with pulmonary arterial load. This ventriculo-vascular coupling can be measured with the PV loop analysis in a multibeat, a single-beat or volumetric measurements.[27] The multibeat PV loops require PV loops to be obtained at decreasing levels of preload, while in the single-beat method, the RV waveform tracing is utilized to estimate the maximum isovolumetric pressure. The volumetric method estimates Ees as the ratio of ESP/ESV and Ea as ESP/SV. However, all of these methods have limitations that need to be considered, especially in advanced RV failure/PH. Noninvasive methods by echocardiography and cardiac MRI also have their share of ambiguities and limitations.[27] RV efficiency can be estimated by PV loops, and ventricular oxygen supply can be estimated by direct measurement of coronary blood flow and the arterio-venous O_2 difference calculated. HFpEF patients typically present with RV dysfunction in the setting of coronary artery disease with microvascular involvement and endothelial dysfunction, fibrosis, RV dyssynchrony,

Table 1
Hemodynamic parameters derived from right heart catheterization

Parameter	Equation	Normal Range
Right atrial pressure (RAP)		2–6 mm Hg
Right ventricular pressure (RVP)	Systolic (RVSP) diastolic (RVDP)	15–25 mm Hg 0–8 mm Hg
Pulmonary artery pressure	Pulmonary artery systolic (PASP) Pulmonary artery diastolic (PADP)	15–25 mm Hg 8–15 mm Hg
Mean pulmonary artery pressure (MPAP)	PASP +(2 × PADP)/3	10–20 mm Hg
Pulmonary artery wedge pressure (PAWP)		6–12mrnHg
Diastolic pulmonary gradient	PADP-PCWP	<7 mm Hg
PAC	Stroke volume/pulmonary artery pulse pressure	3.8–12 mL/mm Hg
PAPi	(PASP-PADP)/RAP	>2.0
Transpulmonary gradient	MPAP-PCWP	<12 mm Hg
Cardiac output (CO)	HR × SV/1000	4.0–8.0 L/min
Cardiac index (CI)	CO/BSA !	2.5–4.0 L/min/m²
Stroke volume (SV)	CO/HR × 1000	60–100 mL/beat
Stroke volume index (SVI)	CI/HR × 1000	33–47 mL/m²/beat
SVR	80 × (MAP-RAP)/CO	800–1200 dyn.sec.cm⁵
SVR index (SVRI)	80 × (MAP-RAP)/CI	1970–2390 dyn.s/cm⁵/m²
PVR	80 × (MPAP- PAWP)/CO	<250 dyn.s/cm⁵
PVR index (PVRI)	80 × (MPAP-PAWP)/CI	255–285 dyn.s/cm⁵/m²
RVSW	SV × (MPAP-RAP) × 0.0136	8–16 gm-m/beat
RVSWI	SVI × (MPAP-RAP) × 0.0136	5–10 gm-m/m²/beat

and atrial fibrillation. Additionally, diastolic dysfunction contributes to RV failure in HFpEF patients. The RV structure/function relationship will need further investigation with invasive and noninvasive methods to refine risk characteristics in this population.

RVSWI is an invasive parameter assessed by right heart catheterization as shown in **Table 1**. It is derived from pressure and flow indices. The RWSWI is used to predict RV failure after LV assist device placement.[31] However, higher RVSWI in HFpEF patients was noted to have an inverse relationship with glomerular filtration rate consistent with worsening kidney function. This association has been found only in HFpEF patients who have combined post- and precapillary PH (Cpc-PH). Increased RVSWI also predicted worse outcomes because of increased stiffness of the pulmonary arterial system caused by structural remodeling of the pulmonary vascular bed. Precapillary PH exists in this group as shown by the increased PVR and DPG. This sheds light on the fact that vascular remodeling and consequent higher RV workload drive worsening renal function in this population of HFpEF patients.[32–35] Patients may benefit from targeted PH therapy as per some studies in the current literature.[32,33]

DPG is a parameter that correlates with pulmonary vascular remodeling. However, in HFpEF patient with Cpc-PH, DPG did not show any specific difference with 5′phosphodiesterase inhibitor therapy with sildenafil/tadalafil.[36] Additionally, it has been suggested that the pulmonary arterial stiffness in HFpEF may be higher than in those with reduced ejection fraction but DPG did not emerge as a strong predictor of survival compared with pulmonary arterial compliance.[37]

PULMONARY ARTERY COMPLIANCE AND PULMONARY VASCULAR RESISTANCE

The Windkessel model is the simplest way to define RV afterload. The 3 components of this model are resistance, compliance, and impedance, represented by PAC, PVR, and input impedance. The small distal pulmonary arteries define PVR. Applying Poiseuille law, resistance is inversely proportional to radius[4] of the vessel and directly proportional to the vessel length and the viscosity of the blood. PVR is the static resistance accounting for three-fourths of the RV afterload and does not account for the pulsatile aspect of the afterload. PAC constitutes the compliance aspect of the Windkessel model and the pulsatile aspect of RV afterload, accounting for 25% of the total RV afterload, In the pulmonary circulation, compliance is distributed throughout the pulmonary bed because of the branching vessels. Fifteen percent to 20% of the total PAC is contributed by the main, proximal left, and right pulmonary arteries. A large portion of the resistance and compliance in the pulmonary circulation is contributed by the distal pulmonary arterial bed. The proximal pulmonary arteries are involved in RV ejection and RV–PA coupling. PAC is used with PVR to evaluate RV afterload. Input impedance of the proximal pulmonary arteries is not used in assessing afterload of the RV, because the contribution made by impedance is insignificant.[38–42]

Of all the methods proposed to determine PAC, right heart catheterization appears to be the simplest, as shown in **Table 1**. It is simple to perform but has limitations in that it can overestimate PAC. However, PAC values obtained by right heart catheterization appear to correlate well with that obtained based on the Windkessel model. PAC determined by echocardiography may be less accurate because of several approximations done in the calculations to derive PAC.[42]

PAC is a strong/independent predictor of mortality in patients with PH.[42,43] PAC has also been implicated in proliferative vasculopathy that leads to irreversible remodeling. In animal models, reduction of PAC precedes disruption of elastic lamina, followed by the smooth muscle proliferation in the continuum of events leading to proliferative vasculopathy. Decrease in Pac has been noted in mild PH, suggestive of a prominent role for PAC in PH progression.[44–48] Hence, PAC is an important parameter to assess and monitor in this population.

PAPi is a parameter calculated by right heart catheterization as shown in **Table 1**. PAPi has been shown to be have a significant association with worsening renal function in the long term in a small study of 81 HFpEF patients.[49] PAPi has been shown to be a better marker of RV dysfunction in another study consisting of HF patients with reduced ejection fraction undergoing LV assist device surgery.[50] Another important parameter used to predict renal dysfunction HFpEF patients is the ratio of RAP to PCWP. This relationship does not yet appear to be significantly better than PAPi in predicting renal dysfunction in HFpEF patients but appears to be a significant predictor of renal dysfunction in patients with a reduced EF. PAPi measures RV systolic function and is not hemodynamically influenced by the left-sided hemodynamics. PAPi may therefore be a more sensitive hemodynamic marker in detecting long-term renal dysfunction secondary to RV dysfunction in HFpEF. RV failure has been implicated as a major factor in the deterioration of renal function progressively in this population. In the ESCAPE trial, RAP was the most useful predictor of renal dysfunction.[51] Many possible mechanisms including activated systemic inflammation and endothelial dysfunction for RV function deterioration and renal failure have been postulated in HFpEF patients. However among the most significant mechanisms has been increased central venous pressure and the consequent decreased renal perfusion.[49]

PULMONARY VASCULAR RESISTANCE AND PRECAPILLARY PULMONARY VASCULAR RESISTANCE IN HEART FAILURE WITH PRESERVED EJECTION FRACTION

Prevalence of PH has been found to be high in HFpEF, with consequent increased mortality. Precapillary PH occurs in HFpEF and can be easily distinguished by estimating the PVR during right heart catheterization. Increases in PVR are consistent with pulmonary vascular remodeling and PH even if the LV filling pressure remains low and predisposes HFpEF patients to increased mortality. Systemic dysregulation of vascular tone because of imbalances between nitric oxide (NO) and endothelin (ET) has been shown to contribute to both increased PVR in the pulmonary arteries and increased pulse wave velocity (PWV) in the arteries of systemic circulation.[52]

PH with increased PVR has been noted to predict adverse clinical outcomes such as worsening HF and acute coronary syndrome in patients with HFpEF in addition to increased mortality. Association between increased PVR and increased systemic arterial stiffness may explain the lack of effectiveness in altering prognosis by just treating diastolic dysfunction in the HFpEF population. Such observations suggest that structural remodeling and consequent functional abnormality result from impaired endothelium-dependent vasodilation, increased smooth muscle tone, and medial hypertrophy associated with nitric oxide availability in the vascular bed. In the pulmonary and systemic arteries, the endothelium controls arterial tone through the fine balance between nitric oxide and endothelin levels. Imbalance between nitric oxide and endothelin levels possibly results in high PVR. Additionally, other comorbidities such as dyslipidemia, diabetes, and systemic hypertension can all contribute to increased PVR and the consequent adverse effects.[52–54]

Many invasive parameters derived by right heart characterization can be used to follow progression of HFpEF. **Fig. 2** shows the different invasive hemodynamic parameters that drive progression of HFpEF. Decreased PAC, increased PVR, and increased DPG have all been implicated in proliferative pulmonary vasculopathy.[29,42,43] A decrease in PAPi appears to be consistent with RV failure, while higher RVSWI predicts pulmonary arterial stiffness secondary to structural remodeling. RAP is noted to increase in HFpEF patients with combined PH.[55] Increases in mean pulmonary artery pressure (MPAP) and PCWP have been noted with progression of HFpEF.[56] Invasive

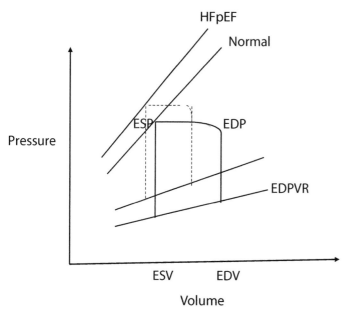

Fig. 2. Invasive hemodynamic parameters implicated in the progression of HFpEF.

hemodynamics can therefore be used as a window to understand pathophysiology and follow progression of HFpEF.

FUTURE DIRECTIONS

Defined clinical trials are needed to test clinical effectiveness and efficacy of pulmonary vasodilatory therapies in HFpEF. The selection of the study population has to be stringent, and studies should define the patient population to reduce heterogeneity. Invasive hemodynamics can be used to risk stratify patients. Newer invasive hemodynamic parameters such as DPG, PAPi, and PAC should be used to identify study groups to create homogenous populations. The value of combining different invasive parameters should be assessed in HFpEF patients with and without PH to develop better diagnostic and therapeutic strategies. The role of pulmonary vasodilators in HFpEF patients remains less defined at this time, and this is an area that requires further investigation. Hemodynamic profiling of study populations is important when attempting clinical investigations. Such well-characterized populations will enhance the reliability of outcomes from clinical studies.

SUMMARY

Profiling of patients using invasive hemodynamic parameters will lead to better patient selection for clinical research. Incorporating PAPi, DPG, PAC, and other parameters into current risk models will significantly improve patient selection for defining advanced therapies and clinical outcomes in this population. Invasive hemodynamics can be used to diagnose and stage HFpEF and characterize patient populations with other etiologies for dyspnea. Invasive hemodynamics can also be used to standardize parameters obtained from implantable devices used in remote monitoring of fluid status in HFpEF patients.

CLINICS CARE POINTS

- Aggressive control of hypertension in HFpEF patients has been shown to reduce HF-related hospitalizations.
- Although atrial dilation is seen in HFpEF patients with atrial fibrillation, the evidence showing benefits of rhythm

control is lacking at present in this population.
- Monitoring of hemodynamic parameters that signal progression of HFpEF such as increased pulmonary arterial wedge pressure, diastolic pulmonary gradient, and increased PVR, and alterations in pulmonary arterial compliance should be done aggressively, as these parameters contribute to proliferative vasculopathy and vascular remodeling worsening the prognosis.
- PAC should be used with pulmonary vascular resistance to evaluate RV afterload.
- Pulmonary arterial pulsatility index measures RV systolic function but is not influenced by the left-sided hemodynamics. It may therefore be a more sensitive hemodynamic marker in detecting long-term renal dysfunction secondary to RV dysfunction in HFpEF.
- RV function using invasive hemodynamic parameters like RVSWI should be monitored, as worsening RV function correlates with worsening renal function.
- Invasive hemodynamics should be used to detect and estimate magnitude of interatrial shunts. Interatrial shunts closed using mechanical devices help unload the left atrium and decrease pulmonary arterial capillary wedge pressures. The patients with interatrial shunt devices should be followed using invasive hemodynamics to assess right-sided pressures.
- Measurement of right atrial pressure and pulmonary capillary wedge pressure in imperative in managing fluid overload when titrating diuretic treatments.
- Wireless monitoring of devices placed in the pulmonary artery to assess fluid overload measures pulmonary artery pressures forming a basic component of fluid management in HFpEF patients.
- The role of pulmonary vasodilators in HFpEF patients remains less defined at this time and requires further investigation.
- Hemodynamic profiling of study populations is important when attempting clinical investigations, because well-characterized populations will enhance the reliability of outcomes from clinical studies.

DISCLOSURE

Dr N. Nair has no disclosures with relevance to this work.

REFERENCES

1. Virani S, Alonzo A, Benjamin E, et al. Heart disease and stroke statistics—2020 update: a report from the American Heart Association. Circulation 2020; 141:e139–596.

2. McKee P, Castelli W, McNamara P, et al. The natural history of congestive heart failure: the Framingham study. N Engl J Med 1971;285:1441–6.

3. Eriksson H, Caidaul K, Larsson B, et al. Cardiac and pulmonary causes of dyspnoea—validation of a scoring test for clinical-epidemiological use: the study of men born in 1913. Eur Heart J 1987;8:1007–14.

4. Carlson K, Lee D, Goroll A, et al. An analysis of physicians' reasons for prescribing long-term digitalis therapy in outpatients. J Chronic Dis 1985;38:733–9.

5. Ponikowski P, Voors A, Anker S, et al, ESC Scientific Document Group. ESC guidelines for the diagnosis and treatment of acute and chronic heart failure: the task force for the diagnosis and treatment of acute and chronic heart failure of the European Society of Cardiology (ESC). Developed with the special contribution of the Heart Failure Association (HFA) of the ESC. Eur Heart J 2016;37:2129–200.

6. Bielinski S, Pathak J, Carrell D, et al. A Robust e-Epidemiology tool in phenotyping heart failure with differentiation for preserved and reduced ejection fraction: the Electronic Medical Records and Genomics (eMERGE) Network. J Cardiovasc Translational Res 2015;8:475–83.

7. Blecker S, Katz S, Horwitz L, et al. Comparison of approaches for heart failure case identification from electronic health record data. JAMA Cardiol 2016;1:1014–20.

8. Andersen M, Borlaug B. Invasive hemodynamic characterization of heart failure with preserved ejection fraction. Heart Fail Clin 2014;10:435–44.

9. Abudiab M, Redfield M, Melenovsky V, et al. Cardiac output response to exercise in relation to metabolic demand in heart failure with preserved ejection fraction. Eur J Heart Fail 2013;15:776–85.

10. Schwartzenberg S, Redfield M, From A, et al. Effects of vasodilation in heart failure with preserved or reduced ejection fraction implications of distinct pathophysiologies on response to therapy. J Am Coll Cardiol 2012;59:442–51.

11. Pfeffer M, Shah A, Borlaug B. Heart failure with preserved ejection fraction in perspective. Circ Res 2019;124:1598–617.

12. Borlaug B. The pathophysiology of heart failure with preserved ejection fraction. Nat Rev Cardiol 2014; 11:507–15.

13. Borlaug B, Jaber W, Ommen S, et al. Diastolic relaxation and compliance reserve during dynamic exercise in heart failure with preserved ejection fraction. Heart 2011;97:964–9.

14. Penicka M, Bartunek J, Trakalova H, et al. Heart failure with preserved ejection fraction in outpatients with unexplained dyspnea: a pressure-volume loop analysis. J Am Coll Cardiol 2010;55:1701–10.

15. Borlaug B, Nishimura R, Sorajja P, et al. Exercise hemodynamics enhance diagnosis of early heart failure with preserved ejection fraction. Circ Heart Fail 2010;3:588–95.

16. Borlaug B, Lam C, Roger V, et al. Contractility and ventricular systolic stiffening in hypertensive heart disease insights into the pathogenesis of heart failure with preserved ejection fraction. J Am Coll Cardiol 2009;54:410–8.

17. Borlaug B, Olson T, Lam C, et al. Global cardiovascular reserve dysfunction in heart failure with preserved ejection fraction. J Am Coll Cardiol 2010;56:845–54.

18. Maeder M, Thompson B, Brunner-La Rocca H, et al. Hemodynamic basis of exercise limitation in patients with heart failure and normal ejection fraction. J Am Coll Cardiol 2010;56:855–63.

19. Lam C, Roger V, Rodeheffer R, et al. Pulmonary hypertension in heart failure with preserved ejection fraction: a community-based study. J Am Coll Cardiol 2009;53:1119–26.

20. Lam C, Roger V, Rodeheffer R, et al. Cardiac structure and ventricular-vascular function in persons with heart failure and preserved ejection fraction from Olmsted County, Minnesota. Circulation 2007;115:1982–90.

21. Borlaug B, Paulus W. Heart failure with preserved ejection fraction: pathophysiology, diagnosis, and treatment. Eur Heart J 2011;32:670–9.

22. Borlaug B, Kass D. Ventricular-vascular interaction in heart failure. Heart Fail Clin 2008;4:23–36.

23. Deferm S, Bertrand P, Verbrugge F, et al. Atrial functional mitral regurgitation: JACC review topic of the week. J Am Coll Cardiol 2019;73:2465–76.

24. Ikoma T, Obokata M, Okada K, et al. Impact of right atrial remodeling in heart failure with preserved ejection fraction. J Cardiac Fail 2020;Dec 29:1–8.

25. Bayes-Genis A, Bisbal F, Núñez J, et al. Transitioning from preclinical to clinical heart failure with preserved ejection fraction: a mechanistic approach. J Clin Med 2020;9:1110.

26. Hoeper M, Humbert M, Souza R, et al. A global view of pulmonary hypertension. Lancet Respir Med 2016;4:306–22.

27. Bernardo R, Haddad F, Couture E, et al. Mechanics of right ventricular dysfunction in pulmonary arterial hypertension and heart failure with preserved ejection fraction. Cardiovasc Diagn Ther 2020;10(5):1580–603.

28. Ghio S, Gavazzi A, Campana C, et al. Independent and additive prognostic value of right ventricular systolic function and pulmonary artery pressure in

patients with chronic heart failure. J Am Coll Cardiol 2001;37:183–8.

29. Gerges C, Gerges M, Lang MB, et al. Diastolic pulmonary vascular pressure gradient: a predictor of prognosis in "out-of-proportion" pulmonary hypertension. Chest 2013;143:758–66.

30. Zakeri R, Mohammed SF. Epidemiology of right ventricular dysfunction in heart failure with preserved ejection fraction. Curr Heart Fail Rep 2015;12:295–301.

31. Imamura T, Kinugawa K, Kinoshita O, et al. High pulmonary vascular resistance in addition to low right ventricular stroke work index effectively predicts biventricular assist device requirement. J Artif Organs 2016;19:44–53.

32. Rosenkranz S, Gibbs J, Wachter R, et al. Left ventricular heart failure and pulmonary hypertension. Eur Heart J 2016;37:942–54.

33. Vachiéry L, Adir Y, Barberà J, et al. Pulmonary hypertension due to left heart diseases. J Am Coll Cardiol 2013;62:D100–8.

34. Stevens G, Garcia-Alvarez A, Sahni S, et al. RV dysfunction in pulmonary hypertension is independently related to pulmonary artery stiffness. JACC Cardiovasc Imaging 2012;5:378–87.

35. Kanjanahattakij N, Sirinvaravong N, Aguilar F, et al. High right ventricular stroke work index is associated with worse kidney function in patients with heart failure with preserved ejection fraction. Cardiorenal Med 2018;8:123–9.

36. Kramer T, Dumitrescu D, Gerhardt F, et al. Therapeutic potential of phosphodiesterase type 5 inhibitors in heart failure with preserved ejection fraction and combined post- and pre-capillary pulmonary hypertension. Int J Cardiol 2019;283:152–8.

37. Adir Y, Guazzi M, Offer A, et al. Pulmonary hemodynamics in heart failure patients with reduced or preserved ejection fraction and pulmonary hypertension: similarities and disparities. Am Heart J 2017;192:120–7.

38. Saouti N, Westerhof N, Helderman F, et al. Right ventricular oscillatory power is a constant fraction of total power irrespective of pulmonary artery pressure. Am J Respir Crit Care Med 2010;182:1315–20.

39. Saouti N, Westerhof N, Postmus PE, et al. The arterial load in pulmonary hypertension. Eur Respir Rev 2010;19:197–203.

40. Vonk-Noordegraaf A, Haddad F, Chin KM, et al. Right heart adaptation to pulmonary arterial hypertension: physiology and pathobiology. J Am Coll Cardiol 2013;62(25, Suppl):D22–33.

41. Saouti N, Westerhof N, Helderman F, et al. RC time constant of single lung equals that of both lungs together: a study in chronic thromboembolic pulmonary hypertension. Am J Physiol Heart Circ Physiol 2009;297:H2154–60.

42. Thenappan T, Prins K, Pritzker M, et al. The critical role of pulmonary arterial compliance in pulmonary hypertension. Ann Am Thorac Soc 2016;13:276–84.

43. Al-Naamani N, Preston I, Paulus J, et al. Pulmonary arterial capacitance is an important predictor of mortality in heart failure with a preserved ejection fraction. JACC Heart Fail 2015;3:467–74.

44. Sanz J, Kariisa M, Dellegrottaglie S, et al. Evaluation of pulmonary artery stiffness in pulmonary hypertension with cardiac magnetic resonance. JACC Cardiovasc Imaging 2009;2:286–95.

45. Lau E, Chemla D, Godinas L, et al. Reduced distensibility of the pulmonary circulation during exercise in early pulmonary vascular disease. Am J Respir Crit Care Med 2015;191:A4787.

46. Mullin C, Damico R, Kolb T, et al. Resting compliance and stroke volume is associated with abnormal pulmonary vascular response to exercise in systemic sclerosis. Am J Respir Crit Care Med 2015;191:A4790.

47. Todorovich-Hunter L, Dodo H, Ye C, et al. Increased pulmonary artery elastolytic activity in adult rats with monocrotaline-induced progressive hypertensive pulmonary vascular disease compared with infant rats with nonprogressive disease. Am Rev Respir Dis 1992;146:213–23.

48. Maruyama K, Ye C, Woo M, et al. Chronic hypoxic pulmonary hypertension in rats and increased elastolytic activity. Am J Physiol 1991;261:H1716–26.

49. Lo K, Mezue K, Ram P, et al. Echocardiographic and hemodynamic parameters associated with diminishing renal filtration among patients with heart failure with preserved ejection fraction. Cardiorenal Med 2019;9:83–91.

50. Morine K, Kiernan M, Pham D, et al. Pulmonary artery pulsatility index predicts right ventricular failure following LVAD surgery. Circulation 2014;130(Suppl 2):A19195.

51. Nohria A, Hasselblad V, Stebbins A, et al. Cardiorenal interactions: insights from the ESCAPE trial. J Am Coll Cardiol 2008;51:1268–74.

52. Nakamura T, Uematsu M, Deyama J, et al. Pulmonary vascular resistance is associated with brachial-ankle pulse-wave velocity and adverse clinical outcomes in patients with heart failure with preserved ejection fraction. J Card Fail 2019;25:725–32.

53. Tomiyama H, Yamashina A. Noninvasive vascular function tests: their pathophysiological background and clinical application. Circ J 2010;74:24–33.

54. Moraes D, Colucci W, Givertz M. Secondary pulmonary hypertension in chronic heart failure: the role of the endothelium in pathophysiology and management. Circulation 2000;102:1718–23.

55. Gorter T, Obokata M, Reddy Y, et al. Exercise unmasks distinct pathophysiologic features in heart failure with preserved ejection fraction and pulmonary vascular disease. Eur Heart J 2018;39:2825–35.

56. Lai Y, Wang L, Gladwin M. Insights into the pulmonary vascular complications of heart failure with preserved ejection fraction. J Physiol 2019;597:1143–56.

Noninvasive Hemodynamic Evaluation at Rest in Heart Failure with Preserved Ejection Fraction

Morten Sengeløv, MD[a,b], Tor Biering-Sørensen, MD, MPH, PhD[a,b,c,d],*

KEYWORDS

• Echocardiography • Noninvasive • HFpEF • Doppler imaging • Risk assessment

KEY POINTS

• Echocardiography is an essential tool in the noninvasive evaluation of HFpEF patients that confers diagnostic and prognostic information.
• Several studies have emphasized the importance of echocardiography without the use of invasive and functional testing.
• Doppler echocardiography remains the preferred image modality to evaluate the hemodynamic profile in HFpEF patients, but novel methods are emerging.
• A complete noninvasive hemodynamic assessment of HFpEF patients includes thorough investigation of the left heart, right heart, and pulmonary function.

INTRODUCTION

Heart failure with preserved ejection fraction (HFpEF) has in recent decades been established as an important phenotype within the heart failure syndrome. However, the diagnosis of HFpEF remains clinically challenging because no gold standard is universally acknowledged. An area of research interest has been the underlying hemodynamic physiology, which is inherently tied to the definition of heart failure, where the heart fails to adequately meet the metabolic demand of the body.[1] The hemodynamic profile of the HFpEF patient is interesting because it arises from a complex interplay of cardiac function, neurohumoral activation, arterial vascular tree, and pulmonary circulation; all of which are affected in this heterogenous syndrome.

With growing concerns of increasing prevalence and high morbidity and mortality,[2,3] a substantial proportion of patients is to be expected in the outpatient setting. This warrants cheap and readily available investigations of hemodynamics and intracardiac volume status to minimize the use of invasive measures and functional testing. It is important because many patients with dyspnea go undiagnosed for long periods of time. Although the gold standard for hemodynamic assessment is

Conflicts of interest: none.
[a] Department of Cardiology, Copenhagen University Hospital Gentofte, Hjertemedicinsk Forskning 2, Gentofte Hospital, Gentofte Hospitalsvej 8, 3. sal, Post 835, 2900 Hellerup, Copenhagen, Denmark; [b] Department of Biomedical Sciences, Faculty of Health and Medical Sciences, University of Copenhagen, Denmark; [c] Department of Biomedical Sciences, Faculty of Health and Medical Sciences, University of Copenhagen, Copenhagen, Denmark; [d] Cardiovascular Non-Invasive Imaging Research Laboratory, Department of Cardiology, Herlev & Gentofte Hospital, Copenhagen, Denmark
* Corresponding author. Department of Cardiology, Copenhagen University Hospital Gentofte, Hjertemedicinsk Forskning 2, Gentofte Hospital, Gentofte Hospitalsvej 8, 3. sal, Post 835, 2900 Hellerup, Copenhagen, Denmark.
E-mail addresses: Tor.Biering-Soerensen@regionh.dk; tor.biering.sorensen@alumni.harvard.edu; tobs@sund.ku.dk

Heart Failure Clin 17 (2021) 423–434
https://doi.org/10.1016/j.hfc.2021.02.006
1551-7136/21/© 2021 Elsevier Inc. All rights reserved.

heart catherization, and functional testing is essential in unmasking insufficient response to exercise, important information is to be gained from a noninvasive hemodynamic assessment of HFpEF at rest. Transthoracic echocardiography remains the most important investigation and, as evident from the name of the disease, is essential in the initials steps to establish the diagnosis.

The application of Doppler modality allows for a thorough hemodynamic evaluation of the left ventricle (LV), right ventricle (RV), and pulmonary function (**Fig. 1**, **Table 1**). In addition, the investigation is safe without adverse risk, whereas invasive measures are associated with an increased risk of infection and cardiac complications, such as perforation and tamponade. Moreover, not all patients are able to complete functional exercise testing. Thus, this review focuses on contemporary trends in the hemodynamic evaluation of HFpEF with focus being on measures attainable through transthoracic echocardiography.

SYSTOLIC PULMONARY ARTERY PRESSURE AND PULMONARY HYPERTENSION

It is well established that pulmonary hypertension (PH) is prevalent in HFpEF and is associated with an unfavorable prognosis.[4,5] It is now commonly referred to as PH associated with left heart disease, or group 2 PH,[6] where HFpEF represents a distinct clinical phenotype within this group.[7] This group has been identified as being older with several comorbidities and a higher symptomatic burden.[8] Hemodynamic measures obtained by echocardiography are relevant when screening pulmonary function through the right heart (RV)

and has shown good reliability with invasive monitoring.[9]

PH is evaluated based on pressure estimates from the right heart and has historically been defined as having a mean pulmonary artery pressure (mPAP) of 25 mm Hg or a systolic pulmonary artery pressure (sPAP) greater than 35 mm Hg.[6] The pressure gradient across the tricuspid valve is approximated by continuous wave Doppler measuring the maximal tricuspid regurgitation (TR) jet velocity using the simplified Bernoulli equation.[10] Adding the right atrial (RA) pressure to the gradient across the tricuspid valve allows for the calculation of the systolic artery pressure if no pulmonic stenosis is present, which is then also equal to the RV systolic pressure. A simplified approach is using the maximum TR velocity as the main variable to approximate the likelihood of an increased sPAP and thus PH, which is recommended in the 2015 European Society of Cardiology/European Respiratory Society guidelines for the diagnosis of PH.[6] If the value is greater than 3.4 m/s, no other supplementary measures are needed for the diagnosis.

The diagnosis of PH is usually reported by the mPAP from invasive assessments. This measure can also be obtained noninvasively through the velocity time integral (VTI) from the TR velocity or using empirical formulas (mPAP = 0.61* sPAP + 2 mm Hg).[11] However, a common problem is that a suitable TR jet is not obtainable during the echocardiographic examination. A measure that might aid in this situation is the pulmonary artery acceleration time measured in the RV outflow tract by pulsed wave Doppler. From the acceleration time, mPAP can them be calculated from the Mahan equation.[12] A value of less than 100 ms is indicative elevated

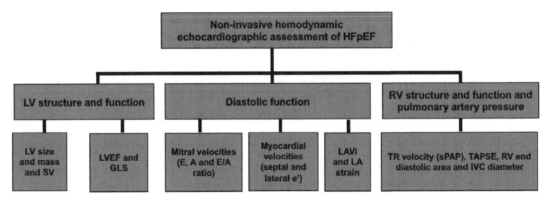

Fig. 1. Echocardiographic measures in the assessment of HFpEF at rest. A suggestion for a simple approach for evaluating HFpEF patients with measures that provide diagnostic and prognostic information in combination with novel indices. A, peak transmitral late diastolic inflow velocity; E, peak transmitral early diastolic inflow velocity; e', average peak early diastolic mitral annular velocity; GLS, global longitudinal strain; LA, left atrial; LAVI, left atrial volume index; LVEF, left ventricular ejection fraction; sPAP, systolic pulmonary artery pressure; SV, stroke volume; TAPSE, tricuspid annular plane systolic excursion; TR, tricuspid regurgitation.

Table 1
Prevalence and prognostic information of selected reviewed echocardiographic measures related to hemodynamic assessment in HFpEF

Measures	Hemodynamic Remark	Abnormal Investigation	Prevalence in HFpEF[a]	Diagnostic Property	Prognostic Remarks
mPAP	mPAP = .61*sPAP + 2 mm Hg or using TR VTI.	>20–25 mm Hg	—	PH-HFpEF	Associated with mortality when obtained invasively[16]
sPAP	sPAP = 4 (TR velocity)^2 + RAP Can also be approximated by PAAT	>35 mm Hg	25%–83%[5,15]	PH-HFpEF	Associated with combined end point of CV death and hospitalization[15] and all-cause mortality[5]
TR velocity	RV/RA gradient + RAP = sPAP	>2.8–2.9 m/s	31%–36%[15,44]	DD and PH	Associated with hospitalization and CV death[15,36]
TAPSE/sPAP	Index of RV to pulmonary circulation coupling	<0.35 mm/mm Hg (the lower tertile associated with worse outcome[17])	—	Pulmonary artery compliance	Associated with combined end point of death and hospitalization[17]
EPLAR	TRvmax/(E/e') index of transpulmonary gradient	—	—	Isolated postcapillary PH[18]	—
IVC diameter	Used for estimation of RAP	>2.1 cm and collapse <50% = RAP 15 mm Hg (range, 10–15)	19%[15]	sPAP; PH-HFpEF	Associated with total hospitalization and CV death, but not incident[15]
LA reservoir strain	Equal to peak longitudinal LA strain	Reservoir <22.7%	—	LA chamber stiffness	Associated with combined end point including death[46,47]
RVEDA	—	>24 (men); >20 (women)	39%[15]	RV pressure overload	Associated with combined end point of CV death and hospitalization[15]

(continued on next page)

Table 1
(continued)

Measures	Hemodynamic Remark	Abnormal Investigation	Prevalence in HFpEF[a]	Diagnostic Property	Prognostic Remarks
RV wall thickness	—	>5 mm	34%[21]	RV hypertrophy and overload	Associated with CV hospitalization and death[21]
TAPSE	Measure of global systolic RV function	<16 mm	28%–31%[4,15]	RV dysfunction	Univariably associated with outcome in meta-analysis,[4] not associated with outcome in PARAGON fully adjusted model[15]
GLS	Angle independent measure of global systolic function	≤16%	54.3%[22]	Systolic dysfunction	Associated with all-cause mortality in acute HFpEF[23]
SV	Derived from the LVOT VTI in combination with LVOT diameter	<35 mL/m²	37%[28]	Low-flow phenotype	VTI LVOT associated with worse outcome in hospitalized patients[28]
E wave	Marker of early diastolic LV suction	—	—	DD and LAP	Associated with combined end point of CV death and hospitalization[15]
A wave	Marker of atrial kick in late diastole	—	—	DD and LAP	Associated with combined end point of CV death and hospitalization[15]
E/e'	LAP calculated empirically: 1.9 + 1.24 E/e'	>14	53%[15]	DD and LAP	Lateral and septal E/e' associated with combined end point of CV death and hospitalization.[15]
RV E/e'	mRAP surrogate marker of LV filling pressure	—	—	—	Associated with outcome in patients with indeterminate LV filling pressure[39]

LAVi	Marker of LAP	>58 (men); >52 (women)	46%–59%[15,44]	DD and LAP	Not associated with outcome in PARAGON[15]
LVMi	Measures used to obtain LVMi can further classify into concentric or eccentric LV hypertrophy	>115 (men); >95 (women)	52%[44]	LV hypertrophy	Associated with outcome in PARAGON and I-PRESERVE[15,28]

Abbreviations: A, peak transmitral late diastolic inflow velocity; CV, cardiovascular; DD, diastolic dysfunction; E, peak transmitral early diastolic inflow velocity; e′, average peak early diastolic mitral annular velocity; ePLAR, echocardiographic pulmonary to left atrial ratio; FAC, fractional area change; HFpEF, heart failure with preserved ejection fraction; IVC, inferior vena cava; LA, left atrial; LAP, left atrial pressure; LAVi, left atrial volume index; LV, left ventricular; LVMi, left ventricular mass index; LVOT, Left ventricular outflow tract; mPAP, mean pulmonary artery pressure; mRAP, mean RA pressure; PAAT, pulmonary artery acceleration time; PH, pulmonary hypertension; RA, right atrial; RAP, right atrial pressure; RV, Right ventricular; RVEDA, right ventricle end-diastolic area; sPAP, systolic pulmonary artery pressure; SV, stroke volume; TAPSE, tricuspid annular plane systolic excursion; TR, tricuspid regurgitation; VTI, velocity time integral.

^a Reported by echocardiography.

pulmonary arterial (PA) pressure[12] and it has also been shown to be associated with sPAP estimated from the TR velocity.[13] Thus, because the measure is routinely obtained without difficulties, it may be a reliable way to estimate the pulmonary pressure in HFpEF. However, there has not been a specific study looking to validate the measure in large HFpEF cohorts.

PREVALENCE OF PULMONARY HYPERTENSION IN HEART FAILURE WITH PRESERVED EJECTION FRACTION BY ECHOCARDIOGRAPHY

Different reports have estimated the prevalence of PH in HFpEF by using noninvasive echocardiographic measures. Lam and colleagues[5] found that 83% had PH defined as having sPAP greater than 35 mm Hg in 244 HFpEF patients.[5]

It is well established that PA pressure increases with age and other comorbidities.[14] Nevertheless, in a subanalysis in the study from Lam and colleagues,[5] the authors found that HFpEF patients had high measures of sPAP even when excluding patients with chronic pulmonary obstructive disease and adjusting for age. In addition, increasing sPAP was associated with higher mortality. In contrast, results from approximately 500 HFpEF patients from the PARAGON study found a lower prevalence estimate of PH of 25%.[15] However, a definition of PH was used with sPAP greater than 39 mm Hg. The true prevalence is probably somewhere between those estimates, which is confirmed by a meta-analysis by Gorter and colleagues[4] who found a PH prevalence of 68%. Thus, PH must be considered a common finding by Doppler echocardiography and this is also replicated when conducting invasive right heart catherization.[16]

NOVEL MEASURES IN PULMONARY HYPERTENSION AND HEART FAILURE WITH PRESERVED EJECTION FRACTION

It has been suggested to combine sPAP with the tricuspid annular systolic plane excursion (TAPSE) to quantify the RV pulmonary circulation coupling, and it has been shown that a lower ratio of TAPSE/sPAP is independently associated with worse outcome in HFpEF.[17] It is a potential useful measure because it combines RV contractile function with pulmonary hemodynamic estimates. Another measure that has been proposed to identify PH of left-sided origin or postcapillary, is the echocardiographic pulmonary to left atrial (LA) ratio (TR velocity/[E/e']). In 133 patients with PH (including HFpEF patients), lower value of echocardiographic pulmonary to LA ratio was associated with isolated postcapillary PH,[18] which is the form thought to be present in HFpEF. This may be useful to separate patients that have PH because of pathology of the pulmonary vasculature from HFpEF patients with PH originating because of backward failure of the LV.

CENTRAL VENOUS PRESSURE

Estimation of the central venous pressure, corresponding to the RA pressure, is an important component in the noninvasive hemodynamic assessment of HFpEF. In addition, it is used for the calculation of the pulmonary artery pressures previously discussed.

It is most commonly calculated by measuring the diameter of the inferior vena cava and registering the presence of inspiratory collapse. A dilated inferior vena cava that does not collapse on inspiration is suggestive of increased RA pressure. In the acute setting, insights from the MEDIA-DHF study showed that patients with exacerbations of HFpEF have venous congestion similar to those with heart failure with reduced ejection fraction (HFrEF) as evident of enlarged inferior vena cava diameter and right atria.[19] In contrast, a study by Thenappan and colleagues[8] found that PH-related HFpEF patients have less frequent right atrial enlargement compared with having pure pulmonary artery hypertension.

RIGHT VENTRICLE STRUCTURE AND FUNCTION

Although not directly related to hemodynamic measures, an evaluation of right heart chamber dilation and septal flattening should be made to gauge the likelihood of underlying chronic pathology and RV overload. Reports have shown that RV diastolic area can increase 21% in 4 years in HFpEF patients, and that this increase is associated with higher sPAP and RV dilation at baseline.[20] Furthermore, RV diastolic area was among the measures that were associated with the composite end point of heart failure hospitalization and cardiovascular death in the echocardiographic study of the PARAGON trial.[15] In addition, RV free wall thickness (>5 mm) has been shown to be prevalent and strongly associated with outcome.[21] Although the role of RV diastolic function in HFpEF is less clear, RV dysfunction is frequently seen. A meta-analysis of 38 studies found abnormal TAPSE to be the most common marker of RV dysfunction with a prevalence of 28% and significantly associated with outcome.[4]

Thus, an evaluation of right heart beyond quantifying PA pressures is advisable.

SYSTOLIC LEFT VENTRICLE FUNCTION AND HEART FAILURE WITH PRESERVED EJECTION FRACTION

The systolic function of the LV must be considered closely related to the hemodynamic profile in HFpEF. Strain analysis by two-dimensional speckle tracking has gained attention in recent decades because it allows for more subtle detection of LV abnormalities. Specifically, the measure global longitudinal strain (GLS) has been applied to HFpEF patients with success in detecting LV dysfunction and has been shown to be related to poor outcome.[22,23] Thus, the notion that systolic function is normal in HFpEF has been abandoned through these reports. The physiologic properties of strain analysis were investigated by Biering-Sørensen and coworkers in 85 patients with unexplained dyspnea, and showed that lower absolute values of GLS at rest was associated with higher LV pressures during exercise measured invasively.[24] In contrast, higher value of circumferential strain at rest was associated with greater increase in filling pressures during exercise. Intriguingly, the ratio between longitudinal and circumferential strain was the strongest predictor of PH during exercise.

Although the clinical applicability of the strain deformation imaging is not completely accounted for, the technique holds promise with novel multilayer strain assessments, which allows for even more precise detection of regional systolic abnormalities.

SYSTOLIC FUNCTION BY DOPPLER ECHOCARDIOGRAPHY

Systolic function as assessed by noninvasive Doppler echocardiography is less widely applied at rest. A hallmark of HFpEF is exercise intolerance and indeed invasive studies have shown a blunted increase in cardiac output and stroke volume in response to exercise stimulation with no difference at rest.[25] At rest, stroke volume and cardiac output are easily obtained from the Doppler VTI of the left ventricular outflow tract (LVOT) in combination with the LVOT diameter and heart rate. One advantage with this method is that one can also quantify the AV velocity from the continuous wave VTI, which has been shown to be a prognosticator in HPpEF.[15]

Stroke volume has been reported within the normal range when obtained through Doppler echocardiography at rest in HFpEF.[26] However, cardiac output obtained invasively has been shown to differentiate patients with PH-related HFpEF from pulmonary arterial hypertension.[8] In addition, insights from the RELAX trial identified a low-flow phenotype of HFpEF as defined by a stroke volume less than 35 mL/m^2 with a prevalence of 37% among the study participants.[27] This was further investigated in a study population of 214 hospitalized HFpEF patients where lower VTI of the LVOT at admission was associated with worse outcome.[28] Thus, the measures might become more relevant in the future where therapy may be guided in accordance to the specific phenotype of HFpEF.[29]

DIASTOLIC DYSFUNCTION

Diastolic dysfunction (DD) is largely defined as the heart's inability to fill sufficiently because of impaired relaxation and/or increased stiffness of the cardiac chamber walls.[30,31] The diagnosis of HFpEF has previously interchangeably been referred to as "diastolic heart failure" or "heart failure with DD,"[32] and DD has been viewed as the causal factor in the presence of preserved systolic function.[33] We now recognize DD as a separate entity in the HFpEF disease spectrum that often, but not always, is prevalent. Ultimately, it is still an important part of the hemodynamic assessment that presents diagnostic and prognostic information.

Estimating filling pressures has been a primary focus in the evaluation of diastolic function. Noninvasive left-sided filling pressures, such as the LV end-diastolic pressure, is estimated through diastolic Doppler measurements. The corresponding invasive measurement is the pulmonary artery wedge pressure, which is also equivalent to the LA pressure if no significant valve stenosis or insufficiency is present in the LV.

The mitral inflow velocities are obtained through pulsed wave Doppler. The peak early diastolic filling (E wave), caused by the rapid filling of the LV from unloading potential energy stored during systole, represents the pressure gradient between the LA and LV during early diastole. Similarly, the diastolic atrial filling from the atrial contraction represents the pressure gradient between the LA and LV in late diastole. Derivative measures, such as the E/A ratio and deacceleration time of the E-wave, are used to identify filling patterns.[34] As a consequence of impaired relaxation, the E-wave has a lower velocity and higher deacceleration time, the velocity of the atrial kick is increased, and the E/A ratio is subsequently increased. This process transpires naturally in the aging heart but may be problematic if filling pressures increases concomitantly. In HFpEF, however, it has been shown that these mitral velocities were not well correlated with LV filling pressure.[35]

TISSUE DOPPLER IMAGING AND LEFT ATRIAL FILLING PRESSURES

A modality of interest has been tissue Doppler imaging. Instead of looking at blood flow velocities, the method allows for the assessment of tissue velocities at the mitral annulus during the whole cardiac cycle, where the early relaxation and late diastolic velocities is annotated e' (e prime) and a' (a prime), respectively. The process of "active" relaxation is mirrored in the e' measure, which is followed by the aforementioned E wave. Thus, a low E wave velocity coupled with high e' tissue velocity is under normal circumstances indicative of a healthy heart. However, when the LV function starts to decline and filling pressures rise, the normal early relaxation is inhibited, and the pressure is propagated into the left atrium, and the movement of blood across the mitral valve into the LV becomes an active process powered by the left atrium. Thus, the E/e' is higher in patients with DD and higher filling pressures. An E/e' less than eight is normal and an E/e' greater than 14 is considered abnormal. Filling pressures naturally rise with age, which poses a challenge when evaluating patients with HFpEF, which is predominately a disease of the elderly. One advantage of E/e' is that the measure is less age-dependent that other diastolic measures,[34] and it is clinically widely applied as the primary noninvasive measure of LV filling pressure. In addition, the measure is also frequently associated with outcome in HFpEF.[36]

DIAGNOSIS OF DIASTOLIC DYSFUNCTION

The diagnosis of diastolic dysfunction and grading is under constant renewal and improvement. In 2016, the American Society of Echocardiography and the European Association of Cardiovascular Imaging released an updated recommendation.[34] Two schemes are presented, one for diagnosing DD when LV ejection fraction is normal and no cardiac disease is suspected, the other to diagnose DD and estimate LV filling pressures (LA pressure) in patients with depressed or preserved LV ejection fraction and concurrent cardiac disease (**Fig. 2**). In HFpEF, the algorithm has subsequently been proven useful for estimating the risk of hospitalizations and cardiac mortality.[37]

One challenge with the diastolic grading algorithm is that it places some patients in the category of indeterminate LA pressure.[34] In these patients it might be useful to assess the mean RA pressure, which is estimated with reasonable accuracy through tissue Doppler imaging by using early tricuspid inflow velocity in relation to the lateral RV annulus myocardial velocity (E/e' for RV).[38] Mele and colleagues[39] have suggested to reclassify these patients based on the mean RA pressure, because they show this measure is associated with outcome in hospitalized HF patients with in indeterminate LA pressure, but not in patients with normal or increased LA pressure.

Recently, a meta-analysis sought to investigate the evidence behind the diastolic parameters recommended in currents guidelines, and they showed that E/e' was most established, but contrary to previous reports, the relationship with

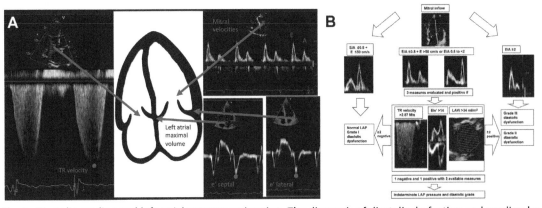

Fig. 2. Diastolic grading and left atrial pressure estimation. The diagnosis of diastolic dysfuction and grading by the recommendation of the American Society of Echocardiography and the European Association of Cardiovascular Imaging. (*A*) Echocardiographic target areas for the measures used in the algorithm. (*B*) Examples to help follow the diagnosis and grading diastolic dysfunction and left atrial pressure are presented following the algorithm. A, peak transmitral late diastolic inflow velocity; E, peak transmitral early diastolic inflow velocity; e', average peak early diastolic mitral annular velocity; LAP, left atrial pressure; LAVi, left atrial volume index.

fillings pressures was only shown to be modest.[40] However, a novel method of estimating the filling pressure by using the ratio of the early diastolic strain rate tissue velocity obtained by speckle tracking echocardiography has shown promising results by being an independent prognosticator in HFrEF[41] and is associated with LV filling pressure.[42] This measure might also prove to be a useful prognosticator in HFpEF, although this has not yet been investigated in this population.

PREVALENCE OF DIASTOLIC DYSFUNCTION IN HEART FAILURE WITH PRESERVED EJECTION FRACTION

When estimating the prevalence of DD in the literature, the fact that the grading of diastolic function has changed over time becomes a challenge. Insights from the echocardiographic substudy of CHARMES have shown that only around two-thirds of patients with HFpEF have DD.[43] Nevertheless, more severe grading of DD was associated with poor prognosis. These finding are supported in data from the TOPCAT trial that found 66% of the population with HFpEF had DD[44] and 69% in the I-PRESERVE study.[26] However, common for these studies is that they used gradings criteria for DD that relied mainly on mitral inflow and filling patterns. The prevalence must be held in comparison with contemporary analyses in the general population. In the ARIC-study of community-dwelling elders older than the age of 65 and free of HF, the prevalence of having at least one abnormal diastolic measure among e', E/e', and LA volume index (LAVi) was found to be 96% based on guidelines-specific cutoffs.[45]

However, using age-specific cutoff derived from the cohort reclassified 46% of the participants as having normal diastolic function. Thus, taking age into account when evaluating DD is advisable to prevent falsely overestimating the prevalence.

ATRIAL STRAIN IN HEART FAILURE WITH PRESERVED EJECTION FRACTION

Atrial strain by speckle tracking is performed in HFpEF patients and gives information of the three LA functions of (1) pump, (2) reservoir, and (3) conduit. It has been shown in a meta-analysis that all three functions are depressed compared with healthy control subjects as assessed by atrial strain.[46] In addition, a study by Freed and colleagues[47] found especially reservoir function associated with outcome in fully adjusted multivariable models including measures of LV function. However, a study by Santos and colleagues[48] found the prognostic role less clear when adjusting

for LV systolic function and filling pressure, which seem to eliminate the prognostic signal from atrial strain in their HFpEF cohort.

LEFT HEART CARDIAC CHAMBERS

The morphology of LV cardiac chambers gives away important information related to chronic and acute pathology in HFpEF. The left atrium is subject to increased filling pressures, which results in subsequent remodeling and expansion of the cardiac chamber.[34] The echocardiographic measure of LAVi is part of suggested diagnostic criteria for HFpEF together with LV mass index (LVMi),[49] and both were used as inclusion criteria in the PARAGON trial.[15] As evident, LAVi holds an important place in the diagnostic work-up, but has generally not been reported as a significant prognosticator.[15,36] Contrarily to the LA, when looking at the LV, the usual finding is a nondilated chamber. Nevertheless, concentric hypertrophy of the LV is prevalent in HFpEF and increased LVMi was found to be 52% in the TOPCAT trial.[44]

DIAGNOSTIC ALGORITHMS OF HEART FAILURE WITH PRESERVED EJECTION FRACTION

Diagnostic algorithms that estimate the probability of having HFpEF have in recent years been proposed to aid in the diagnosis.[50,51] Common for these algorithms is that they all include a practical assessment of right and left heart measures by echocardiography. In 2019, the Heart Failure Association of the European Society of Cardiology released a consensus recommendation presenting the HFA–PEFF diagnostic algorithm.[50] A standard echocardiography to assess LV ejection fraction is included in this first step. The second step entails comprehensive echocardiography functional hemodynamic measures including the septal and lateral e', E/e' ratio, TR velocity, sPAP, and morphologic measures including LAVi and LVMi. Interestingly, the deformation parameter GLS is included as a minor criterium. Depending on the calculated score, HFpEF is either reliably diagnosed or further advanced functional or invasive testing is needed. A more simplistic approach is found in the H_2FPEF algorithm, which relies on six variables to assign a score ranging from 0 to 9 corresponding to the probability of having HFpEF. Two hemodynamic parameters are included: E/e', where a ratio of greater than nine elicits one-point; and an sPAP greater than 35 mm Hg elicits one point. Both diagnostic algorithms has been validated in the ARIC cohort and shown to be predictive of poor outcome,[52] and may therefore be a useful tool in clinical practice.

SUMMARY

Echocardiography holds a central place in the evaluation of HFpEF patients. The attainable measures of the hemodynamic profile provide information that aids in establishing the diagnosis of HFpEF and gives valuable prognostic information. Although a vast amount of literature exists on the topic of noninvasive evaluation of HFpEF patients at rest, it is important to emphasize the complexity of the syndrome, which often warrants multiple investigations across clinical, paraclinical, and imaging modalities. In addition, studies with head-to-head comparison of conventional and novel echocardiographic parameters are warranted to elucidate the prognosticators of highest value in HFpEF.

CLINICS CARE POINTS

- Pulmonary hypertension is highly prevalent, and systolic pulmonary artery pressure is a strong prognosticator in HFpEF
- Estimation of filling pressure by E/e' still holds a central place in the grading of diastolic dysfunction and is included in all suggested diagnostic algorithms for HFpEF
- Measures of systolic function beyond LV ejection fraction has proven useful in phenotyping and risk assessment
- Structural abnormalities as an indicator of maladaptive response to hemodynamic alterations is found in the right and left heart

DISCLOSURE

T. Biering-Sørensen: Steering Committee member of the Amgen financed GALACTIC-HF trial. Advisory Board: Sanofi Pasteur. Advisory Board: Amgen. Speaker Honorarium: Novartis. Speaker Honorarium: Sanofi Pasteur; Research grant: GE Healthcare (Norway). Research grant: Sanofi Pasteur. M. Sengeløv: None.

REFERENCES

1. Denolin H, Kuhn H, Krayenbuehl HP, et al. The definition of heart failure. Eur Heart J 1983;4(7):445–8.
2. Bhatia RS, Tu JV, Lee DS, et al. Outcome of heart failure with preserved ejection fraction in a population-based study. N Engl J Med 2006; 355(3):260–9.
3. Owan TE, Hodge DO, Herges RM, et al. Trends in prevalence and outcome of heart failure with preserved ejection fraction. N Engl J Med 2006; 355(3):251–9.
4. Gorter TM, Hoendermis ES, van Veldhuisen DJ, et al. Right ventricular dysfunction in heart failure with preserved ejection fraction: a systematic review and meta-analysis. Eur J Heart Fail 2016;18(12): 1472–87.
5. Lam CSP, Roger VL, Rodeheffer RJ, et al. Pulmonary hypertension in heart failure with preserved ejection fraction: a community-based study. J Am Coll Cardiol 2009;53(13):1119–26.
6. Galiè N, Humbert M, Vachiery J-L, et al. 2015 ESC/ERS guidelines for the diagnosis and treatment of pulmonary hypertension: the Joint Task Force for the Diagnosis and Treatment of Pulmonary Hypertension of the European Society of Cardiology (ESC) and the European Respiratory Society (ERS) Endorsed by Association for European Paediatric and Congenital Cardiology (AEPC), International Society for Heart and Lung Transplantation (ISHLT). Eur Respir J 2015;46(4):903–75.
7. Vachiéry J-L, Tedford RJ, Rosenkranz S, et al. Pulmonary hypertension due to left heart disease. Eur Respir J 2019;53(1). https://doi.org/10.1183/13993003.01897-2018.
8. Thenappan T, Shah SJ, Gomberg-Maitland M, et al. Clinical characteristics of pulmonary hypertension in patients with heart failure and preserved ejection fraction. Circ Heart Fail 2011;4(3):257–65.
9. de Scordilli M, Pinamonti B, Albani S, et al. Reliability of noninvasive hemodynamic assessment with Doppler echocardiography: comparison with the invasive evaluation. J Cardiovasc Med 2019; 20(10):682–90.
10. Rudski LG, Lai WW, Afilalo J, et al. Guidelines for the echocardiographic assessment of the right heart in adults: a report from the American Society of Echocardiography endorsed by the European Association of Echocardiography, a registered branch of the European Society of Cardiology, and the Canadian Society of Echocardiography. J Am Soc Echocardiogr 2010;23(7):685–713 [quiz: 786–8].
11. Chemla D, Castelain V, Humbert M, et al. New formula for predicting mean pulmonary artery pressure using systolic pulmonary artery pressure. Chest 2004;126(4):1313–7.
12. Dabestani A, Mahan G, Gardin JM, et al. Evaluation of pulmonary artery pressure and resistance by pulsed Doppler echocardiography. Am J Cardiol 1987;59(6):662–8.
13. Yared K, Noseworthy P, Weyman AE, et al. Pulmonary artery acceleration time provides an accurate estimate of systolic pulmonary arterial pressure during transthoracic echocardiography. J Am Soc Echocardiogr 2011;24(6):687–92.

14. Armstrong DW, Tsimiklis G, Matangi MF. Factors influencing the echocardiographic estimate of right ventricular systolic pressure in normal patients and clinically relevant ranges according to age. Can J Cardiol 2010;26(2):e35–9.

15. Shah AM, Cikes M, Prasad N, et al. Echocardiographic features of patients with heart failure and preserved left ventricular ejection fraction. J Am Coll Cardiol 2019;74(23):2858–73.

16. Vanderpool RR, Saul M, Nouraie M, et al. Association between hemodynamic markers of pulmonary hypertension and outcomes in heart failure with preserved ejection fraction. JAMA Cardiol 2018;3(4):298–306.

17. Guazzi M, Dixon D, Labate V, et al. RV contractile function and its coupling to pulmonary circulation in heart failure with preserved ejection fraction. JACC Cardiovasc Imaging 2017;10(10):1211–21.

18. Scalia GM, Scalia IG, Kierle R, et al. ePLAR: the echocardiographic pulmonary to left atrial ratio. A novel non-invasive parameter to differentiate pre-capillary and post-capillary pulmonary hypertension. Int J Cardiol 2016;212:379–86.

19. Van Aelst LNL, Arrigo M, Placido R, et al. Acutely decompensated heart failure with preserved and reduced ejection fraction present with comparable haemodynamic congestion. Eur J Heart Fail 2018;20(4):738–47.

20. Obokata M, Reddy YNV, Melenovsky V, et al. Deterioration in right ventricular structure and function over time in patients with heart failure and preserved ejection fraction. Eur Heart J 2019;40(8):689–97.

21. Burke MA, Katz DH, Beussink L, et al. Prognostic importance of pathophysiologic markers in patients with heart failure and preserved ejection fraction. Circ Heart Fail 2014;7(2):288–99.

22. Kraigher-Krainer E, Shah AM, Gupta DK, et al. Impaired systolic function by strain imaging in heart failure with preserved ejection fraction. J Am Coll Cardiol 2014;63(5):447–56.

23. Park JJ, Park J-B, Park J-H, et al. Global longitudinal strain to predict mortality in patients with acute heart failure. J Am Coll Cardiol 2018;71(18):1947–57.

24. Biering-Sørensen T, Santos M, Rivero J, et al. Left ventricular deformation at rest predicts exercise-induced elevation in pulmonary artery wedge pressure in patients with unexplained dyspnoea. Eur J Heart Fail 2017;19(1):101–10.

25. Abudiab MM, Redfield MM, Melenovsky V, et al. Cardiac output response to exercise in relation to metabolic demand in heart failure with preserved ejection fraction. Eur J Heart Fail 2013;15(7):776–85.

26. Zile MR, Gottdiener JS, Hetzel SJ, et al. Prevalence and significance of alterations in cardiac structure and function in patients with heart failure and a preserved ejection fraction. Circulation 2011;124(23):2491–501.

27. Patel KV, Mauricio R, Grodin JL, et al. Identifying a low-flow phenotype in heart failure with preserved ejection fraction: a secondary analysis of the RELAX trial. ESC Heart Fail 2019;6(4):613–20.

28. Omote K, Nagai T, Iwano H, et al. Left ventricular outflow tract velocity time integral in hospitalized heart failure with preserved ejection fraction. ESC Heart Fail 2019;7(1):167–75.

29. Shah Sanjiv J, Kitzman Dalane W, Borlaug Barry A, et al. Phenotype-specific treatment of heart failure with preserved ejection fraction. Circulation 2016;134(1):73–90.

30. Borlaug BA, Kass DA. Mechanisms of diastolic dysfunction in heart failure. Trends Cardiovasc Med 2006;16(8):273–9.

31. Brutsaert DL, Sys SU, Gillebert TC. Diastolic failure: pathophysiology and therapeutic implications. J Am Coll Cardiol 1993;22(1):318–25.

32. Vasan RS, Levy D. Defining diastolic heart failure. Circulation 2000;101(17):2118–21.

33. Zile MR, Baicu CF, Gaasch WH. Diastolic heart failure: abnormalities in active relaxation and passive stiffness of the left ventricle. N Engl J Med 2004;350(19):1953–9.

34. Nagueh SF, Smiseth OA, Appleton CP, et al. Recommendations for the evaluation of left ventricular diastolic function by echocardiography: an update from the American Society of Echocardiography and the European Association of Cardiovascular Imaging. J Am Soc Echocardiogr 2016;29(4):277–314.

35. Yamamoto K, Nishimura RA, Chaliki HP, et al. Determination of left ventricular filling pressure by Doppler echocardiography in patients with coronary artery disease: critical role of left ventricular systolic function. J Am Coll Cardiol 1997;30(7):1819–26.

36. Shah AM, Claggett B, Sweitzer NK, et al. Cardiac structure and function and prognosis in heart failure with preserved ejection fraction: findings from the echocardiographic study of the Treatment of Preserved Cardiac Function Heart Failure with an Aldosterone Antagonist (TOPCAT) Trial. Circ Heart Fail 2014;7(5):740–51.

37. Torii Y, Kusunose K, Yamada H, et al. Updated left ventricular diastolic function recommendations and cardiovascular events in patients with heart failure hospitalization. J Am Soc Echocardiogr 2019;32(10):1286–97.e2.

38. Nageh MF, Kopelen HA, Zoghbi WA, et al. Estimation of mean right atrial pressure using tissue Doppler imaging. Am J Cardiol 1999;84(12):1448–51.

39. Mele D, Pestelli G, Molin DD, et al. Right atrial pressure is associated with outcomes in patients with heart failure and indeterminate left ventricular filling pressure. J Am Soc Echocardiogr 2020;33(11):1345–56.

40. Nauta JF, Hummel YM, van der Meer P, et al. Correlation with invasive left ventricular filling pressures

and prognostic relevance of the echocardiographic diastolic parameters used in the 2016 ESC heart failure guidelines and in the 2016 ASE/EACVI recommendations: a systematic review in patients with heart failure with preserved ejection fraction. Eur J Heart Fail 2018;20(9):1303–11.

41. Lassen MCH, Sengeløv M, Qasim A, et al. Ratio of transmitral early filling velocity to early diastolic strain rate predicts all-cause mortality in heart failure with reduced ejection fraction. J Card Fail 2019. https://doi.org/10.1016/j.cardfail.2019.07.007.

42. Wang J, Khoury DS, Thohan V, et al. Global diastolic strain rate for the assessment of left ventricular relaxation and filling pressures. Circulation 2007; 115(11):1376–83.

43. Persson H, Lonn E, Edner M, et al. Diastolic dysfunction in heart failure with preserved systolic function: need for objective evidence: results from the CHARM Echocardiographic Substudy–CHARMES. J Am Coll Cardiol 2007;49(6):687–94.

44. Shah AM, Shah SJ, Anand IS, et al. Cardiac structure and function in heart failure with preserved ejection fraction: baseline findings from the echocardiographic study of the Treatment of Preserved Cardiac Function Heart Failure with an Aldosterone Antagonist trial. Circ Heart Fail 2014;7(1): 104–15.

45. Shah AM, Claggett B, Kitzman D, et al. Contemporary assessment of left ventricular diastolic function in older adults: the atherosclerosis risk in communities study. Circulation 2017;135(5):426–39.

46. Khan MS, Memon MM, Murad MH, et al. Left atrial function in heart failure with preserved ejection fraction: a systematic review and meta-analysis. Eur J Heart Fail 2020;22(3):472–85.

47. Freed BH, Daruwalla V, Cheng JY, et al. Prognostic utility and clinical significance of cardiac mechanics in heart failure with preserved ejection fraction. Circ Cardiovasc Imaging 2016;9(3):e003754.

48. Santos ABS, Roca GQ, Claggett B, et al. The prognostic relevance of left atrial dysfunction in heart failure with preserved ejection fraction. Circ Heart Fail 2016; 9(4). https://doi.org/10.1161/CIRCHEARTFAILURE. 115.002763.

49. Ponikowski P, Voors AA, Anker SD, et al. 2016 ESC guidelines for the diagnosis and treatment of acute and chronic heart failure. The Task Force for the diagnosis and treatment of acute and chronic heart failure of the European Society of Cardiology (ESC) Developed with the special contribution of the Heart Failure Association (HFA) of the ESC. Eur Heart J 2016;37(27):2129–200.

50. Pieske B, Tschöpe C, de Boer RA, et al. How to diagnose heart failure with preserved ejection fraction: the HFA–PEFF diagnostic algorithm: a consensus recommendation from the Heart Failure Association (HFA) of the European Society of Cardiology (ESC). Eur Heart J 2019;40(40):3297–317.

51. Reddy YNV, Carter RE, Obokata M, et al. A simple, evidence-based approach to help guide diagnosis of heart failure with preserved ejection fraction. Circulation 2018;138(9):861–70.

52. Selvaraj S, Myhre PL, Vaduganathan M, et al. Application of diagnostic algorithms for heart failure with preserved ejection fraction to the community. JACC Heart Fail 2020;8(8):640–53.

Stress Testing in Heart Failure with Preserved Ejection Fraction

Chi Young Shim, MD, PhD

KEYWORDS

- Heart failure - Preserved ejection fraction - Stress - Echocardiography

KEY POINTS

- Stress testing provides crucial information for the diagnosis of heart failure (HF) with preserved ejection fraction (EF) before the advanced stage.
- Among various stress tests, noninvasive supine bicycle diastolic stress echocardiography has provided the most evidence for diagnosing and predicting the prognosis of HF with preserved EF by evaluating exercise E/e′ and exercise pulmonary artery systolic pressure.
- Preload augmentation by passive leg raising or treadmill exercise echocardiography can be used as an alternative method for supine bicycle diastolic stress echocardiography.
- During the subclinical stage of HF, the assessment of diastolic functional reserve is helpful for the early detection and intervention of the risk of future HF.

INTRODUCTION

Heart failure (HF) is a clinical syndrome that reduces cardiac output and/or elevates the intracardiac pressures at rest or during exercise.[1] There are 4 stages in HF. Stage A is the risk of HF, whereas stage D is end-stage disease.[1,2] The classification of such a stage corresponds to HF with reduced ejection fraction (EF) as well as HF with preserved EF. There are no identified treatments that improve the outcome of HF with preserved EF. The lack of treatments may be related to the diagnostic challenges of HF with preserved EF and its frequent diagnosis at a late stage. In addition, exercise intolerance and exertional dyspnea are not specific to HF with preserved EF. Therefore, it is important to diagnose HF with preserved EF precisely, differentiate it from other disease states, and control its risk factors before it progresses to the advanced stage. In this respect, stress testing provides crucial information about the diagnosis and prognosis of HF with preserved EF before it reaches the advanced stage.

THE RATIONALE FOR STRESS TESTING TO DIAGNOSE HEART FAILURE WITH PRESERVED EJECTION FRACTION

Patients with HF with preserved EF have symptoms that are related predominantly to left ventricular (LV) diastolic dysfunction. Several alternative and complementary mechanisms are present in HF, however, with preserved EF, including longitudinal LV systolic dysfunction, pulmonary hypertension, abnormal ventricular-vascular coupling, abnormal exercise-induced vasodilation, and chronotropic incompetence.[3–5] In recent years, there have been efforts to classify HF with preserved EF into several phenotypes and to apply tailored treatment strategies.[6–9] Among the phenotypes classified based on clinical presentation, the phenotype of exercise-induced elevation of the LV filling pressure cannot be detected by resting echocardiography alone.[5,6] Moreover, several problems of resting echocardiography for diagnosing HF with preserved EF are encountered.[5,10,11] Grade 1 diastolic dysfunction on resting echocardiography is highly prevalent in

Division of Cardiology, Severance Cardiovascular Hospital, Yonsei University College of Medicine, 50-1 Yonsei-ro, Seodaemun-gu, Seoul 03722, Republic of Korea
E-mail address: cysprs@yuhs.ac

Heart Failure Clin 17 (2021) 435–445
https://doi.org/10.1016/j.hfc.2021.02.007
1551-7136/21/© 2021 Elsevier Inc. All rights reserved.

the middle-aged and elderly population.[11] Moreover, in the early stage, the left atrial pressure is elevated only when it is under exertion.[11] Even in subjects with identical impaired relaxation in resting conditions, the myocardial performance and intracardiac pressures vary during exercise.[11] In the graph showing the association between the LV end-diastolic volume and pulmonary capillary wedge pressure (LV filling pressure) suggested by Kitzman and colleagues,[12] patient A and patient B displayed very different responses during exercise, although they had similar pressure-volume relationships at rest (**Fig. 1**A). Patient A is a healthy control, whereas patient B is a patient with HF with preserved EF.[12] Compared with patient A, patient B experienced a steep increase in the pulmonary capillary wedge pressure. The LV diastolic volume does not increase any more due to impaired LV compliance.[12] In patient B, a dramatic change in the mitral inflow Doppler pattern during exercise can be confirmed on a diastolic stress echocardiogram (see **Fig. 1**B).

The second rationale for stress testing is that the mechanisms responsible for exertional dyspnea or exercise intolerance often is associated with noncardiac conditions, such as pulmonary disease; systemic disease, including anemia, systemic inflammatory disease, and neuromuscular disorder; obesity and deconditioning; and psychological disease (**Fig. 2**).[11] In particular, various causes tend to be combined in the elderly population. Therefore, it is helpful to know the main mechanisms for treatment in each individual. A comprehensive analysis of exercise hemodynamics and cardiac performance can be used to distinguish whether the cause of exertional dyspnea is due to an increase in LV filling pressure during exercise or other causes.[5,11] Therefore, performing a diastolic stress test using exercise is needed when a patient's symptoms cannot be explained completely with resting echocardiography or exercise-induced hemodynamic changes compatible with HF with preserved EF confirmed.

APPLICATION OF APPROPRIATE STRESS METHODS

Various methods of noninvasive stress tests already have been used in the field of cardiology. These methods typically are used to diagnose ischemic heart disease.[13] Noninvasive stress testing is divided into a physiologic stress testing with exercise and a pharmacologic stress testing using dobutamine, dipyridamole, or adenosine.[13] Exercise tests are more physiologic than are pharmacologic stress tests. These exercise tests are not able to unmask diastolic abnormalities that are not evident under resting conditions.[13–15] The exercise methods include treadmill exercise, upright bicycle exercise, and supine bicycle exercise. Among these methods, supine bicycle exercise echocardiography was introduced approximately 15 years ago to assess the exercise LV filling pressure noninvasively, which is the main indicator for HF with preserved EF.[11] Bicycle exercise echocardiography can reproduce patients' symptoms in daily life due to physiologic stress and detect LV diastolic dysfunction during exercise through

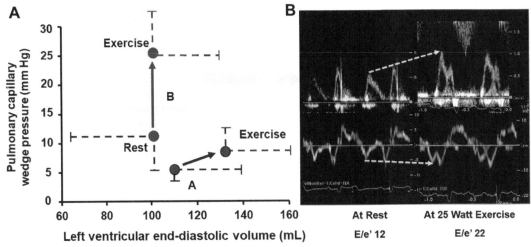

Fig. 1. LV filling pressure at rest and during exercise. (*A*) The relationship between LV end-diastolic volume and pulmonary capillary wedge pressure at rest and during exercise. (*B*) Mitral inflow and mitral annular velocities at rest and during exercise showing a remarkable increase of exercise E/e'. ([A] *Adapted from* Kitzman DW, Higginbotham MB, Cobb FR et al. Exercise intolerance in patients with heart failure with preserved left ventricular systolic function: failure of the Frank-Starling mechanism. J Am Coll Cardiol 1991:17(5);1065-72; with permission.)

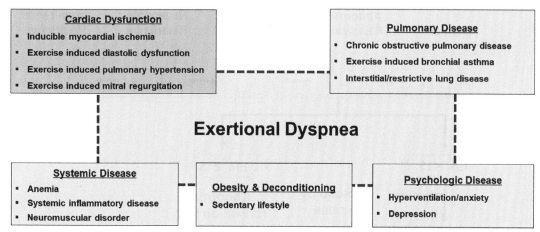

Cardiac Dysfunction
- Inducible myocardial ischemia
- Exercise induced diastolic dysfunction
- Exercise induced pulmonary hypertension
- Exercise induced mitral regurgitation

Pulmonary Disease
- Chronic obstructive pulmonary disease
- Exercise induced bronchial asthma
- Interstitial/restrictive lung disease

Exertional Dyspnea

Systemic Disease
- Anemia
- Systemic inflammatory disease
- Neuromuscular disorder

Obesity & Deconditioning
- Sedentary lifestyle

Psychologic Disease
- Hyperventilation/anxiety
- Depression

Fig. 2. Diverse etiologies of exertional dyspnea requiring differentiation from HF with preserved EF.

continuous imaging.[11] In addition, because the supine position increases myocardial wall tension and oxygen demand, it is suitable for diastolic stress.[11] An invasive stress test of exercise cardiac catheterization also can be used to diagnose HF with preserved EF using high-fidelity pressure catheters.[16–18] It is not used widely, however, given its invasive nature. In the recently released recommendations for diagnosis of HF with preserved EF, an invasive hemodynamic stress test is recommended in cases of remaining diagnostic uncertainty after stress echocardiography.[19]

ALTERNATIVE METHODS TO SUPINE BICYCLE STRESS ECHOCARDIOGRAPHY
Patients Who Have Difficulty Doing Bicycle Exercise: Preload Augmentation by Passive Leg Raising

Many patients with suspected HF with preserved EF are elderly or obese women.[20,21] Patients often are encountered who have difficulty with bicycle exercising due to knee or hip problems. Other patients are unfamiliar with the bicycle exercise itself, which makes it difficult to test their cardiac status. The passive leg-raising method is a simple way of provoking LV filling pressure elevation by preload augmentation and differentiating impaired relaxation vulnerable for HF from stable impaired relaxation (**Fig. 3**).[22] For preload augmentation, a patient's legs should be passively elevated until the femoral ischial joint is at a 60o angle for 3 minutes.[22] In a previous study, patients with E/e′ less than 15 at rest but increased E/e′ greater than 15 in the leg-raised state were older, more frequently female, had a lower diastolic functional reserve to exercise, and had lower exercise capacity compared with patients with persistent E/e′ less than 15.[22] Therefore, preload reserve can be assessed using a simple, 3-minute, passive leg-raising method. Patients with lower

preload reserves have easily increased LV filling pressures without an incremental increase in stroke volume in response to preload augmentation (such as volume loading or exercise), which induces an increase in venous return.[22]

Instiues Without Facilities of Bicycle Ergometer: Treadmil Exercise Stress Echocardiography

Stress echocardiography using a treadmill has a disadvantage in that it cannot measure the change in diastolic function at each stage of exercise. In contrast, the treadmill exercise has the advantage of detecting myocardial ischemia (a form of exercise-induced diastolic dysfunction), because the exercise workload is stronger than the supine bicycle exercise.[23,24] With regard to treadmill exercise, exercise diastolic function usually is evaluated immediately after exercise, although some studies have demonstrated data from peak treadmill exercise echocardiography. It is important to minimize the time delay in postexercise imaging of treadmill exercise echocardiography, because the diastolic dysfunction in patients without ischemia tends to normalize quickly after exercise. **Table 1** shows comparisons of the characteristics between treadmill stress echocardiography and supine bicycle exercise echocardiography for diastolic stress tests.

STRESS TESTING FOR DIAGNOSING HEART FAILURE WITH PRESERVED EJECTION FRACTION IN CONSENSUS RECOMMENDATIONS

In 2016, the American Society of Echocardiography (ASE) and the European Association of Cardiovascular Imaging (EACVI) published recommendations for evaluating LV diastolic function using echocardiography.[14] In this recommendation, a diastolic stress test was discussed,

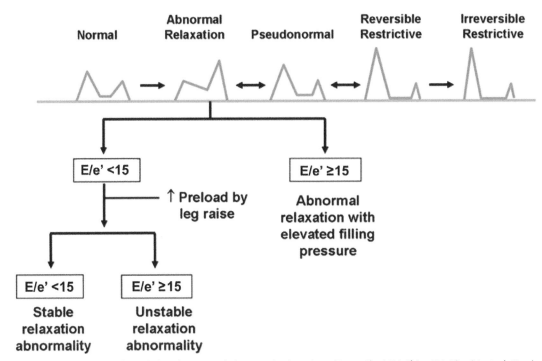

Fig. 3. Passive leg raise for subclassification of abnormal relaxation. (*From* Choi EY, Shim CY, Kim SA et al. Passive leg-raise is helpful to identify impaired diastolic functional reserve during exercise in patients with abnormal myocardial relaxation. J Am Soc Echocardiogr 2010; 23(5):523-20; with permission.)

including its indications, performance, interpretation, and detection of early myocardial disease and prognosis. The main statements were as follows: (1) diastolic stress testing is indicated in patients with dyspnea and grade 1 diastolic dysfunction at rest; (2) at rest, mitral E and annular e' velocities should be recorded, along with the peak velocity of tricuspid regurgitation (TR) jet from multiple windows. The same parameters are recorded during exercise, and 1 minute to 2 minutes after the exercise finished when E and A velocities are not merged. This result can be explained by the fact that the increased filling pressures unusually persist for a few minutes. In addition, (3) the test is considered positive when all of the following 3 conditions are met during exercise: average E/e' 14 or septal E/e' ratio greater than 15, peak TR velocity greater than 2.8 m/s, and septal e' velocity less than 7 cm/s (**Fig. 4**).[14] The results are normal when the average (or septal) E/e' was less than 10 with exercise, and the peak TR velocity was less than 2.8 m/s with exercise.[14] In another recommendation for the clinical use of stress echocardiography in nonischemic heart

Table 1
Comparisons between treadmill stress echocardiography and supine bicycle exercise echocardiography for diastolic stress tests

	Treadmill Exercise Echo	Supine Bicycle Exercise Echo
Exercise workloads	Average 9–10 METs Vigorous intensity activities: running, calisthenics, jumping	Average 5–7 METs Moderate-intensity activities: walking, jogging
Myocardial ischemia	Frequent and more extensive	Less frequent
Exercise diastolic function	Immediate after exercise	Each stage of exercise (3-min interval, 25-W increments)
Effect of position	Upright—preload ↓	Supine—preload ↑ (myocardial well tension ↑ oxygen demand ↑)

Abbreviations: METs; metabolic equivalents.

disease from the EACVI and the ASE, exercise using a supine bicycle is the recommended modality for diastolic stress tests to detect impaired LV diastolic function reserve and the resulting increase in LV filling pressure in patients with unexplained dyspnea or subclinical diastolic dysfunction (**Fig. 5**).[15]

In 2020, a consensus recommendation from the Heart Failure Association (HFA) of the European Society of Cardiology provided a practical diagnostic algorithm by using stress testing to diagnose HF with preserved EF.[19] This recommendation provides a new stepwise diagnostic process for HF with preserved EF, as follows: step 1 (P = pretest assessment), step 2 (E = echocardiography and natriuretic peptides score), step 3 (F_1 = functional testing), and step 4 (F_2 = final etiology).[19] During this diagnostic process, stress testing plays a role in steps 1 and 3. Step 1 (P) should be performed in any patient who presents with symptoms and/or signs that are compatible with a diagnosis of HF. In the first step of the HF diagnostic work-up, 1 of the following diagnostic tests should be considered: a bicycle or treadmill exercise test; dobutamine stress echocardiography; cardiac magnetic resonance imaging or myocardial scintigraphy; or an anatomic approach using coronary computed tomography angiography or invasive angiography if coronary artery disease (CAD) is suspected.[19] A

stress test provides information about exercise capacity, and the blood pressure and heart rate responses to exercise. Step 3 is performed when the HFA-PEFF score (obtained by combining the results from resting echocardiogram and natriuretic peptide in step 2) is unable to diagnose HF with preserved EF.[19] Exercise echocardiography should be considered abnormal if the average E/e' at peak stress increases to greater than or equal to 15, with or without a peak TR velocity greater than 3.4 m/s.[19] An isolated increase in TR velocity should not be used to diagnose HF with preserved EF, because it can be caused simply by a normal hyperdynamic response to exercise (with increased pulmonary blood flow) in the absence of LV diastolic dysfunction. An average E/e' during exercise of greater than or equal to 15 adds 2 points to the HFA-PEFF score.[19] An average E/e' greater than or equal to 15 with a peak TR velocity greater than 3.4 m/s adds 3 points to the previous score from step 2 (E).[19] If the combined score from step 2 (E) and step 3 (F_1) is greater than or equal to 5 points, then the diagnosis of HF with preserved EF can be confirmed.[19] Exercise right heart catheterization generally is recommended if a patient has a diagnostic uncertainty from step 2 (E) or if diastolic stress echocardiography is inconclusive or not feasible when there is a high index of suspicion that HF with preserved EF is present.[19] A steep increase in pulmonary capillary wedge

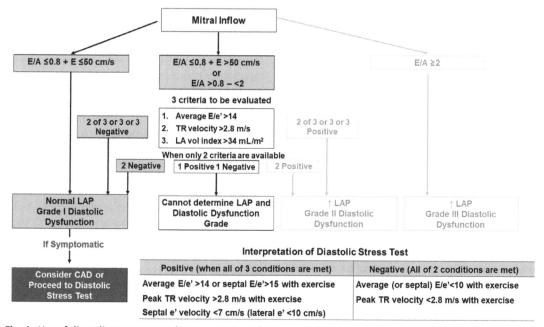

Fig. 4. Use of diastolic stress test and interpretation of the results. LAP, left atrial pressure. (*Adapted from* Nagueh SF, Smiseth OA, Appleton CP et al. Recommendations for the Evaluation of the Left ventricular Diastolic Function by Echocardiography: An Update form the American Society of Echocardiography and the European Association of Cardiovascular Imaging. J Am Soc Echocardiogr 2016; 29(4):277-314; with permission.)

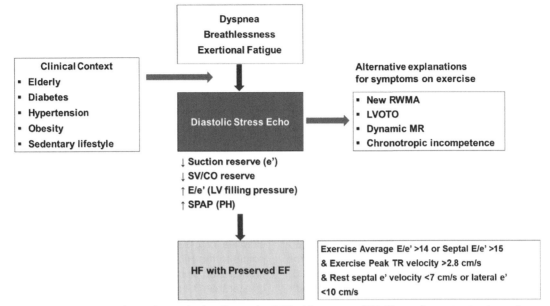

Fig. 5. Diastolic stress echocardiography for diagnosis of HF with preserved EF. CO, cardiac output; echo, echocardiography; LVOTO, left ventricular outflow tract obstruction; MR, mitral regurgitation; PH, pulmonary hypertension; RWMA, regional wall motion abnormality; SPAP, systolic pulmonary artery pressure; SV, stroke volume. (*Adapted from* Lancellotti P, Pellikka PA, Budts W et al. The Clinical Use of Stress Echocardiography in Non-Ischaemic Heart Disease: Recommendations from the European Association of Cardiovascular Imaging and the American Society of Echocardiography. J Am Soc Echocardiogr 2017; 30(2):101-38; with permission.)

pressure during exercise is a typical hemodynamic response in HF with preserved EF. Patients with values less than 25 mm Hg during peak exercise are classified as having noncardiac dyspnea.[19]

THE PROTOCOL OF DIASTOLIC STRESS ECHOCARDIOGRAPHY

The protocol of the noninvasive diastolic stress test is slightly different at each institution. The general rules, however, are similar across institutions. After obtaining standard parasternal and apical view rest images, multistage supine bicycle exercise testing is performed with a variable-load bicycle ergometer.[11] The subjects pedaled at a constant speed beginning at a workload of 25 W, with an incremental workload of 25 W every 3 minutes until the patient's ability was limited by the his/her symptoms.[11] All of the measurements are taken at rest and at each stage in the same sequence.[11] Because the images of a predetermined protocol must be acquired for a given 3 minutes, some images may need to be added or subtracted depending on the purpose of the examination and the patient's cardiac disease. Because mitral inflow and mitral annular velocity are the most important parameters that tend to be summated during exercise, these should be measured first. After these measurements, Doppler parameters, such as the TR velocity and

LV outflow tract pulsed wave Doppler, are evaluated. In order to determine inducible myocardial ischemia during exercise, regional wall motion abnormalities should be observed through parasternal short-axis and apical views. When it is difficult to measure the exercise-induced mitral regurgitation at every stage, it can be observed at baseline and peak exercise through color Doppler imaging. Exercise-induced mitral regurgitation is not common in patients with preserved EF but important in patients with mild to moderate mitral regurgitation combined with an inferior wall motion abnormality. A 12-lead electrocardiogram is registered continuously to exclude significant myocardial ischemia. Peripheral blood pressures are measured at the end of each stage of exercise on the left arm using a blood pressure monitoring device. The exercise workload is defined by the total metabolic equivalents achieved. Peak V_{O_2} is defined as the highest 10-second average of oxygen uptake in the last minute of exercise.

INTERPRETATION OF MAIN PARAMETERS FROM DIASTOLIC STRESS ECHOCARDIOGRAPHY
Exercise E/e′ and Exercise Left Ventricular Filling Pressure

A validation study of 37 patients by Burgess and colleagues showed a reasonable correlation between invasively measured LV filling pressures and the Doppler-derived E/e′ ratio during exercise.[25] A cutoff value of 13 identified patients with an LV diastolic pressure of greater than 15 mm Hg, which allowed for the accurate classification of patients into those with high or low filling pressure during exercise. Another validation study in 12 patients by Talreja and colleagues[26] revealed that an E/e′ ratio greater than 15 during exercise is associated with a significant elevation in the pulmonary artery wedge pressure greater than 20 mm Hg. Therefore, exercise E/e′ can be used reliably for the diagnosis of HF in patients with normal or mildly abnormal diastolic parameters at rest.

Obokata and colleagues[10] showed that currently proposed diagnostic guidelines for HF with preserved EF are poorly sensitive in simultaneous echocardiographic-catheterization studies at rest and during exercise in subjects with HF with preserved EF and those with noncardiac dyspnea. This group identified greater than 34% to 60% of subjects with proved HF with preserved EF based on resting echocardiographic data alone.[10] The addition of an exercise E/e′ ratio greater than 14 improved sensitivities to 90% and the negative predictive value but compromised specificity (71%). These results suggest that exercise echocardiography may help to rule out HF with preserved EF.[10]

Exercise E/e′ not only has additional value in the diagnosis of HF with preserved EF but also has implications in predicting clinical outcomes. Holland and colleagues[27] investigated 522 patients who were referred to exercise echocardiography and showed that elevated exercise E/e′ is associated independently with subsequent cardiovascular hospitalization over a median of 13.2 months. This finding was independent of and incremental to inducible myocardial ischemia.[27] A recent study in 156 patients with chronic kidney disease suggested that exercise E/e′ can unmask latent diastolic dysfunction in those with normal or indeterminate resting E/e′.[28] A raised exercise E/e′ of greater than 13 in patients with chronic kidney disease was an independent predictor of cardiovascular outcome over a follow-up period of 41.4 months.[28]

Exercise Pulmonary Artery Systolic Pressure and Exercise-Induced Pulmonary Hypertension

The pulmonary artery systolic pressure (PASP) increase during exercise is highly variable and can be influenced by an exercise-induced increase in cardiac output and left atrial pressure, and blunted pulmonary vasodilation.[29] Exercise-induced pulmonary hypertension is thought to be an early and mild phase that precedes pulmonary hypertension.[30] In contrast, it might be related to an enhanced cardiac output response in physiologic conditions.[31] Therefore, in current guidelines for the diastolic stress test, an isolated increase in the exercise peak TR velocity must be interpreted cautiously, because normal subjects can have a significant increase in the peak TR velocity related to increased pulmonary blood flow.[14,15] The exercise workload at peak exercise varies according to the individual. Therefore, it is necessary to determine if the exercise-induced pulmonary hypertension occurred from a low workload or high workload, and if it is related to LV filling pressure elevation during exercise. In a previous study of 396 subjects referred for exercise echocardiography, it was demonstrated that exercise-induced pulmonary hypertension (defined as present if PASP >50 mm Hg at 50 W of exercise) was common, even in subjects with normal LVEF (**Fig. 6**).[32] Exercise-induced pulmonary hypertension was associated strongly with E/e′, TR velocity, age, female sex, and systolic blood pressure during exercise.[32] In a longitudinal outcome study of 498 subjects with preserved LVEF, the author and colleagues[29] demonstrated that exercise-induced pulmonary hypertension was associated with worse outcomes during a median follow-up of 41 months. When exercise-induced pulmonary hypertension was associated with an increase in estimated LV filling pressure with exercise, there were poorer clinical outcomes in subjects with exercise-induced pulmonary hypertension.[29]

Diastolic Functional Reserve

Diastolic functional reserve is the ability of the LV to augment diastolic function with exercise, and it may be impaired in patients with risk factors for HF with preserved EF.[33–35] Various methods of evaluating diastolic functional reserve during a diastolic stress echo have been introduced over the past decade. The diastolic functional reserve can be evaluated simply by the change in e′ from resting to each stage of exercise (**Fig. 7**). It also is assessed by calculating the indices corrected to the e′ value at rest. The clinical significance of the diastolic functional reserve has been proved in several clinical situations, including hypertension, diabetes mellitus, and hypertrophic cardiomyopathy.[35–40] Lower diastolic functional reserve was associated with reduced exercise capacity.[34,38] Among the various risk factors for HF with preserved EF, diabetes mellitus is an important disease group in the detection

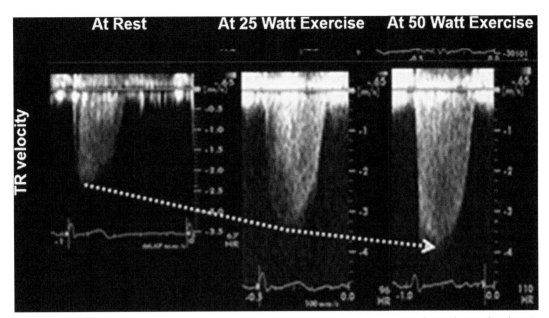

Fig. 6. Exercise-induced pulmonary hypertension. TR velocities on diastolic stress echocardiography showing normal estimated PASP at rest but remarkable elevation of estimated PASP during exercise.

of subclinical LV dysfunction and prevention of HF by evaluating the diastolic functional reserve.[35,40] When patients were classified into 2 groups according to the median delta change of e' velocity (from rest to 25 W of exercise and from rest to 50 W of exercise), patients with a lower delta change had significantly worse outcomes than did those with a higher value.[40] A recent randomized placebo-controlled trial proved the effects of a sodium-glucose cotransporter 2 inhibitor on LV diastolic function in patients with diabetes mellitus by assessing LV diastolic functional reserve on diastolic stress echocardiography at baseline and 24 weeks.[41] Evaluation of diastolic functional reserve in stress testing, therefore, is important in assessing the risk and prognosis of HF at a subclinical stage and for early therapeutic intervention.

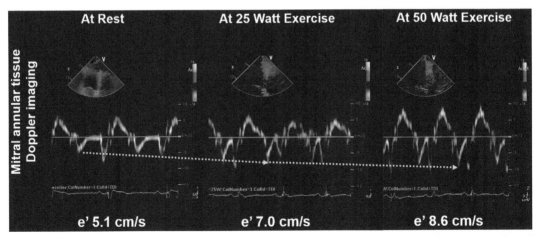

Fig. 7. Diastolic functional reserve. The e' velocity at rest and its changes at each stage of exercise on diastolic stress echocardiography.

SUMMARY

The use of stress tests is crucial, especially when there is no clear diagnostic information from resting echocardiography. Among various stress tests, noninvasive supine bicycle diastolic stress echocardiography has provided the most evidence for diagnosis and predicting the prognosis of HF with preserved EF by evaluating exercise E/e′ and exercise PASP. At the subclinical stage of HF, assessment of the diastolic functional reserve is helpful for early detection and intervention of the risk of future HF.

CLINICS CARE POINTS

- Resting echocardiography is poorly sensitive for diagnosing HF with preserved EF.
- Even in subjects with identical impaired relaxation in resting conditions, the myocardial performance and intracardiac pressures vary during exercise.
- Exercise E/e′ not only has added value in the diagnosis of HF with preserved EF but also has implications in predicting clinical outcomes.
- Exercise-induced pulmonary hypertension combined with an elevation of exercise E/e′ is associated with poor clinical outcome.
- Evaluation of diastolic functional reserve in supine bicycle exercise echocardiography is useful in assessing the risk of HF at a subclinical stage.

CONFLICT OF INTEREST

The author has nothing to disclose.

ACKNOWLEDGMENT OF GRANT SUPPORT

None.

REFERENCES

1. Ponikowski P, Voors AA, Anker SD, et al. 2016 ESC guidelines for the diagnosis and treatment of acute and chronic heart failure: The Task Force for the diagnosis and treatment of acute and chronic heart failure of the European Society of Cardiology (ESC) Developed with the special contribution of the Heart Failure Association (HFA) of the ESC. Eur Heart J 2016;37(27):2129–200.

2. Yancy CW, Jessup M, Bozkurt B, et al. 2017 ACC/AHA/HFSA focused update of the 2013 ACCF/AHA guideline for the management of heart failure: a report of the American College of Cardiology/American Heart Association Task Force on Clinical Practice Guidelines and the Heart Failure Society of America. Circulation 2017;136(6):e137–61.

3. Oktay AA, Shah SJ. Diagnosis and management of heart failure with preserved ejection fraction: 10 key lessons. Curr Cardiol Rev 2015;11(1):42–52.

4. Pfeffer MA, Shah AM, Borlaug BA. Heart failure with preserved ejection fraction in perspective. Circ Res 2019;124(11):1598–617.

5. Shim CY. Heart failure with preserved ejection fraction: the major unmet need in cardiology. Korean Circ J 2020;50(12):1051–61.

6. Shah SJ, Katz DH, Deo RC. Phenotypic spectrum of heart failure with preserved ejection fraction. Heart Fail Clin 2014;10(3):407–18.

7. Shah SJ, Kitzman DW, Borlaug BA, et al. Phenotype-specific treatment of heart failure with preserved ejection fraction: a multiorgan roadmap. Circulation 2016;134(1):73–90.

8. Lewis GA, Schelbert EB, Williams SG, et al. Biological phenotypes of heart failure with preserved ejection fraction. J Am Coll Cardiol 2017;70(17):2186–200.

9. Silverman DN, Shah SJ. Treatment of heart failure with preserved ejection fraction (HFpEF): the phenotype-guided approach. Curr Treat Options Cardiovasc Med 2019;21(4):20.

10. Obokata M, Kane GC, Reddy YNV, et al. Role of diastolic stress testing in the evaluation for heart failure with preserved ejection fraction: a simultaneous invasive-echocardiographic study. Circulation 2017;135(9):825–38.

11. Ha JW, Oh JK, Pellikka PA, et al. Diastolic stress echocardiography: a novel noninvasive diagnostic test for diastolic dysfunction using supine bicycle exercise Doppler echocardiography. J Am Soc Echocardiogr 2005;18(1):63–8.

12. Kitzman DW, Higginbotham MB, Cobb FR, et al. Exercise intolerance in patients with heart failure with preserved left ventricular systolic function: failure of the Frank-Starling mechanism. J Am Coll Cardiol 1991;17(5):1065–72.

13. Pellikka PA, Arruda-Olson A, Chaudhry FA, et al. Guidelines for performance, interpretation, and application of stress echocardiography in ischemic heart disease: from the American Society of Echocardiography. J Am Soc Echocardiogr 2020;33(1):1–41.e8.

14. Nagueh SF, Smiseth OA, Appleton CP, et al. Recommendations for the evaluation of the left ventricular function by echocardiography: an update form the American Society of Echocardiography and the European Association of Cardiovascular Imaging. J Am Soc Echocardiogr 2016;29(4):277–314.

15. Lancellotti P, Pellikka PA, Budts W, et al. The clinical use of stress echocardiography in non-ischemic heart disease: recommendations from the European Association of Cardiovascular Imaging and the American Society of Echocardiography. J Am Soc Echocardiogr 2017;30(2):101–38.

16. Ha JW, Andersen OS, Smiseth OA. Diastolic stress test: invasive and noninvasive testing. JACC Cardiovasc Imaging 2020;13(1 Pt 2):272–82.

17. Borlaug BA, Nishimura RA, Sorajja P, et al. Exercise hemodynamics enhance diagnosis of early heart failure with preserved ejection fraction. Circ Heart Fail 2010;3(5):588–95.

18. Hong SJ, Shim CY, Kim D, et al. Dynamic change in left ventricular apical back rotation: a maker of diastolic suction with exercise. Eur Heart J Cardiovasc Imaging 2018;19(1):12–9.

19. Pieske B, Tschöpe C, de Boer RA, et al. How to diagnose heart failure with preserved ejection fraction: the HFA-PEFF diagnostic algorithm: a consensus recommendation from the Heart Failure Association (HFA) of the European Society of Cardiology (ESC). Eur Heart J 2019;40(40):3297–317.

20. Shim CY, Park S, Choi D, et al. Sex differences in central hemodynamics and their relationship to left ventricular diastolic function. J Am Coll Cardiol 2011;57(10):1226–33.

21. Shim CY, Yang WI, Park S, et al. Overweight and its association with aortic pressure wave reflection after exercise. Am J Hypertens 2011;24(10):1136–42.

22. Choi EY, Shim CY, Kim SA, et al. Passive leg-raise is helpful to identify impaired diastolic functional reserve during exercise in patients with abnormal myocardial relaxation. J Am Soc Echocardiogr 2010;23(5):523–30.

23. Peteiro J, Bouzas-Mosquera A, Estevez R, et al. Head-to-head comparison of peak supine bicycle exercise echocardiography and treadmill exercise echocardiography at peak and at post-exercise for the detection of coronary artery disease. J Am Soc Echocardiogr 2012;25(3):319–26.

24. Caiati C, Lepera ME, Carretta D, et al. Head-to-head comparison of peak upright bicycle and post-treadmill echocardiography in detecting coronary artery disease: a randomized, single-blind crossover study. J Am Soc Echocardiogr 2013;26(12):1434–43.

25. Burgess MI, Jenkins C, Sharman JE, et al. Diastolic stress echocardiography: hemodynamic validation and clinical significance of estimation of ventricular filling pressure with exercise. J Am Coll Cardiol 2006;47(9):1891–900.

26. Talreja D, Nishimura RA, Oh JK. Estimation of left ventricular filling pressure with exercise by Doppler echocardiography in patients with normal systolic function: a simultaneous echocardiographic-cardiac catheterization study. J Am Soc Echocardiogr 2007;20(5):477–9.

27. Holland DJ, Prasad SB, Marwick TH. Prognostic implications of left ventricular filling pressure with exercise. Circ Cardiovasc Imaging 2010;3(2):149–56.

28. Gan GCH, Kadappu KK, Bhat A, et al. Exercise E/e' is a determinant of exercise capacity and adverse cardiovascular outcomes in chronic kidney disease. JACC Cardiovasc Imaging 2020;13(12):2485–94.

29. Shim CY, Kim SA, Choi D, et al. Clinical outcomes of exercise-induced pulmonary hypertension in subjects with preserved left ventricular ejection fraction: implication of an increase in left ventricular filling pressure during exercise. Heart 2011;97(17):1417–24.

30. Tolle JJ, Waxman AB, Van Horn TL, et al. Exercise-induced pulmonary arterial hypertension. Circulation 2008;118(21):2183–9.

31. Bossone E, Rubenfire M, Bach DS, et al. Range of tricuspid regurgitation velocity at rest and during exercise in normal adult men: implications for the diagnosis of pulmonary hypertension. J Am Coll Cardiol 1999;33(6):1662–6.

32. Ha JW, Choi D, Park S, et al. Determinants of exercise-induced pulmonary hypertension in patients with normal left ventricular ejection fraction. Heart 2009;95(6):490–4.

33. Borlaug BA, Olson TP, Lam CSP, et al. Global cardiovascular reserve dysfunction in heart failure with preserved ejection fraction. J Am Coll Cardiol 2010;56(11):845–54.

34. Ha JW, Choi D, Park S, et al. Left ventricular diastolic functional reserve during exercise in patients with impaired myocardial relaxation at rest. Heart 2009;95(5):399–404.

35. Ha JW, Lee HC, Kang ES, et al. Abnormal left ventricular longitudinal functional reserve in patients with diabetes mellitus: implication for detecting subclinical myocardial dysfunction using exercise tissue Doppler echocardiography. Heart 2007;93(12):1571–6.

36. Choi EY, Ha JW, Yoon SJ, et al. Increased plasma aldosterone-to-renin ratio is associated with impaired left ventricular longitudinal functional reserve in patients with uncomplicated hypertension. J Am Soc Echocardiogr 2008;21(3):251–6.

37. Ha JW, Ahn JA, Kim JM, et al. Abnormal longitudinal myocardial functional reserve assessed by exercise tissue Doppler echocardiography in patients with hypertrophic cardiomyopathy. J Am Soc Echocardiogr 2006;19(11):1314–9.

38. Choi EY, Ha JW, Rim SJ, et al. Incremental value of left ventricular diastolic function reserve index for predicting exercise capacity in patients with hypertrophic cardiomyopathy. J Am Soc Echocardiogr 2008;21(5):487–92.

39. Moon J, Hong YJ, Kim YJ, et al. Extent of late gadolinium enhancement on cardiovascular magnetic

resonance imaging and its relation to left ventricular longitudinal functional reserve during exercise in patients with hypertrophic cardiomyopathy. Circ J 2013;77(7):1742–9.

40. Kim SA, Shim CY, Kim JM, et al. Impact of left ventricular longitudinal diastolic functional reserve on clinical outcome in patients with type 2 diabetes mellitus. Heart 2011;97(15):1233–8.

41. Shim CY, Seo J, Cho I, et al. Randomized, controlled trial to evaluate the effect of dapagliflozin on left ventricular diastolic function in patients with type 2 diabetes mellitus: the IDDIA trial. Circulation 2021; 143(5):510–2.

Comprehensive Assessment of Heart Failure with Preserved Ejection Fraction Using Cardiac MRI

Julián Vega-Adauy, MD[a,b], Ozge Ozden Tok, MD[c],*, Ahmet Celik, MD[d], Ahmet Barutcu, MD[e], Mani A. Vannan, MBBS[f]

KEYWORDS

- Heart failure with preserved ejection fraction • Diastolic dysfunction • Cardiac magnetic resonance
- Cardiac filling pressures

KEY POINTS

- The diagnostics process of heart failure with preserved ejection fraction (HFpEF) is complex and generally imprecise.
- Allocating heart failure phenotypes based on a discrete marker of cardiac function as the ejection fraction by the Simpson biplane method can be misleading.
- Echocardiography is a first-line imaging technique to characterize HFpEF but suffers inherent limitations related to ultrasound capabilities.
- Cardiac magnetic resonance (CMR) provides superior anatomic and functional assessment and enables tissue characterization, providing unprecedented diagnostic precision.
- CMR refinements that incorporate advanced cardiac mechanics and tissue characterization will redefine the imaging boundaries in HFpEF.

INTRODUCTION

Heart failure (HF) with preserved ejection fraction (HFpEF) accounts for nearly half of the HF burden and its prevalence is increasing because of population aging. Its diagnostic process is challenging and generally imprecise because of the absence of a single diagnostic marker to adjudicate this condition, the complex and multiparametric echocardiography evaluation involved, and the broad spectrum of causes encompassed in HFpEF.[1]

Guidelines have historically referred to this condition as diastolic HF because of the frequent associated diastolic dysfunction (DD). However, the presence of DD does not imply HFpEF, so these 2 conditions do not always go together.

In 1998, the European study group on "diastolic heart failure" suggested diagnostic criteria detaching this entity from systolic or congestive HF.[2]

Regarding the ejection fraction (EF) criteria, a pragmatic and arbitrary approach divided HF with preserved left ventricular ejection fraction

[a] Chilean Institute of Cardiac Imaging, Santiago de Chile, Chile; [b] Millennium Nucleus in Cardiovascular Magnetic Resonance, Cardio MR, Pontificia Universidad Católica de Chile-Campus San Joaquín, Vicuña Mackenna 4860, Macul, Santiago, Chile; [c] Department of Cardiology, Memorial Bahcelievler Hospital, Istanbul, Turkey; [d] Department of Cardiology, Mersin University Medical Faculty, Mersin, Turkey; [e] Department of Cardiology, Onsekizmart University Medical Faculty, Canakkale, Turkey; [f] Marcus Heart Valve Center, Piedmont Heart Institute, Atlanta, GA, USA
* Corresponding author.
E-mail address: ozgeozdenctf@hotmail.com
Twitter: @ecocardio_cl (J.V.-A.); @drzgezdentok1 (O.O.T.); @drheartfailure (A.C.); @AhmetBarutcu (A.B.); @ManiVannanheart (M.A.V.)

Heart Failure Clin 17 (2021) 447–462
https://doi.org/10.1016/j.hfc.2021.03.006

(LVEF) more than 50% and reduced LVEF less than 40%, leaving in between an awkward mid-range phenotype of HF.[3] This snapshot approach's main problem is that it generates an artificial division of a likely continuous phenomenon based on a very discrete ventricular function marker, such as the LVEF by Simpson's biplane method.

Current diagnostic criteria give a central role to imaging (mainly echocardiography), demonstrating LVEF more than 50% and relevant structural heart disease to which the symptoms could be attributable. However, it also incorporates clinical features, such as HF signs and symptoms, and biomarker evidence of elevated intracardiac pressures represented by increased brain natriuretic peptide.

The caveat with this definition is that it only encompasses symptomatic patients (stages C and D of ACC/AHA classification), excluding patients at risk of HF (stage A) or asymptomatic patients with structural alterations, such as left ventricular hypertrophy (LVH) (stage B), which is precisely the most frequent scenario to encounter in clinical practice.

Furthermore, recent diagnostic scores systems, such as the H2FPEF and the HFA-PEFF, intend to solve the diagnosis challenge by giving distinct consideration to clinical data, biomarkers, and imaging, but with large discrepancies in adjudicating this condition,[4] highlighting the complexities in HFpEF diagnosis and underscoring the need for a robust imaging technique to characterize this disease.

This review describes cardiac magnetic resonance (CMR) capabilities in HFpEF, focusing on differential diagnosis, and portrays CMR as a one-stop shop for HF.

Considerations in Heart Failure with Preserved Ejection Fraction Imaging

Echocardiographic evaluation of the heart cavities was mainly anatomic and static until Nishimura's publications on left ventricular (LV) diastolic function in 1997, portraying the diastolic evaluation as the clinicians' "Rosetta Stone."[5] Since then, echocardiography has come a long way, implementing an algorithmic evaluation that grades DD into stages and incorporates cardiac mechanics (strain).[6] Recently arising are advanced cardiac work indexes assembled from the LV pressure-strain loops, such as global work, index, waste, and efficiency. Notwithstanding all these refinements, inadequate acoustic windows and the impossibility of performing tissue characterization are the main limiting factors for this widespread technique.

In contrast, CMR is a comprehensive diagnostic tool that combines anatomic, functional, and tissue characterization capabilities, being better suited for evaluating a broad disease, such as HFpEF. CMR is the gold standard for size and function in cardiac chambers, providing functional information using flow sequences (2-dimensional [2D] or 4-dimensional [4D]). Most remarkably allows performing tissue characterization via parametric mapping (T1, extracellular volume [ECV], T2) and gadolinium (GAD) enhancement. Furthermore, novel CMR sequences, such as fast strain-encoded CMR (fast SENC), and postprocessing techniques, such as feature tracking, enable accurate cardiac mechanics evaluation. Moreover, on the immediate horizon is high-quality coronary angiography with flow acquisition, automatic quantitative stress myocardial perfusion, and fingerprinting CMR that allows for nongated real-time simultaneous acquisition of mapping and CINE images,[7] enhancing detection of underlying alterations that could ultimately be a game-changer in cardiac imaging.

HEART FAILURE WITH PRESERVED EJECTION FRACTION IMAGING

HF with reduced ejection fraction frequently presents with LV dilatation and ejection fraction (EF) less than 40% to 50%; on the other side, gross imaging characteristics of HFpEF include normal or near-normal systolic LV function (LVEF >50%), cardiac structural alterations, mainly in the form of LVH or left atrial enlargement (LAE) and variable degrees of DD. Unfortunately, these features are common to a conundrum of disorders,[8] such as arterial hypertension, myocardial ischemia, obstructive sleep apnea, diabetes, chronic kidney disease, obesity, early stages of hypertrophic cardiomyopathy (HCM), and the broad spectrum of restrictive cardiomyopathies, including storage and infiltrative that present LV thickening.

The main advantage of CMR over echocardiography is the ability of CMR to integrate anatomic, functional, and tissue characterization, offering unprecedented diagnostic precision. Notwithstanding CMR capabilities, echocardiography, because of its widespread access and well-validated features, is the first-line imaging technique in HFpEF.

Imaging Objectives

Aiming to improve patient prognostic imaging in HFpEF, should provided:

a. Cardiac chamber size and systolic function

b. Diastolic function, cardiac filling pressures, and pulmonary hypertension (PH)

c. Likely cause of HF

d. Associated findings

Cardiac chamber size and systolic function

Left ventricle LV wall thickness magnitude and distribution using 2D mode (or B mode) are generally reliably. Common echocardiography pitfalls are missing apical lateral hypertrophy because of poor visualization and overestimating basal septum thickness by including in the measurement the right ventricle (RV) moderator band's insertion. Because of its high in-plane spatial resolution, CMR can accurately measure wall thickness in a short-axis plane, reassuring that the measure is orthogonal to the long-axis plane.

Regarding echocardiography LV mass calculation, its assessment is quite deficient because echocardiography indirectly assesses the mass by sampling one point of the anteroseptal septum and the posterior wall, extrapolating it and assuming an ellipsoid shape. In contrast, CMR calculates LV mass directly without geometric assumptions by tracing the epicardial and endocardial contours in a complete short-axis stack of the heart.

LV systolic function is calculated in echocardiography by the modified Simpson's biplane method of disk summation, which is a marker of how much blood is retained and expelled in the LV systole. In preserved EF, the LV should eject at least half of its filling volume. This simplistic approach for evaluating LV function has stood over time, but it is insufficient and limited to comprehensively assess LV function. Furthermore, significant LVH can be associated with severely reduced LV longitudinal excursion, a scenario in which Simpson's methods do not reflect the real LV systolic function, overestimating EF because of geometric confounders.[9] Another shortcoming is the presence of limited acoustic windows and the foreshortening of the LV, which causes a dramatic underestimation of LV volumes. These issues portray some of the serious limitations of Simpson's EF in adjudicating LV function.

Deformation imaging, such as strain, partially overcomes these limitations. Still, it is highly dependent on acoustic windows, adequate temporal resolution, and operator experience, not to mention it is time-consuming and presents significant variabilities depending on the vendor's software. Consequently, in daily practice, LVEF by Simpson's method is an imperfect best choice.

Regarding CMR, evaluation of LV volumes uses a short-axis cine stack that covers the entire heart. Modern cine sequences use breath-hold, electrocardiographic-gating, and segmented steady-state free precession (SSFP), delivering images with a high spatial and temporal resolution, which are far superior to other cardiac imaging modalities.

Left atrium Left atrium (LA) enlargement is the chronic expression of LV diastolic function. As DD progresses, LA filling pressure increases, affecting its reservoir, conduit, and pumping or contractile properties.

Atrial volume and function constitute reliable indicators of the duration and severity of DD independent of loading conditions and provide prognostic information.

There is a large amount of data supporting maximal LA volume use at LA end-diastole, but also minimal LA volume at end-systole has prognostic significance.[10]

Regarding LA volume estimation by echocardiography, it is performed in a 2-chamber and 4-chamber view and then indexed by body surface area. This variable, termed left atrium volume index (LAVI), is presented as the standard. However, this method is known to underestimate LA volume, and also its normal limit that started at 28 mL/m^2 and is now on 34 mL/m^2 may be still a moving target.[10]

CMR evaluation of LA volume is the gold standard (**Fig. 1**). This calculation is performed in a short-axis stack of the whole LA (see **Fig. 1B**), contouring the end-diastolic area of the LA for each slice. As slice thickness and gap are known, an accurate anatomic 3-dimensional (3D) model of the LA can be constructed (see **Fig. 1C**). The pitfalls of this approach are it is time consuming, and cumbersome. A more practical but less academic approach calculates the LAVI using a biplane (see **Fig. 1A**) or triplane view, which yields significantly higher values than echocardiography.

In addition, CMR enables advanced mechanical assessment of the LA, using feature tracking to measure LA strain and strain rate, variables that are impaired in HFpEF and associated with exercise intolerance,[11] whereas on the other end, endurance athletes' evidence increased LA contractile function evaluated by strain,[12] highlighting the central role of LA function besides its size.

LA enlargement in HFpEF is the hallmark of the disease. It should be proportionate to the rest of the cardiac anatomic and functional findings. For example, mild LVH generally goes with type I DD and with mild or moderate LA enlargement. If severe LA enlargement is identified in this setting,

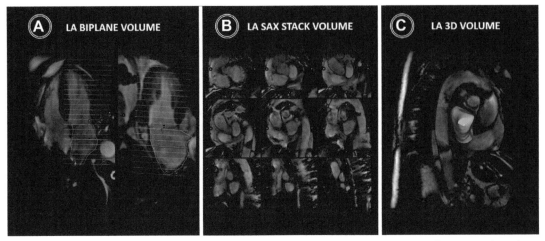

Fig. 1. Quantification of left atrial volume using CMR. (*A*) The biplane method measures the LA area in 4-chamber and 2-chamber view and integrates a volume by using a disk or mesh method. (*B*) Standard procedure for LAV assessment in CMR. The LA area is traced at each slice of a short-axis stack covering it entirely. (*C*) LA 3D volume. Because slice thickness and gap are known, an accurate 3D model is constructed using panel B information.

other causes of LA dilatation should be considered (atrial fibrillation or mitral valve disease). Conversely, it is not advisable to pursue an HFpEF diagnosis in the presence of confirmed normal size LA, suggesting other causes of dyspnea, such as pulmonary disease, be addressed (**Table 1**).

Right ventricle RV function is a crucial prognostic element in HF and relevant to assess in the presence of advanced DD causing PH.

The RV is a crescent-shaped structure with 3 distinct sections, an inlet, a trabeculated apex, and an outlet. Because of this particular shape, LV evaluation parameters, such as Simpson's biplane, are not applicable.

Echocardiography has traditionally settled for surrogate markers of right ventricular ejection fraction (RVEF), such as markers of regional and longitudinal function. These markers are measure at the lateral tricuspid annulus, and consist on the tricuspid annular plane systolic excursion (TAPSE) and the systolic annular velocity using tissue Doppler index (TDI).

Serious limitations of these local parameters are as follows: being dependent on volume changes and pericardial integrity and reflecting a small portion of the RV function. Other so-called global indexes, such as fractional area change and myocardial performance index by TDI, are also discrete surrogates for RVEF.

CMR is the only technique that can directly and confidently estimate RVEF without surrogate markers or geometric assumptions. Furthermore, CMR can also evaluate DD using the RV filling curve and flow parameters and perform strain analysis.

Table 1
Differentials of heart failure with preserved ejection fraction (mimics of heart failure with preserved ejection fraction)

Group	Etiology	Tests
Respiratory	Pulmonary hypertension primary or secondary (obstructive sleep apnea, chronic obstructive pulmonary disease)	Pulmonary function test, 6-min walking test, high-resolution computed tomography, overnight respiratory polygraphy
Extracardiac volume overload	Liver and kidney disease, nephrotic syndrome	Liver and kidney ultrasound and MRI, liver fibroscan
High-output state	Anemia, hyperthyroidism, extracardiac shunts	Laboratory test, echocardiography bubble test with late acquisition
Others	Obesity, physical deconditioning, venous insufficiency	6-min walking test, treadmill, Lower extremity Doppler ultrasound

Diastolic function, filling pressures, and pulmonary hypertension

Diastolic function is a complex process that requires the orchestrated contribution of ventricular relaxation and suction in the early phase and a brisk atrial contraction and filling in the later stage. Noninvasive evaluation of diastolic function is performed by echocardiography using a series of different parameters, mainly pulsed-wave Doppler measurements that assess the filling of the LA and LV, and tissue Doppler that interrogates myocardial velocities.

DD initiates classically as an LV relaxation impairment condition associated with normal filling pressures, DD progress elevating LV and LA filling pressures, and finally, severely compromising left atrial function and its contribution to LV filling.

Echocardiography evaluation of DD specifically uses Doppler to evaluate transmitral inflow, pulmonary veins flow, and mitral annular velocities (E′), among other more complex indexes. The main caveat of echocardiographic DD evaluation is that it uses elements that occur late in diastole, such as parameters of LV filling or atrial contraction, therefore, not accounting for the isovolumetric LV relaxation occurring in early diastole, which is one of the earliest and essential determinants of diastolic function.

Adding more complexity, flow-derived variables, such as mitral inflow, are subject to a phenomenon known as "pseudonormalization," which generates a normal aspect of the mitral inflow pattern with increasing LA pressure.

Finally, the mitral inflow pattern is more reliable in the presence of reduced LVEF and should not be interpreted solely in preserved LVEF.[6]

Diastolic function assessed by cardiac magnetic resonance CMR using flow sequences accurately provides flow information averaged over numerous cardiac cycles, delivering curves that resemble Doppler echocardiography. Moreover, CMR can also measure mitral annular velocities (e') using low-speed phase-contrast sequences, but it is far more practical to rely on echocardiography in this arena.

An interesting approach to assess LV function via CMR is calculating volume-time curves (**Fig. 2**), which is done by tracing LV volume in the short axis (see **Fig. 2**A), ideally with full heart coverage (see **Fig. 2**C, D). For each slice, contours are traced throughout the cardiac cycle (typically, 1 RR interval includes 30 frames per slice). This LV volume-time curve (see **Fig. 2**E) allows calculating a myriad of parameters representing systolic and diastolic function, such as systolic indexes: peak ejection rate (PER), peak ejection time, and diastolic indexes: peak filling rate (PFR), peak filling time (PFT). Both PER and PFR can be normalized to end-diastolic volume (EDV), giving 2 other derived indexes PER/EDV and PFR/EDV, that can also be calculated for the RV (see **Fig. 2**F).

The classic drawback with this approach is that it requires manual tracing of a massive set of images that could easily exceed 500 images for both ventricles.

To overcome this challenge, state-of-the-art dedicated CMR software that incorporates artificial intelligence can deliver fully automatic whole-heart biventricular contour tracing throughout the cardiac cycle, thus rendering this method attractive (see **Fig. 2**).

Moreover, dedicated advanced cardiac software that processes a whole-heart 4D flow can semiautomatically track the 4 cardiac valves, thus performing a comprehensive quantitation of intracardiac flow, providing automatically classical indexes of diastolic function for both atrioventricular valves, such as E- and A-wave velocity, E/A ratio, e' velocity, and E/e' ratio (**Fig. 3**); however, this module is currently for research only.

Filling pressures LV filling pressure is assessed based on the early mitral inflow wave (E) in relation to the mitral annulus early velocity (e') at the lateral and septal locations. The general concept is that myocardial disease reduces e' velocities, and a stiff LV has diminished early filling time, augmenting the E velocity because the same amount of volume has less time to transit from the LA to the LV. These changes increase the E/e' ratio; in echocardiography, an average of the septal and lateral E/e' over 14 reflects LV augmented filling pressures.

Other useful elements indicating augmented LV and LA filling pressures that CMR identify include the following:
- High-velocity flow during diastasis (termed L wave), which reflects elevated LA pressure forcing flow to enter the LV in middiastole
- Pulmonary vein flow pattern with a marked diastolic predominance and an augmented atrial reversal wave, denoting a vigorous LA contraction to overcome increased LV pressure
- Mitral regurgitation with a diastolic component (in the absence of electric conduction abnormalities), evidencing elevated LV pressure at end-diastole, that overcomes LA pressure, producing premature mitral regurgitation

Pulmonary hypertension Regarding PH, besides calculating pulmonary arterial pressures (PAP), imaging techniques should address its source as

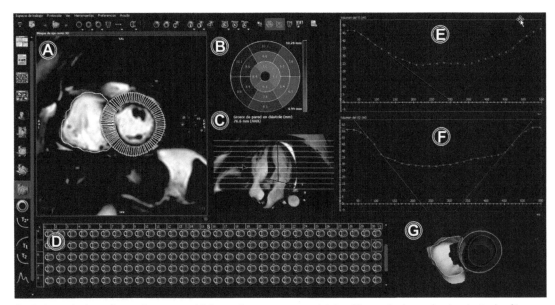

Fig. 2. Ventricular volume-time curves. Volume-time curves are obtained by analyzing a short-axis stack of images with complete coverage of both ventricles. (*C*) A 4-chamber view of the heart that demonstrates full coverage of the short-axis stack containing 10 slices. (*A*) One slice of this stack (slice 5/10) located at the midlevel of the ventricles. In this slice, endocardial contours for the right and left ventricle are traced, repeating this procedure throughout the entire cardiac cycle (typically involving 30 frames inside 1 RR interval) (*D*). This manual process is incredibly enhanced by CMR dedicated software with artificial intelligence border detection. This software accurately and rapidly (in <10 seconds) traces more than 800 images, including contours of the LV endocardium and epicardium and the RV endocardium, a process that would be manually unbearable. With this information, volume-time curves are constructed for the LV (*E*) and the RV (*F*), providing systolic and diastolic indexes of cardiac function, such as systolic PER, systolic PFT, diastolic PFR, and diastolic PFT. Of note, PER and PFR need to be indexed by EDV. Also, this software performs automatic thickness measurement of each LV myocardial segment (*B*) and provides a live 3D model of the whole heart over the entire cardiac cycle (*G*).

cardiac or extracardiac. In the former, echocardiography using Doppler is far superior to CMR in estimating PAP because CMR estimation of PAP uses cumbersome indirect formulas applied to pulmonary flow. What CMR can offer in this area is a better anatomic and functional evaluation of the pulmonary vasculature, including advanced flow dynamics (vortexes, energy loss, branches flow asymmetry, among others) and assessment of extracardiac causes of PH, such as shunts and pulmonary and vascular diseases.

Likely cause of ventricular thickening and heart failure

In the presence of LVH, the imaging goal is to pinpoint its cause at an early stage. An ideal imaging technique should distinguish between adaptation or load-related LVH, such as in hypertensive cardiomyopathy, aortic stenosis, and athletes' hearts, versus a pathologic LV thickening not associated with loading conditions, for example, infiltrative cardiomyopathy or HCM.

Echocardiography provides clues regarding LVH patterns and some red flags (**Table 2**), suggesting pathologic LVH. Unfortunately, most of these red-

flag features are only evident at later stages of the disease. Thus, echocardiography cannot confidently distinguish between the mentioned scenarios.

Conversely, because of its tissue characterization capabilities, CMR can identify distinct LV wall-thickening phenotypes and depict myocardial fibrosis and other features, such as lipid and iron deposition, providing unmatched diagnostic precision.

Table 3 summarizes the imaging objectives in HFpEF and compares the performance of echocardiography versus CMR.

Associated alterations and findings

CMR can provide clues of extracardiac findings that can be a valuable piece in solving the diagnostic puzzle. For example, CMR can accurately quantify hepatic iron overload and confirm the diagnosis of iron overload cardiomyopathy. In amyloidosis, besides LVH (**Fig. 4**A) associated with myocardial T1 and ECV elevation (**Fig. 4**B), marked renal T1 and ECV elevation (**Fig. 4**C) could link renal failure and HF together, whereas mediastinal pathologic lymph nodes or axillary lymph

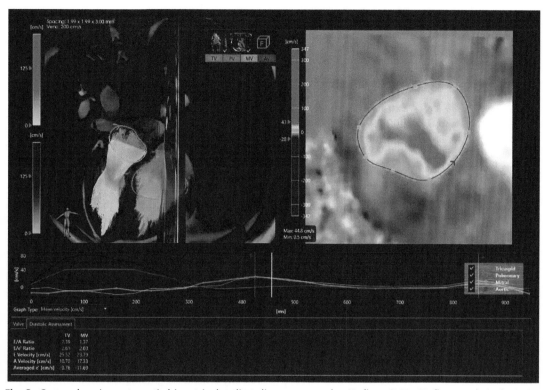

Fig. 3. Comprehensive automatic biventricular diastolic assessment by 4D flow CMR. 4D flow analysis depicting biventricular inflow; flow patterns are analyzed in the 4 cardiac valves with the aid of valve tracking, obtaining accurate biventricular time-volume curves, filling velocities early (E), and late (A) for mitral and tricuspid inflow along with annular velocities (e'). Also, E/A and E/e' ratios are given, delivering an automatic integral evaluation of diastolic function.

nodes, especially when more than 3 cm, may suggest sarcoidosis.

Other useful extracardiac findings are signs of chronic liver and kidney disease that can produce volume overload and thus mimic or contribute to the HFpEF pathophysiology.

Cardiac Magnetic Resonance Evaluation in Heart Failure with Preserved Ejection Fraction

Gross basic concepts

MRI uses the potential body magnetism related to the hydrogen molecule abundant in the human body. To do so, the patient is position inside a powerful static magnetic field (MF), generally with a strength of 1.5 or 3.0 T, which corresponds to nearly 30,000 times the earth's MF. This basal MF (M_z) aligns hydrogen atoms that start swirling around the main axis, phenomena termed precession, and the cornerstone of CMR, which is very similar to a spin rotating. This basal and resting magnetization needs to be manipulated in order to be measured. Manipulation of hydrogen molecules or spins uses intermittent radiofrequency pulses (RF) that are rapidly switched on and off

in sequence (producing a periodic loud and awkward sound). Every time the RF pulse is turned off, spins return to their basal precession condition, exhibiting 2 main components, namely the longitudinal relaxation (T1) and the transverse relaxation (T2), each of these components is measured at a specific time-point, giving the known T1 and T2 relaxation times in milliseconds.

T1 and T2 times are unique for each tissue and depend on the size of the molecule and its relation to surrounding structures (lattice).

CMR uses 2 basic types of sequences, spin echo sequences that provide morphologic and anatomic assessment, and gradient echo sequences that give functional information. GAD-based contrast agents allow scar or fibrosis detection and are also used for myocardial perfusion.

CMR is a method with high reproducibility and good spatial and temporal resolution, and because of its nonionizing nature, it is incredibly safe and green.

On the downside, CMR requires expertise in scanning and reporting and presents patient limitations, such as claustrophobia, poor breath holders, irregular heart rhythm, tachycardia, glomerular

Table 2
Red flags for specific cardiomyopathies

	Feature
Clinical	• Young age at presentation • Extracardiac clinical findings, such as speech or intellectual impairment, muscle weakness • Visual impairment (retinitis pigmentosa) • Evidence of multisystemic affection
Auxiliary examinations and laboratory tests	• ECG with short PR or Wolff • High liver enzymes • High skeletal muscle creatine kinase owing to myopathy
Echocardiography	• Atrial septal thickening • Diffuse valvular thickening • Presence of thrombus without wall motion alteration • Marked reduction of longitudinal function with apparent preserved LVEF • Pericardial effusion • Advanced systolic or diastolic dysfunction at young age

Table 3
Imaging objectives in HFpEF and comparison of the performance of echocardiography versus CMR

Variable	CMR	Echo
Cause of HF	+++	−
LV volume and function	+++	++
RV volume and function	+++	+
Valvular alterations	+++	++
Estimating filling pressures	+	++
Grading DD	+	++
Pulmonary hypertension	+	++
Extracardiac findings	++	−

(+++), optimal; (++), adequate; (+), discrete; (−), insufficient.

filtration rate less than 30 mL/min, which precludes GAD administration and the presence of incompatible implanted metal objects (brain clips, cochlear implants, external bone tutors).

Cardiac magnetic resonance basic protocol for heart failure with preserved ejection fraction

A basic CMR protocol is detailed in **Table 4** and includes anatomic, functional, and tissue characterization information; this protocol can be accomplished in 45 minutes of magnet.

Specific sequences and uses

Flow patterns by cardiac magnetic resonance CMR evaluates flow using 2 distinct sequences: the traditional one is called phase contrast, consisting of a 2D flow acquisition at a specific point, with the inherent anatomic and plane orientation limitations. The second alternative is an advanced sequence called 4D flow, which constructs a volumetric image with 3D flow information attached. Both sequences need an input of maximum velocity to analyze (called velocity encoding or VENC), which behaves exactly as the Nyquist limit in echocardiography. Notably, the well-validated Doppler velocity criteria for grading DD should not be used in CMR, as these velocities are underestimated by phase-contrast CMR.[13] Nevertheless, flow curve morphology, flow direction, and velocities ratios (such as E/A ratio) are reliable and validated and in line with echocardiography flow patterns.[13]

For example, a mitral inflow pattern with an early velocity (E wave) less than three-quarters of the atrial filling (A wave) is consistent with a typical Doppler pattern of impaired relaxation (type I) and thus concordant with normal filling pressures. Opposite to this, a triphasic mitral inflow pattern with a high-velocity middiastolic (diastasis) filling flow, termed L wave, is diagnostic of elevated LV and LA - filling pressures

Regarding RV DD, the tricuspid filling is highly variable depending on the respiratory cycle and the loading conditions. Hence, tricuspid inflow pattern is not as reliable as mitral inflow for evaluating DD. So other elements must be used to assess RV DD, such as antegrade pulmonary arterial flow in late diastole throughout the respiratory cycle and an increase in atrial reversal at the superior vena cava. Elements that are superiorly appraised by 4D flow CMR, enabling infinite flow measurements in any plane or orientation, providing comprehensive simultaneous flow and functional analysis.

Respective to CMR flow information, it is displayed as flow over time in milliliters per second; but, maximum and mean velocities and gradients can also be displayed.

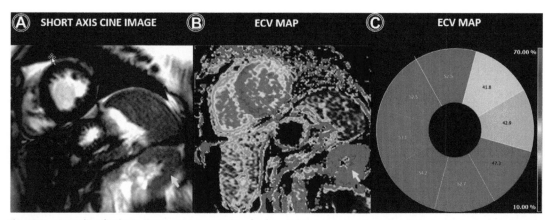

Fig. 4. Extracardiac findings in HFpEF. Extracardiac finding linking renal and cardiac failure. (*A*) A short axis of the heart showing moderate LVH. (*B*) The ECV map depicting extremely high EVC values in the LV septum and inferior walls and the left kidney (*arrow*). (*C*) The numerical value of the ECV in a bull's-eye plot. The final diagnosis was cardiac and renal amyloidosis.

Figs. 5 and **6** portray LV and RV diastolic restrictive physiology analyzed using 4D flow.

Tissue characterization and fibrosis assessment
Although different pathophysiological mechanisms are involved in HFpEF, including myocyte, interstitium, microvascular, and metabolic causes, it remains unclear whether HFpEF is a separate clinical entity, a result, or a part of a clinical syndrome. Adding more complexity is the fact that various pathologic conditions accompany HFpEF.[8] The most crucial benefit of CMR is

Table 4
Standard cardiac magnetic resonance imaging protocol in heart failure with preserved ejection fraction

CMR Sequence	Objective
1. Localizers	Study planning
2. Bright blood and black blood anatomic axial stacks	Thoracic anatomic evaluation
3. Fast-speed, low-quality SFFP CINE pilots	Study planning
4. Long-axis SSFP CINE (4C, 2C, 3C)	Visual assessment of size and function and longitudinal strain analysis
5. T1 map native	Interstitial fibrosis evaluation
6. T2 map	Edema evaluation
Contrast Administration	
7. First-pass perfusion imaging	Resting perfusion defect
8. Short-axis CINE stack	Measurement of ventricular wall thickness, function, volumes, and mass. Radial and circumferential strain
9. Phase contrast pulmonary vein flow	Grading of diastolic function and estimated filling pressures
10. Phase contrast mitral inflow (ideally analysis performed with valve tracking)	Grading of diastolic function and estimate filling pressures
11. Other flow sequences according to specific pathologic condition	Evaluation of valvular alterations
12. T1 map post-GAD	Estimation of extracellular volume
13. Late gadolinium enhancement (single shot and segmented in short and long axis)	Detection of replacement fibrosis
14. Whole-heart 4D flow optional (if 4DF is performed phase contrast sequences are skipped)	Comprehensive analysis of cardiac and vascular flow

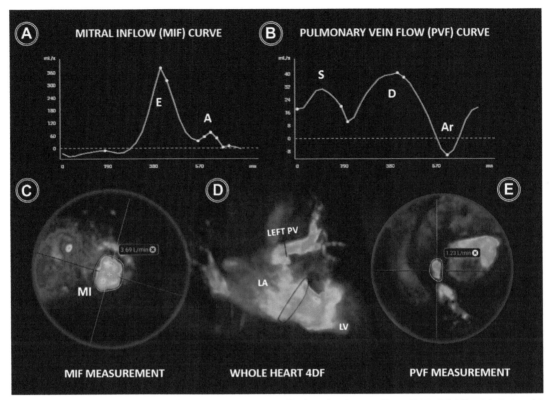

Fig. 5. LV restrictive filling by 4D flow. Severe LV DD is displayed using 4D flow CMR. (*A*) Mitral inflow with marked E-wave predominance over A wave. (*B*) Pulmonary venous flow with diastolic predominance and marked atrial reversal (Ar). (*C*) Mitral inflow measurement in multiplanar reconstruction (MPR). (*D*) The 4D flow volume center in the LV and LA. (*E*) Flow assessment of the left pulmonary trunk in MPR.

detecting the underlying pathologic condition of DD and revealing structural changes. Several diseases with similar clinical presentations may have the same clinical phenotype as the HFpEF condition, termed phenocopy, beclouding the diagnostic process.

GAD is a paramagnetic contrast agent that is rapidly washed out from normal myocardium. In the presence of replacement fibrosis, which corresponds to a scar with high collagen content, GAD is retained inside this scar, presenting a slow and late washout, reducing T1 relaxation time in this area and generating a bright or hyperintense signal in inversion recovery sequences. GAD distribution can be easily detected in the LV myocardium but is more challenging to see in thinner structures, such as the RV free wall or the atrias, where a 3D late gadolinium enhancement (LGE) high-resolution sequence is preferred.

Patterns of LGE can be separated into the following 2 groups (**Fig. 7**):

1. **Ischemic pattern** is the LGE pattern that follows anatomic coronary distribution, starting from the subendocardium and progressing in transmurality from endocardium to epicardium. LGE involving less than 50% of wall thickness is termed subendocardial and is deemed viable. Conversely, LGE comprising more than 50% of wall thickness is termed transmural and is reckoned not viable, meaning that those segments have a very low probability of recovering contractile function following revascularization. Sometimes small focal and subendocardial infarctions could be spotted in patients with HFpEF and are considered a "bystander" myocardial infarction not responsible for the clinical picture.

2. **Nonischemic pattern** is a group of distinct LGE patterns that include midwall, epicardial, and global endocardial (not corresponding to a coronary artery segmentation). In addition, its distribution could be patchy, focal, or diffuse. Specific pathologic conditions tend to affect the myocardium differently, thus presenting distinctive LGE patterns that are key to the differential. For example, amyloidosis can give a global endocardial or a patchy midmyocardial pattern; Anderson-Fabry disease generally presents basal inferolateral epicardial or mid-wall LGE.

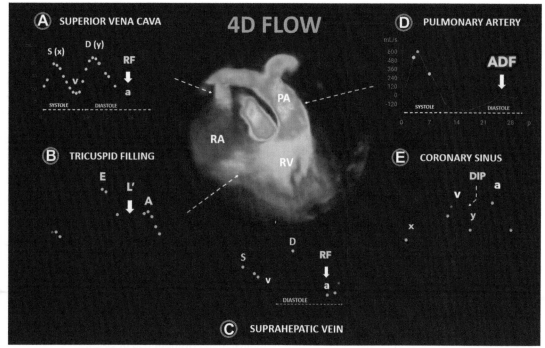

Fig. 6. RV restrictive filling. RV advanced DD, evaluated by a comprehensive set of parameters. Main findings. (*A*) superior vena cava with prominent reversal of flow (RF) corresponding to the "a" wave of the venous pulse. (*B*) Tricuspid inflow with E wave predominance and presence of an L wave, indicating flow from RA to RV during diastasis (hypertensive RA). (*C*) Flow in the suprahepatic vein displaying similar findings to SVC flow. (*D*) The hallmark of restrictive RV physiology evidencing anterograde diastolic flow (ADF) mainly at end-diastole, evidencing increased RV end-diastolic pressure generating premature pulmonary valve opening and ADF. (*E*) Flow in the coronary sinus depicting a DIP and steep curve corresponding to the "y" wave of the venous pulse.

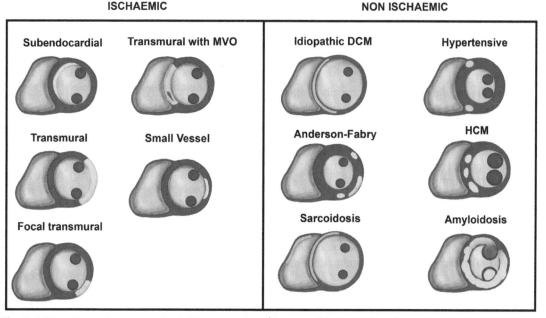

Fig. 7. LGE patterns. Representative LGE patterns in various conditions. In this scheme, 2 main groups are presented: ischemic LGE pattern and no ischemic LGE pattern. These LGE patterns are essential to the differential diagnosis process.

Unspecific patterns, another pattern frequently encountered but highly unspecific, is the affection of RV insertion points (inferior and superior) in the basal and midseptum, which is an expression of cardiac overload and is observed in various conditions, such as hypertensive cardiomyopathy, PH, HCM, and dilated cardiomyopathy.

Late gadolinium enhancement involvement in hypertensive cardiomyopathy Hypertensive cardiomyopathy or hypertensive heart disease (HHD) is among the most frequent conditions associated with HFpEF, so accurate imaging portrayal is crucial. HHD presents a broad spectrum of cardiac involvement ranging from mild LVH with normal systolic function, grade I DD (normal filling pressures), and mild LA enlargement. In this scenario, CMR reveals normal T1 and ECV and the absence of LGE.

In advanced stages, HHD can present moderate to severe LVH, advanced DD (grade II or III) with associated PH, and severe LA enlargement leading to atrial fibrillation. In this latter situation, CMR depicts elevated T1 and ECV and the presence of LGE that can range from the frequent focal involvement of both RV insertion points to the rare case of intense midwall LGE patches; **Fig. 8** portrays evolving stages in HHD summarizing anatomic, functional, and tissue characteristics at each stage.

HCM can present with diverse LVH phenotypes (**Fig. 9**), which could be challenging to differentiate from HHD in the absence of LGE.

Some clues to differential are that HCM can present as follows:

○ LVH generally follows a spiral anticlockwise pattern going from base to apex
○ Mitral valve and papillary muscle abnormalities (elongated leaflets, accessory valvular tissue, anterior displacement, or apical insertion of papillary muscles)
○ Typically has a type I transmitral inflow pattern
○ Can present RV outflow tract obstruction
○ Presence of myocardial crypts
○ When LGE is present in half of the cases, it correlates with the thicker segments

As stated, LGE pattern is central to diagnosis, but the amount of LGE is crucial in terms of prognosis and to predict response to therapy. Because the presence of a higher percentage of LGE (ie, 15% in HCM) relates to worse outcomes in HF, worse DD, sudden cardiac death, and arrhythmias, furthermore higher LGE presence is related to fewer reverse remodeling following medical therapy.

Parametric mapping (T1, ECV, T2 and T2*), relies on each tissue inherent and unique magnetic relaxation properties, allowing CMR tissue characterization by measuring relaxation times (T1 and T2), also known as parametric mapping.

T1 mapping is acquired before contrast (native) and after contrast administration, to estimate ECV, which ideally needs a same-day hematocrit to subtract red blood cell volume. Elevated native T1 values reflect interstitial or microscopic fibrosis that is not visible by LGE. It is essential to mention that native T1 values must be measured in regions without LGE because the objective is to identify microscopic fibrosis. There is no practical point in measuring native T1 in LGE zones where the value is extremely high. Conversely, very low native T1 values suggest lipid infiltration, as seen in Anderson-Fabry disease, fatty metaplasia, or iron deposits.

T2 mapping allows the detection of water and edema, and T2* is used to detect iron overload mainly in the liver when iron deposit is suspected. Both of these sequences only need acquiring native maps (without use of GAD).

In addition, when GAD is contraindicated, a contrast-free CMR can still give tissue characterization by using native T1, T2, and T2*.

Cardiac mechanics (strain)

Strain imaging, which quantitatively assesses myocardial deformation in longitudinal, radial, and circumferential planes, is considered a less load-dependent index of systolic function than LVEF.[14] Strain is a robust deformation marker with a diagnostic and prognostic role for both global and regional LV function. The subendocardial layer of the myocardium is responsible for the long-axis function of the LV, so strain abnormalities may indicate early myocardial dysfunction in the setting of ischemic heart disease, which first affects the endocardium. Also, a reduced longitudinal strain despite an apparent preserved LVEF is predictive of worse outcomes in HFpEF.[15]

Myocardial strain and torsion can be acquired by CMR using dedicated sequences (FAST SENC, or DENSE) or the traditional SSFP CINES using feature tracking, similar to echocardiographic speckle tracking but yielding values not directly comparable. Nonetheless, CMR strain is not routinely performed.

Fig. 10 depicts an HHD with LVH associated with a septal bulge, peak systolic global longitudinal strain is preserved (see **Fig. 10**A, C), but is reduced in the basal anteroseptal segment (see **Fig. 10**B), segments that also have a slight elevation of native T1 (see **Fig. 10**D).

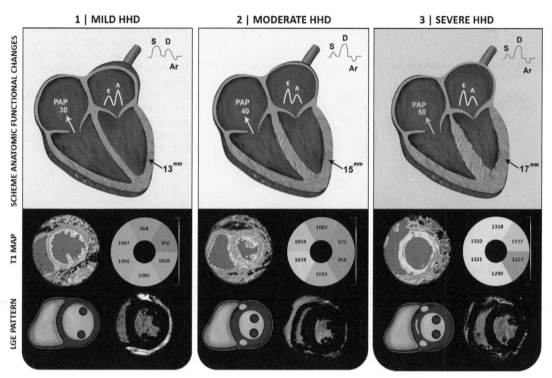

Fig. 8. Stages of HHD. Evolving stages of HHD. (1) Mild HHD, characterized by mild LVH and LAE, frequently presents with type I mitral filling pattern and normal pulmonary venous flow, concordant with normal filling pressures. In this scenario, CMR usually reports average T1 values and absence of LGE. (2) Moderate HHD, usually presents moderate LVH, more LA enlargement, and mitral inflow can be pseudonormalized. Pulmonary venous flow depicts diastolic predominance related to increased LA pressures retrogradely augmenting PAP. CMR, in this case, shows a slight elevation of T1 maps, especially in the thicker segments (septum) and LGE at a single or both insertion points. (3) Severe HHD. In this advanced and less frequent scenario, LVH and LAE are more severe; the mitral filling pattern is restrictive, and pulmonary venous flow shows a deep A-wave inversion. Elevated LV and LA filling pressures generate increasing PAP. CMR evidence of diffuse and higher native T1 elevation and LGE extends beyond insertion points into the LV septum.

Differential diagnosis

A first diagnostic step is to exclude conditions that can mimic HFpEF by causing dyspnea, exercise intolerance, and ankle edema, and are very prevalent, such as obesity, physical deconditioning, lung disease, and venous insufficiency.

A second differential objective should be to rule out specific cardiomyopathies that at early stages could be difficult to tell apart from a pure form of HFpEF. These cardiomyopathies include HCM, amyloidosis, and storage diseases, such as Anderson-Fabry, as previously commented.

Some extracardiac conditions that mimic HFpEF, such as high-output states caused by hyperthyroidism, anemia, extracardiac shunts, and arteriovenous (AV) fistulas, should also be considered.

Finally, any cause that generates extracardiac volume overload can mimic HFpEF, for example, chronic liver and kidney disease and nephrotic syndrome.

NOVEL METHODS AND FUTURE DIRECTIONS

Although increased myocardial stiffness plays an essential role in DD, there is no conventional imaging method to directly measure myocardial stiffness in vivo, as in the liver, where it is measured by transient elastography (Fibroscan). Fibroscan measures shear wave velocity, which corresponds to the sound wave velocity passing through tissues. The more fibrosis, the greater stiffness is present, which enhances sound-wave transmission reaching higher shear wave speed.

The same principle can be performed using 2D and 3D high-frequency magnetic resonance elastographies, which are novel techniques that generate a stiffness map using the same basics of shear wave velocity within tissues. Arani and colleagues[16] demonstrated the feasibility of 3D high-frequency CMR elastography as a contrast agent–free diagnostic imaging technique for quantitatively measuring myocardial stiffness in vivo.

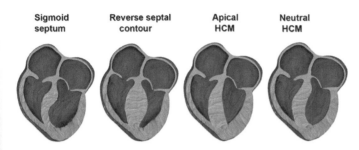

A HCM Hypertrophy patterns

Sigmoid septum   Reverse septal contour   Apical HCM   Neutral HCM

Fig. 9. LVH characteristic in HCM. LVH phenotypes and characteristics can aid in differentiating HCM from HHD. (*A*) LVH phenotypes in HCM. Neutral phenotype can be challenging to differentiate from HHD, especially when no LGE or T1 map alterations are present. (*B*) Counterclockwise spiral rotation of LVH in HCM. Starting from the base to apex, this clue suggests HCM assisting in discriminating between HCM and HHD.

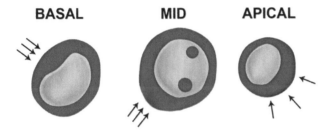

B Counterclockwise spiral rotation of LVH

BASAL   MID   APICAL

Other feature is obesity, which is common in HFpEF and has numerous cardiovascular effects. Obokata and colleagues[17] showed that epicardial adipose tissue has a direct mechanical effect caused by increased pericardial restraint and enhanced ventricular interdependence. Also, a correlation exists between DD and increased epicardial adipose tissue, adding to its classic inflammatory role a potential pathophysiologic one in HFpEF.

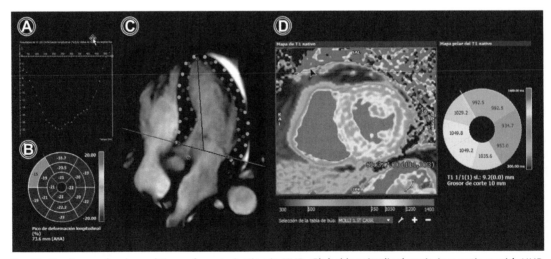

Fig. 10. Cardiac mechanics and tissue characterization in HHD. Global longitudinal strain in a patient with HHD. (*A*) Global strain curve with a preserved peak systolic value at 19.5%. (*B*) A bull's-eye representation of the AHA 17 segment model, evidencing a localized reduction of strain in the basal anteroseptal segment, which corresponds to the thicker segment (septal bulge). (*C*) The boundary points that are traced in the CINE images to estimate strain. (*D*) The native T1 map and its absolute values portraying a slight elevation of T1 values in the thicker segments (septum).

Finally, advanced cardiac flow parameters, such as energy loss index, shear stress, pressure drop, and vortex analysis, are promising elements that can be readily obtained with 4D flow sequences delivering next-level cardiac dynamics assessment.

Machine learning and artificial intelligence are gaining importance in the medical imaging field and are expected to transform clinical practice in the following years. CMR can use machine learning to help guide diagnosis and therapy management. Artificial intelligence is associated with radiomics, which is a novel image analysis technique. In which digital images are converted into numeric data that are analyzed to obtain several numerical quantifiers of shape and tissue characteristics. This radiomics process, when applied to large amounts of cardiac imaging data (as CMR studies store in Biobanks), can automatically identify pathologic clusters of disease that require further workup.[18]

SUMMARY

HFpEF is an etiologically, phenotypically, and clinically heterogeneous syndrome that poses a massive burden on health care systems worldwide. It diagnostic process is challenging; current consensus and guidelines denote the crucial role of cardiac imaging. CMR has emerged as a robust technique in patients with HFpEF, as it provides comprehensive information on most parameters recommended in guidelines. Moreover, CMR integrates anatomic, functional, and tissue characterization capabilities, thus enabling accurate distinction of different phenocopies from a pure form of HFpEF. Classic sequences outperform echocardiography in most aspects, and novel sequences with the aid of artificial intelligence could redefine the imaging boundaries in HFPEF.

CLINICS CARE POINTS

- Heart failure with preserved ejection fraction requires relevant structural heart disease to which the symptoms could be attributable.
- Echocardiography, because of its widespread access and well-validated features, is the first-line imaging technique in heart failure with preserved ejection fraction.
- The diagnostic process is challenging because of the absence of a single diagnostic marker, the complex echocardiography evaluation, and the broad spectrum of entities that cause heart failure with preserved ejection fraction.

- A robust and comprehensive imaging technique, such as cardiac magnetic resonance, is the ideal method to characterize this condition.
- The main advantage of cardiac magnetic resonance over echocardiography is the integration of anatomic, functional, and tissue characterization capabilities, offering unprecedented diagnostic precision.
- Late gadolinium enhancement is central in categorizing heart failure with preserved ejection fraction and has multiple roles, such as aiding diagnosis, by identifying typical late gadolinium enhancement patterns of distinct disease.
- Late gadolinium enhancement patterns are grossly divided into ischemic and nonischemic patterns.
- Total late gadolinium enhancement burden can be quantified, thus providing prognosis information and aiding in predicting response to therapy.
- Hypertensive heart disease presents a broad spectrum of cardiac involvement. Cardiac magnetic resonance findings range from normal T1, extracellular volume, and no late gadolinium enhancement presence, to markedly elevated T1 and extracellular volume and late gadolinium enhancement presence that can go from focal involvement of RV insertion points to intense midwall LGE patches, posing a tremendous diagnostic challenge in differentiating from hypertrophic cardiomyopathy.
- Cardiac magnetic resonance is key to differential diagnosis, separating causes that can mimic heart failure with preserved ejection fraction termed "phenocopies" to a more "pure" form of heart failure with preserved ejection fraction and also identifying extracardiac findings that can orient diagnosis.
- Finally, novel sequences that analyzed cardiac mechanics and advanced intracardiac flow features could reshape the understanding of heart failure with preserved ejection fraction.

DISCLOSURE

The authors have nothing to disclose.

REFERENCES

1. Huis in 't Veld AE, de Man FS, van Rossum AC, et al. How to diagnose heart failure with preserved ejection fraction: the value of invasive stress testing. Neth Heart J 2016;24(4):244–51.

2. Paulus WJ, Brutsaert DL, Gillebert TC, et al. How to diagnose diastolic heart failure. Eur Heart J 1998; 19(7):990–1003.

3. Ponikowski P, Voors AA, Anker SD, et al. 2016 ESC Guidelines for the diagnosis and treatment of acute and chronic heart failure. Eur J Heart Fail 2016; 18(8):891–975.

4. Sanders-van Wijk S, Barandiarán Aizpurua A, Brunner-La Rocca H, et al. The HFA-PEFF and H2FPEF scores largely disagree in classifying patients with suspected heart failure with preserved ejection fraction. Eur J Heart Fail 2019. https://doi.org/10.1002/ejhf.2019.

5. Nishimura RA, Tajik AJ. Evaluation of diastolic filling of left ventricle in health and disease: Doppler echocardiography is the clinician's Rosetta Stone. Depression 1997;30(1):8–18.

6. Nagueh SF, Smiseth OA, Appleton CP, et al. Recommendations for the evaluation of left ventricular diastolic function by echocardiography: an update from the American Society of Echocardiography and the European Association of Cardiovascular Imaging. Eur Heart J Cardiovasc Imaging 2016;17(12): 1321–60.

7. Jaubert O, Cruz G, Bustin A, et al. Free-running cardiac magnetic resonance fingerprinting: joint T1/T2 map and Cine imaging. Magn Reson Imaging 2020;68:173–82.

8. Shah AM, Pfeffer MA. Heart failure: the many faces of heart failure with preserved ejection fraction. Nat Rev Cardiol 2012;9(10):555–6.

9. Stokke TM, Hasselberg NE, Smedsrud MK, et al. Geometry as a confounder when assessing ventricular systolic function: comparison between ejection fraction and strain. J Am Coll Cardiol 2017;70(8): 942–54.

10. Hoit BD. Left atrial size and function: role in prognosis. J Am Coll Cardiol 2014;63(6):493–505.

11. von Roeder M, Rommel KP, Kowallick JT, et al. Influence of left atrial function on exercise capacity and left ventricular function in patients with heart failure and preserved ejection fraction. Circ Cardiovasc Imaging 2017;10(4).

12. Gabrielli L, Herrera S, Contreras-Briceño F, et al. Increased active phase atrial contraction is related to marathon runner performance. Eur J Appl Physiol 2018;118(9):1931–9.

13. Rathi VK, Doyle M, Yamrozik J, et al. Routine evaluation of left ventricular diastolic function by cardiovascular magnetic resonance: a practical approach. J Cardiovasc Magn Reson 2008;10(1):36.

14. Shah AM, Solomon SD. Myocardial deformation imaging: current status and future directions. Circulation 2012;125(2).

15. Shah AM, Claggett B, Sweitzer NK, et al. Prognostic importance of impaired systolic function in heart failure with preserved ejection fraction and the impact of spironolactone. Circulation 2015;132(5):402–14.

16. Arani A, Arunachalam SP, Chang ICY, et al. Cardiac MR elastography for quantitative assessment of elevated myocardial stiffness in cardiac amyloidosis. J Magn Reson Imaging 2017;46(5):1361–7.

17. Obokata M, Reddy YNV, Pislaru Sv, et al. Evidence supporting the existence of a distinct obese phenotype of heart failure with preserved ejection fraction. Circulation 2017;136(1):6–19.

18. Zheng Q, Delingette H, Fung K, et al. Pathological cluster identification by unsupervised analysis in 3,822 UK Biobank cardiac MRIs. Front Cardiovasc Med 2020;7:539788.

Current Status of Pharmacologic and Nonpharmacologic Therapy in Heart Failure with Preserved Ejection Fraction

Mi-Na Kim, MD, PhD, Seong-Mi Park, MD, PhD*

KEYWORDS

- Heart failure • Preserved ejection fraction • Therapy

KEY POINTS

- Heart failure with preserved ejection fraction (HFpEF) is heterogenous systemic disorder that has various phenotype and multiple comorbidities.
- Several therapies for various phenotypes and pathophysiology of HFpEF have been introduced and studied, although the guideline directed medical therapy of HF with reduced EF had shown a limited clinical benefit.
- Several therapies for various phenotypes and pathophysiology of HFpEF have been introduced and studied, although the guideline directed medical therapy of HF with reduced EF had shown a limited clinical benefit.
- The pressure monitoring was demonetrated to reduced HF hospitalization, and several non-pharmacological therapies that are targeting various phenotype and pathophysiology of HEpEF, such as interatrial septal shunt, pacing therapies, left ventricular expander and pericardiectomy, have been introduced and currently studied.

INTRODUCTION

Heart failure with preserved ejection fraction (HFpEF) is now the most common form of heart failure (HF) and accounts for about half the HF cases.[1] It is a growing burden to the health care system because of the increasing prevalence, substantial comorbidities, and unfavorable prognosis.[2] HFpEF is now one of the greatest unmet needs in cardiology[3] because it lacks proven therapy to reduce mortality and morbidity compared with remarkable developments and revolutionized changes in the treatment of HF with reduced ejection fraction (HFrEF). HFpEF is considered to be a systemic syndrome with diverse phenotypes, various pathophysiologies, and multiple comorbidities. The diagnosis of HFpEF has become more refined and sophisticated. Numerous pharmacologic and nonpharmacologic therapies for each phenotype or pathophysiology have been suggested and investigated in the HFpEF population.[4] This article summarizes pharmacologic and nonpharmacologic therapies and reviews recent clinical trials in patients with HFpEF and also provides therapeutic options for unmanageable HFpEF.

Division of Cardiology, Department of Internal Medicine, Korea University Medicine, Korea University Anam Hospital, Goryeodae-ro 73, Seongbuk-gu, Seoul 02841, Republic of Korea
* Corresponding author.
E-mail address: smparkmd@korea.ac.kr

Heart Failure Clin 17 (2021) 463–482
https://doi.org/10.1016/j.hfc.2021.02.008
1551-7136/21/© 2021 Elsevier Inc. All rights reserved.

DIVERSE PATHOPHYSIOLOGY OF HEART FAILURE WITH PRESERVED EJECTION FRACTION AND ITS PHENOTYPE

HFpEF has been considered a diastolic HF for the past 20 years. Left ventricle (LV) diastolic dysfunction caused by impaired relaxation and increased chamber stiffness leads to an increase in LV filling pressure. Increased LV filling pressure at rest or during exercise promotes the development of dyspnea and exercise intolerance. Numerous efforts to elucidate the pathophysiology and define the phenotype of HFpEF have led to a paradigm shift to a systemic syndrome that results from an interplay of coexisting significant abnormalities, including left atrium (LA) dysfunction, subtle LV systolic dysfunction, pulmonary hypertension with right ventricle (RV) dysfunction, extrinsic restraint by epicardial fat, microvascular dysfunction, chronotropic incompetence, skeletal muscle dysfunction, altered ventriculoarterial coupling, and abnormal cardiorenal relationship, besides LV diastolic dysfunction.[5] These abnormalities might be generated and affected by systemic inflammation, endothelial dysfunction, and oxidative stress induced by multiple risk factors and comorbidities of HFpEF, such as coronary artery disease (CAD), hypertension, obesity, diabetes, atrial fibrillation (AF), anemia, renal dysfunction, sleep apnea, and chronic lung disease.[6–8] The oxidative stress induced by systemic inflammation reduces the bioavailability of nitric oxide (NO) and produces highly reactive superoxide in the endothelium. The endothelium is changed to be favorable for vasoconstriction and prothrombotic status.[7] Impaired NO bioavailability influences the NO–cyclic guanosine monophosphate (cGMP)–protein kinase G (PKG) pathway in the myocardium. Because of decreased PKG activity by downregulation of the NO-cGMP-PKG pathway, cardiomyocytes are stiffened.[6,9] Furthermore, interstitial fibrosis occurs because of increased collagen secretion by myofibroblasts activated by an increased level of transforming growth factor-β (TGF-β) released from macrophage.[10] Moreover, upregulated galetin-3 in HFpEF is another important mediator of myocardial fibrosis.[11] Also, systemic inflammation leads to impaired myocardial energetics via altered structure and impaired function of mitochondria, change in energy metabolism, and intracellular calcium overload. These cardiometabolic abnormalities are regarded as another pathophysiology in HFpEF even though these concepts are derived from studies in HFrEF.[12]

A schematic diagram of comorbidities, pathophysiology, and representative phenotypes of HFpEF is presented in **Fig. 1**.

EFFORTS TO INCREASE THE ACCURACY OF HEART FAILURE WITH PRESERVED EJECTION FRACTION DIAGNOSIS

HF is a clinical syndrome caused by structural or functional impairment of contraction or filling of the heart. According to current guidelines, the diagnosis of HF is based on a combination of the presence of symptoms and signs of HF and increased natriuretic peptide levels. Subsequently, HFpEF is classified according to LV ejection fraction (LVEF).[13–15] However, the diagnostic algorithm of current guidelines is limited when diagnosing HFpEF, a clinical syndrome that has numerous causes and various and distinct phenotypes.[16] Recently, new diagnostic algorithms for providing the probability of HFpEF were proposed.[17,18] The H_2FPEF score is obtained by the sum of scores applicable to 6 variables including 2 echocardiographic (representative of increased LV filling pressure and pulmonary hypertension) and 4 clinical variables that are major comorbidities or causes of HFpEF (age, obesity, hypertension, and AF).[17] The HFA-PEFF diagnostic algorithm suggested by the Heart Failure Association of the European Society of Cardiology approaches the patients in a stepwise process. This 4-step algorithm is composed of pretest assessment, risk stratification by HFA-PEFF score, functional test in patients with intermediate probability, and evaluation of specific cause. The HFA-PEFF score is composed of echocardiographic parameters and the level of natriuretic peptides, which have different cutoff values by rhythm status or age. These new diagnostic algorithms have been reported to be superior to current guidelines.[19,20] The preevaluation before both score calculations was similar to the diagnostic criteria of the 2016 European Society of Cardiology guidelines. The probability of diagnosing HFpEF and recommendation of additional tests, such as exercise stress echocardiography or invasive hemodynamic measurement with and without exercise, in patients with uncertainty are common findings in both diagnostic algorithms. The H_2FPEF score considers comorbidities of HFpEF, and the HFA-PEFF diagnostic algorithm recommends the comprehensive diagnostic process for HFpEF. However, the diagnosis of HFpEF remains challenging in clinical practice. Additional validation, comparison of diagnostic accuracy, and elucidation of reclassified patients who have a different likelihood by new diagnostic systems should be investigated in the future.[21]

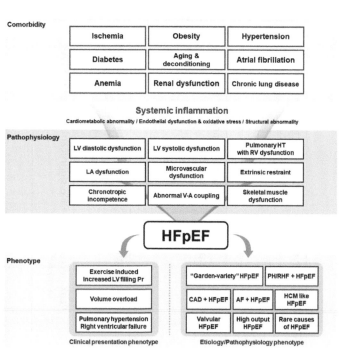

Fig. 1. Comorbidities, pathophysiology, and phenotypes of HFpEF. HCM, hypertrophic cardiomyopathy; HT, hypertension; PH, pulmonary hypertension; Pr, pressure; RHF, right heart failure, V-A, ventriculoarterial.

PHARMACOLOGIC AND NONPHARMACOLOGIC TREATMENT

To date, no treatment has reduced mortality in HFpEF. Therefore, current guidelines recommend an optimal volume control using diuretics for symptom relief and proper management of comorbidities, such as hypertension, obesity, diabetes, and chronic lung disease.[13,22] The blockade of neurohormonal activation, which is a traditional pharmacologic strategy for HFrEF treatment, has failed to reduce mortality in HFpEF. However, many pharmacologic and nonpharmacologic treatment trials targeting specific pathophysiologic phenotypes of HFpEF have been conducted, and a summary of the recent trials is presented in **Table 1**. Ongoing and unreported trials of HFpEF treatment are listed in **Table 2**. The pharmacologic and nonpharmacologic therapies targeted for each pathophysiology of HFpEF are shown in **Fig. 2**.

Pharmacologic Treatment

Conventional medications in heart failure with preserved ejection fraction

Angiotensin-converting enzyme inhibitors and angiotensin-II receptor blockers Inappropriate activation of the renin-angiotensin-aldosterone system (RAAS) is related to the development and progression of HFpEF.[23,24] The RAAS leads to LV hypertrophy and impaired LV diastolic function by increasing arterial and myocardial stiffness.[23] Therefore, several randomized clinical trials have been conducted to evaluate the prognostic value of the RAAS blockade.

The CHARM-preserved (Candesartan in Heart Failure: Assessment of Reduction in Mortality and Morbidity-preserved) trial[25] showed that the primary end point of composite cardiovascular (CV) death or HF hospitalization was not statistically different in candesartan versus placebo (hazard ratio, 0.89; 95% confidence interval [CI], 0.77–1.03; $P = .118$); however, HF hospitalization was significantly reduced by candesartan (hazard ratio, 0.84; 95% CI, 0.07–1.00; $P = .047$). In the PEP-CHF (Perindopril in Elderly People with Chronic Heart Failure) study,[26] perindopril improved HF symptoms and reduced HF rehospitalization at 1-year follow-up, but the benefit of perindopril in HFpEF remains uncertain. Because of the lower event rate than anticipated and the large proportion of withdrawal, the statistical power of the study to show a difference in the primary end point was reduced. The I-PRSERVED (Irbesartan in Heart Failure with Preserved Ejection Fraction) study,[27] irbesartan did not reduce all-cause mortality and CV hospitalization and it did not improve the quality of life (QOL) of HFpEF in long-term follow-up.[28] In conclusion, angiotensin-converting enzyme inhibitors (ACEis) and angiotensin-II receptor blockers (ARBs) did not improve mortality and HF hospitalization in

Table 1
Results of recently reported randomized control trials of pharmacologic and nonpharmacologic therapies of heart failure with preserved ejection fraction

Trials (Number of Patients)	Interventions	Inclusion Criteria	Mean Follow-up (mo)	Primary End Point	Trial Result
Pharmacologic Treatment					
PARAGON-HF[39] 2019, (n = 4822)	Sacubitril-valsartan	NYHA II–IV LVEF ≥ 45% Increased NPs	35	CV death HF hospitalization	No benefit for the primary end point Reduced primary end point in subgroup (patients with LVEF less than median [≤ 57%] and women)
EDIFY[56] 2017, (n = 179)	Ivabradine	NYHA II–III SR with HR ≥ 70 LVEF ≥ 45% Increased NPs	8	E/e′, 6MWD NT-proBNP	No difference in E/e′, 6MWD, and NT-proBNP
NEAT-HFpEF[60] 2015, (n = 110)	Isosorbide mononitrate	LVEF ≥ 50% HF with objective evidence (≥1) • HF hospitalization with congestion, increased LVEDP or PCWP, increased NP, LVDD on ECHO	3	Daily activity level	Decreased activity and worsened QOL
INDIE-HFpEF[66] 2018, (n = 105)	Nebulized inorganic nitrate	Age ≥ 40 y LVEF ≥ 50% HF with objective evidence (≥1) • HF hospitalization with congestion, increased LVEDP or PCWP, increased NP, LVDD on ECHO	3	Peak O$_2$ consumption	No improvement in exercise capacity
RELAX[69] 2016, (n = 216)	Sildenafil	HFpEF with RVD and RV-RA coupling NYHA II–IV LVEF ≥ 50%	6	Peak O$_2$ uptake	No improvement of RV function, exercise capacity, and ventilatory efficiency
DILATE-1[72] 2014, (n = 21)	Riociguat	HFpEF with PH LVEF ≥ 50%, mPAP ≥ 25 mm Hg PAWP >15 mm Hg at rest	6	Peak decrease in mPAP	No significant effect on mPAP

Study	Intervention	Inclusion criteria	Duration (mo)	Primary endpoint	Result
SOCRATES-PRESERVED[73] 2017, (n = 477)	Vericiguat	NYHA II–IV, LVEF ≥ 45%, Increased NPs history of HFH or intravenous diuretics within 4 wk	3	Change of NT-proBNP and LAV	No significant change in NT-proBNP and LAV
CAPACITY HFpEF[74] 2020, (n = 196)	Praliciguat	LVEF ≥ 40%, Impaired peak Vo2, ≥2 condition associated with NO deficiency	3	Peak VO2	No improvement in Peak VO2 consumption
VITALITY-HFpEF[75] 2020, (n = 789)	Vericiguat	NYHA II–III, LVEF ≥ 45%, Recent decompensation within 6 mo	6	KCCQ change	No improvement in KCCQ
EMPERIAL-preserved[98] unpublished, (n = 315)	Empagliflozin	NYHA II–IV, LVEF ≥ 40%	3	6MWD	No improvement in 6MWD
Nonpharmacologic Treatment					
CHAMPION[101] 2011, (n = 119)	Wireless implantable hemodynamic monitoring	HF with NYHA III, LVEF ≥ 40%	6	HF hospitalization	Reduction of HF hospitalization
REDUCELAP-HF I[104] 2018, (n = 94)	Interatrial shunt device	NYHA III, IV, LVEF ≥ 40%, Exercise PCWP ≥ 25 mm Hg, PCWP-RAP gradient ≥ 5 mm Hg	1	Exercise PCWP	Reduction of PCWP during exercise
Ex-DHF[115] 2011, (n = 64)	Endurance/resistance training	Age ≥ 45 y, NYHA II–III, LVEF ≥ 50%, CV risk factor	3	Peak Vo2	Improvement in exercise capacity and QOL
SECRET-1[118] 2016, (n = 200)	Caloric restriction Aerobic exercise training	HF with obesity, Age ≥ 60 y, BMI ≥ 30, LVEF ≥ 50%	1	Peak Vo2 Disease-specific QOL	Increased peak O2uptake both caloric restriction and aerobic exercise training with addictive value

Abbreviations: 6MWD, 6-minute walking distance; BMI, body mass index; CV, cardiovascular; ECHO, echocardiography; HFH, heart failure hospitalization; HR, heart rate; KCCQ, Kansas City Cardiomyopathy Questionnaire; LAV, left atrial volume; LVDD, LV diastolic dysfunction; LVEDP, LV end-diastolic pressure; mPAP, mean peak arterial pressure; NO, nitric oxide; NP, natriuretic peptide; NT-proBNP, N-terminal pro–brain natriuretic peptide; NYHA, New York Heart Association; PAP, pulmonary artery pressure; PAWP, pulmonary artery wedge pressure; PCWP, pulmonary capillary wedge pressure; QOL, quality of life; RA, right atrium; RAP, right atrial pressure; RVD, RV dysfunction; SR, sinus rhythm; VO2, peak oxygen consumption.

Table 2
Ongoing or unreported trials of pharmacologic and nonpharmacologic treatment of heart failure with preserved ejection fraction

Name ClinicalTrials.gov Identifier	Intervention	Study Size	Primary End Point	Study Completion
Pharmacologic Treatment				
SPIRRIT-HFPEF NCT02901184	Spironolactone	3500	CV mortality or HF hospitalization	June 2022
PARAGLIDE-HF NCT03988634	Sacubitril/valsartan	800	Proportional change in NT-proBNP	September 2021
PRISTINE-HF NCT04128891	Sacubitril/valsartan	60	Microvascular function and ischemia	February 2024
NCT03928158	Sacubitril/valsartan	60	6MWD	November 2020
KNO3CK OUT HFPEF NCT02840799	KNO₃ KCl	76	Peak Vo_2	December 2020
PIROUETTE NCT02932566	Pirfenidone	200	Myocardial ECV, measuring using CMR	Complete
Regress-HFpEF NCT02941705	Cardiosphere-derived cells	40	Safety	June 2021
CELLpEF NCT02923609	CD34+ cell	30	Change of E/e'	March 2022
NCT02814097	Elamipretide	46	Change of E/e' during exercise	Complete
NCT02914665	Elamipretide	308	NT-proBNP	Complete
HELP NCT03541603	Levosimendan	38	Exercise PCWP	Complete
ILO-HOPE NCT03620526	Iloprost	34	Exercise pulmonary wedge pressure	NA
DELIVER NCT03619213	Dapagliflozin	6100	CV mortality, HF hospitalization, urgent HF visit	November 2021
EMPEROR-Preserved NCT03057951	Empagliflozin	5988	CV mortality or HF hospitalization	April 2021
PRESERVED-HF NCT03030235	Dapagliflozin	320	KCCQ change	February 2021
EMPERIAL-preserved NCT03448406	Empagliflozin	315	6MWD	Complete

Trial	Intervention	N	Outcome	Completion
FAIR-HFpEF NCT03074591	Ferric carboxymaltose	200	6MWD	July 2021
Nonpharmacologic Treatment				
GUIDE-HF NCT03387813	CardioMEMS HF system	3600	HF hospitalization, intravenous diuretics visit, all-cause mortality	April 2023
REDUCE LAP-HF II NCT03088033	Interatrial septal shunt	608	CV mortality, stroke, HF hospitalization, or worsening QOL	August 2027
RAPID-HF NCT02145351	Rate-adaptive pacing CRT	30	Exercise capacity	May 2021
PREFECTUS NCT03338374	Rate response pacing CRT	10	Diastolic reserve index	June 2020
CCM-HFpEF NCT03240237	CCM	60	KCCQ change	December 2023
LEAD NCT01618981	Left atrial pacing	NA	NA	Complete
NCT02499601	CORolla	10	All-cause mortality, Serious adverse events	September 2024
NCT03923673	Pericardiotomy	4	Major adverse CV event	May 2022

Abbreviations: 6MWD, 6-minute walking distance; CD, cluster of differentiation; CCM, cardiac contractility modulation; CMR, cardiac magnetic resonance; CRT, cardiac resynchronization threapy; CV, cardiovascular; ECV, extracellular volume; HF, heart failure; KCCQ, Kansas City Cardiomyopathy Questionnaire; NA, not available; NT-proBNP, N-terminal pro-brain natriuretic peptide; Peak VO₂, peak oxygen consumption; PCWP, pulmonary capillary wedge pressure; QOL, quality of life.

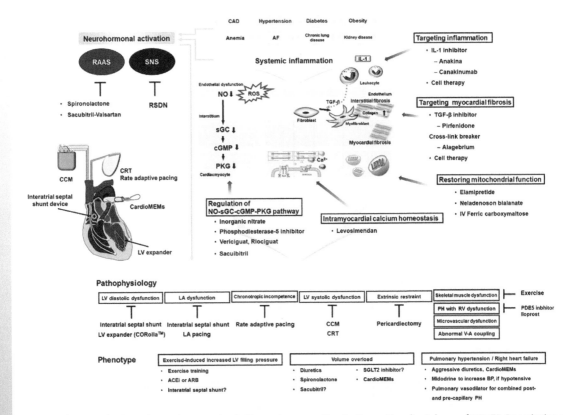

Fig. 2. Pharmacologic and nonpharmacologic therapies according to the pathophysiology of HFpEF. Descriptions of each medication and device therapy are presented in the text. Most of these therapies, except for Cardio-MEMS, are targeted or associated with the pathophysiology of HFpEF. CardioMEMS is implanted in the pulmonary artery and monitors changes in pulmonary arterial pressure. It would be effective to the phenotype of volume overload and pulmonary hypertension with RV dysfunction in HFpEF. CCM, cardiac contractility modulation; CRT, cardiac resynchronization therapy; IL, interleukin; RAAS, renin-angiotensin-aldosterone system; ROS, reactive oxygen species; RSDN, renal sympathetic denervation; PDE, phosphodiesterase; sGC, soluble guanylyl cyclase; SNS, sympathetic nervous system.

patients with HFpEF except for a weak positive result for HF hospitalization by candesartan.

Mineralocorticoid receptor antagonists
Mineralocorticoid receptor antagonists, including spironolactone and eplerenone, are important cornerstones in HFrEF treatment. Aldosterone leads to myocardial fibrosis and results in increased myocardial stiffness and increased ventricular filling pressure. Therefore, aldosterone could be considered a therapeutic target of HFpEF. In the Aldosterone Receptor Blockade in Diastolic Heart Failure (Aldo-DHF) trial, aldosterone showed a positive decrease in LV mass, N-terminal fragment of pro–brain natriuretic peptide (NT-proBNP) level, and improved diastolic function but failed to improve HF symptoms, exercise capacity, and QOL in the HFpEF population.[29] The Treatment of Preserved Cardiac Function Heart Failure With an Aldosterone Antagonist Trial[30] enrolled 3445 patients with HFpEF

(LVEF ≥ 45%) randomly assigned to either spironolactone or placebo. At a mean follow-up of 3.3 years, the primary end points (death from CV causes, aborted cardiac arrest, or HF hospitalization) were not different between the groups (hazard ratio, 0.89; 95% CI, 0.77–1.04; $P = .14$). However, HF hospitalization was moderately decreased in the spironolactone-treated group (hazard ratio, 0.83; 95% CI, 0.69–0.99; $P = .04$). In subgroup and post hoc analysis, the primary outcome was related to increased natriuretic peptide level at baseline[30] and significant regional variation of primary outcome existed between the Americas (United States, Canada, Brazil, and Argentina) and Russia and Georgia.[31] In the Americas, spironolactone reduced primary end points (hazard ratio, 0.82; 95% CI, 0.69–0.98; $P = .026$) but not in Russia or Georgia. The presumed reasons for regional variation were the difference in severity at baseline, determinant of patient enrollment (eg, an increased natriuretic peptide in the Americas vs clinical judgment in Russia and Georgia), and lower medication compliance in Russia and Georgia shown by measuring canrenone, an active metabolite of spironolactone.[32] For this reason, reevaluation of the clinical efficacy of spironolactone is required. The ongoing SPIRRIT (Spironolactone Initiation Registry Randomized Interventional Trial in Heart Failure with Preserved Ejection Fraction; NCT02901184) might clarify the therapeutic efficacy of spironolactone.

Angiotensin receptor neprilysin inhibitors The angiotensin receptor neprilysin inhibitor (ARNI) sacubitril-valsartan is a combination of RAAS blockers and upregulators of the endogenous natriuretic peptide pathway. Sacubitril-valsartan is an upcoming and revolutionizing disease-modifying agent in HFrEF. Inhibition of neprilysin not only augments endogenous natriuretic peptides but also other vasoactive peptides, including cGMP, that are decreased and related to myocardial stiffness in HFpEF.[33] In patients with HFpEF, sacubitril-valsartan was associated with a larger reduction of natriuretic peptide levels, LA reverse remodeling, and greater symptom improvement than valsartan in a phase II study (PARA-MOUNT).[34] This finding might be beneficial to patients with HFpEF. Therefore, the PARAGON-HF[35] (Prospective Comparison of ARNI with ARB Global Outcomes in HF with Preserved Ejection Fraction) trial was conducted to determine the efficacy of sacubitril-valsartan in HFpEF. A total of 4822 patients with New York Heart Association (NYHA) II to IV HF and LVEF greater than or equal to 45% were randomly assigned to sacubitril-valsartan or valsartan. Despite the numerically lower event rate of the primary end points (CV mortality and HF hospitalization), the efficacy of sacubitril-valsartan did not achieve statistical significance (hazard ratio, 0.87; 95% CI, 0.75–1.01; $P = .06$). In subgroup analysis, sacubitril-valsartan showed the benefit of reducing the primary outcome in female patients with LVEF to less than the median ($\leq$57%). In a prespecified analysis of outcomes by sex in the PARAGON-HF trial, the beneficial effect from sacubitril-valsartan to reduce primary composite outcome was greater in women than in men (relative risk [RR], 0.73; 95% CI, 0.59–0.90 in women vs RR, 1.03; 95% CI, 0.84–1.25; P interaction = 0.017).[36] Because of advanced myocardial remodeling even in the same LV systolic function, more progressive age-related arterial stiffening in women, and differences in natriuretic peptide signaling, sacubitril-valsartan might be effective in women, but not in men.[36,37] Recently, the pooled analysis of combined data from PARADIGM-HF (Prospective Comparison of

ARNI With ACEI to Determine Impact on Global Mortality and Morbidity in Heart Failure)[38] and PARAGON-HF[35] trials showed that treatment benefit existed for LVEF less than 42.5% and it was maximized in patients with lower LVEF.[39] Sacubitril-valsartan was effective in women with LVEF less than or equal to 60%; however, the threshold of LVEF to lose efficacy of sacubitril-valsartan was 45% to 50% in men. In post hoc analysis,[8] the effect of sacubitril-valsartan for reduction of the primary end point was maximal in patients recently admitted (within 30 days of prior hospitalization) who had a high risk of rehospitalization and CV death, and it gradually decreased with increasing time from the previous admission. Early administration of sacubitril-valsartan after stabilization within 30 days after hospitalization might have amplified the benefit of sacubitril-valsartan.

The role of RAAS inhibitors in HFpEF is controversial. However, some evidence suggests that RAAS inhibitors might be efficient in HFpEF.[30,35] In a meta-analysis to investigate the efficacy of RAAS inhibitors in HFpEF, only spironolactone reduced HF hospitalization, but it did not decrease mortality.[40] In a recent meta-analysis evaluating the effect of RAAS inhibitors on the outcome of HFpEF that included the five trials mentioned above (CHARM-preserved, PEP-CHF, I-PRE-SERVED, TOPCAT, PARAGON-HF),[41] sacubitril-valsartan was superior to placebo and ARB in reduce HF hospitalization, althouth the RAAS inhibitors did not decrease all-cause mortality and CV mortality. In this context, the ongoing PARAGIDE-HF (Changes in NT-proBNP and Outcomes, Safety, and Tolerability in HFpEF Patients With Acute Decompensated Heart Failure Who Have Been Stabilized During Hospitalization and Initiated In-hospital or Within 30 Days Postdischarge; NCT03988634) study might determine the clinical efficacy of sacubitril-valsartan for HF rehospitalization.

However, the application of RAAS blockade in patients with HFpEF should be made carefully and applied appropriately to each patient. The LVEF cutoff of trials mentioned earlier was greater than or equal to 40% in 2 trials[25,26] and greater than or equal to 45% in 3 trials.[27,30,35] Therefore, a considerable portion of registered patients to trials might belong to HF with mid-ranged EF (HFmrEF) and the proportion of HFmrEF and HFpEF in trials could be different from each other. The RAAS activation is less prominent in HFpEF rather than in HFmrEF and HFrEF and a considerable proportion of patients in trials had already been taking RAAS inhibitors at enrollment due to their comorbidities, hence the effectiveness of

RAAS inhibitors might appear to be limited in HFpEF.

β-Blockers β-Blockers (BBs) are another cornerstone of HFrEF treatment[13] because of improved mortality and HF hospitalization. The increased heart rate (HR) by sympathetic overactivation causes shortening of LV diastolic filling time and leads to increased ventricular filling pressure and exercise intolerance. Thus, HR reduction and reversal of sympathetic overactivation might be beneficial in HFpEF. The increased HR in sinus rhythm, not in AF, is closely associated with poor outcome in HFpEF.[42,43] Thus, several investigations were conducted to evaluate the clinical efficacy of HFpEF. In observational data, BBs showed a modest benefit for survival.[43,44] However, nebivolol did not reduce mortality in patients with HFpEF (LVEF>35%) in prespecified subanalysis of the SENIORS (Study of Effects of Nebivolol Intervention on Outcomes and Rehospitalization in Seniors With Heart Failure).[45] Nebivolol did not improve HF symptoms, exercise capacity, or QOL in the ELANDD (Effects of the Long-term Administration of Nebivolol on the Clinical Symptoms, Exercise Capacity, and Left Ventricular Function of Patients with Diastolic Dysfunction) study.[42] In the Japanese Diastolic Heart Failure (J-DHF) study,[46] carvedilol was not effective in reducing CV death and HF hospitalization in patients with HFpEF (LVEF>40%). In several meta-analyses, the effect of BBs on CV outcome in HFpEF was controversial.[40,47,48] The positive result to reduce mortality in HFpEF was predominantly derived from observational data.[47] In a meta-analysis of 11 randomized controlled trials (RCTs), BBs did not improve prognosis in HFpEF.[48] The prespecified TOPCAT trial to evaluate the effect of BB use on CV outcomes found that BB was associated with increased HF hospitalization and was not associated with CV mortality in HFpEF.[49] A recent meta-analysis revealed that BB had no clear benefit on the severity of HFpEF but it was associated with favorable outcomes in HFpEF with CAD or AF.[50] The conflicting results regarding the efficacy of BB remain to be resolved. These findings might be caused by the differences in the definition of HFpEF, especially LVEF cutoff value, differences in HR at baseline and their changes, and preexisting comorbidities, such as AF and CAD, that could benefit from BB.[51] The use of BB in patients with HFpEF needs to be determined by careful evaluation of the patient conditions and comorbidities.

Ivabradine Ivabradine is a selective blocker of the funny (I_f) channel in the sinoatrial node, thereby decreasing HR. As mentioned earlier, HR reduction might theoretically be beneficial in patients with HFpEF. However, an EDIFY (Preserved Left Ventricular Ejection Fraction Chronic Heart Failure with Ivabradine Study) study[52] found no beneficial effects on LV diastolic function, exercise capacity, and natriuretic peptide level despite HR reduction. In a recently reported meta-analysis, ivabradine also did not show the benefit of improving exercise capacity.[53] The suppression of HR increase during exercise by ivabradine might contribute to the ineffectiveness of ivabradine in HFpEF.[10]

Digoxin Digoxin administration might be considered in patients with HFrEF with sinus rhythm symptoms to decrease the risk of hospitalization and in patients with AF to slow a rapid ventricular rate.[13] However, its utility has been decreasing. In the DIG-PEP (The Effects of Digoxin on Morbidity and Mortality in Diastolic Heart Failure) trial, digoxin did not affect mortality and hospitalization in patients with HFpEF (LVEF>45%) sinus rhythm symptoms.[54]

New disease-modifying treatment
Treatment targeting the nitric oxide–soluble guanylyl cyclase—cyclic guanosine monophosphate–protein kinase G pathway PKGs are intrinsic suppressors of interstitial fibrosis and prevent ventricular hypertrophy via regulation of phosphorylation, structural changes, and oxidation of titin cytoskeletal protein.[4,55] cGMP, a stimulator of PKG, is generated from guanosine triphosphate by guanylyl cyclase (GCs). GCs exist in 2 forms: the soluble form (sGC) stimulated by NO, and the particulate GC (pGC) stimulated by natriuretic peptides.[55]

The downregulation of the NO-sGC-cGMP-PKG pathway is a key mechanism in endothelium-cardiomyocyte signaling altered by systemic inflammation and critical pathophysiology of HFpEF development and progression. Treatments targeting the NO-sGC-cGMP-PKG pathway offer promising therapeutic strategies for HFpEF. Drugs enhancing NO bioavailability, phosphodiesterase-5a (PDE-5) inhibitors, sGC stimulators, and beta 3 adrenergic receptor–selective agonists have been investigated.

Directing nitric oxide donor: organic and inorganic nitrate In the NEAT-HFpEF (Nitrate's Effect on Activity Tolerance in Heart Failure with Preserved Ejection Fraction) trial,[56] organic isosorbide mononitrate did not improve QOL or reduce NT-proBNP level but decreased daily activity and worsened HF symptoms. Excessive hypotension caused by vasodilatation and a decrease in cardiac output by preload reduction[57] were possible causes of the negative outcome of this study. Rapid onset of tolerance and endothelial dysfunction caused by organic nitrates are other possible causes.[58] Inorganic nitrate (NO_3) has a different metabolism of NO via the nitrate-nitrite pathway and might be an important treatment target in HFpEF to improve arterial vasodilatory reserve, increase muscle O_2 delivery, and enhance mitochondrial function in skeletal muscle.[59] In small trials, NO_3 delivered via NO_3-enriched beetroot juice showed an improvement in exercise capacity in the HFpEF population.[60,61] The administration of sodium nitrite via infusion or inhalation improved hemodynamic parameters such as pulmonary artery (PA) pressure during exercise in HFpEF.[59] In contrast with these data, the INDIE-HFpEF (Inorganic Nitrite Delivery to Improve Exercise Capacity in HFpEF) trial[62] showed that inhaled inorganic nitrite failed to improve HF symptoms, exercise capacity, and QOL in patients with HFpEF. Because other administration methods of inorganic nitrite that provide much longer and higher levels of NO achieved positive results, the short-acting nature of inhalation delivery may be the possible cause of the negative result of the INDIE-HFpEF trial. Trials of NO_3 via oral administration in HFpEF, such as KNO3CKOT-HFpEF (Effect of KNO_3 Compared to KCl on Oxygen Uptake in Heart Failure With Preserved Ejection Fraction; NCT02840799) are ongoing.

Phosphodiesterase-5 inhibitors PDE-5 is a metabolizer of NO and cGMP. PDE-5 inhibition is beneficial in HFpEF because of increased cGMP level and cardiac reverse remodeling, and hemodynamic improvement by PDE-5 inhibition has been indicated by experimental and small clinical studies.[63,64] However, in the RELAX (Phosphodiesterase-5 Inhibition to Improve Clinical Status and Exercise Capacity in Heart Failure with Preserved Ejection Fraction) trial,[65] sildenafil did not improve exercise capacity in patients with HFpEF with or without pulmonary hypertension (PH). In patients with HFpEF and postcapillary PH, sildenafil failed to decrease PA pressure and to improve invasive hemodynamics.[66] However, PDE-5 inhibitor is effective in treating precapillary PH and might offer some benefits in combined precapillary and postcapillary PH. Further studies to investigate this possibility are needed.

Soluble guanylyl cyclase stimulators The sGC stimulators (riociguat and vericiguat) enhance cCMP production by acting on NO receptors and are primarily used in the treatment of PH. Recently, a promising result of vericiguat in HFrEF was reported.[67] In HFpEF, sGC stimulators showed limited efficacy in reducing NT-proBNP and LA size in 2 phase 2 trials, DILATE-1 (Acute Hemodynamic Effects of Riociguat in Patients with Pulmonary Hypertension Associated with Diastolic HF)[68] and SOCRATES-PRESERVED (Soluble Guanylate Cyclase Stimulator in Heart Failure Patients with Preserved EF).[69] Furthermore, according to recently reported data (CAPACITY HFpEF [A Study of the Effect of IW-1973 on the Exercise Capacity of Patients With Heart Failure With Preserved Ejection Fraction] trial and VITALITY-HFpEF [Evaluate the Efficacy and Safety of the Oral sGC Stimulator Vericiguat to Improve Physical Functioning in Daily Living Activities of Patients With Heart Failure and Preserved Ejection Fraction] trial), sGC stimulators failed to improve exercise capacity and QOL in the HFpEF population.[70,71]

Other cyclic guanosine monophosphate–protein kinase G–stimulating drugs: sacubitril As mentioned earlier, sacubitril could enhance the production of cGMP and PKG via pGC present in the cell membrane. pGC is stimulated by natriuretic peptides and generates cGMP.[55] The currently reported clinical efficacy of sacubitril-valsartan in HFpEF was described earlier. Although some limited data on sacubitril-valsartan suggest that it may improve hard clinical end points such as mortality, it could also affect so-called soft end points, including reverse cardiac remodeling, improvement of clinical symptoms, exercise capacity, and QOL. Several studies are underway to address these topics (NCT03988634, NCT04128891, and NCT03928158).

Treatment targeting inflammation and myocardial fibrosis

Targeting inflammation: an interleukin-1 inhibitor The interleukin-1 (IL-1) family is one of the major cytokines in chronic systemic inflammation and is an important molecule in the development of HFpEF.[72] In particular, increased IL-1β level affects calcium homeostasis in cardiomyocytes, increases reactive oxygen species (ROS) production, decreases energy production, and impairs myocardial contractility.[72] In a pilot study, D-HART (Diastolic Heart Failure Anakinra Response Trial), anakinra, a recombinant IL-1 antagonist, administered for 2 weeks improved peak oxygen consumption in a small number of patients with HFpEF.[73] However, this favorable outcome was not proved in expanded D-HART2 (Diastolic Heart Failure Anakinra Response Trial 2). Anakinra failed to improve aerobic exercise capacity or ventilatory efficiency even though it reduced C-reactive protein (CRP) levels for 12 weeks.[74] In the Cardiovascular Risk Reduction

Study [education in recurrent major CV disease events], which was a large RCT to investigate the efficacy of canakinumab in patients with myocardial infarction and inflammation (CRP level ≥ 2 mg/L),[75] canakinumab, an IL-1β monoclonal antibody, reduced HF-related hospitalization and mortality in a dose-dependent manner.[76] Further studies are required to elucidate the clinical impact of IL-1 blockade in HFpEF.

Targeting myocardial fibrosis Because interstitial fibrosis and myocyte hypertrophy caused by abandoned deposition of collagen is the major axis of HFpEF pathophysiology, it was hypothesized that antifibrotic therapy used to treat idiopathic pulmonary fibrosis might affect HFpEF.[77] Pirfenidone is an inhibitor of the TGF-β signaling pathway that has shown a favorable effect in IPF[78] by preventing ventricular fibrosis and dysfunction in preclinical tests.[79] The PIROUETTE (Pirfenidone in Patients With Heart Failure and Preserved Left Ventricular Ejection Fraction; NCT02932566) trial evaluating the clinical efficacy of pirfenidone in the HFpEF population has been completed but the results have not been published yet.

Other agents affecting myocardial fibrosis target advanced glycation end products (AGEs). AGEs are molecules formed by nonenzymatic reactions between proteins and carbohydrates.[80] Excessive AGE accumulation in myocardial tissue induces cross-linking with other matrix proteins, such as collagen, and leads to interstitial stiffness and progression of myocardial stiffness. Therefore, AGEs are considered a therapeutic target in HFpEF.[80] Alagebrium is an AGE cross-link breaker that improved LV hypertrophy and LV diastolic dysfunction in patients with diastolic HF.[80]

Cell therapy Cell therapy may be used to decrease inflammation and prevent myocardial fibrosis in HFpEF. In a murine experiment and a pilot study, cell therapy using cardiosphere-derived cells or cluster of differentiation (CD) 34+ cells improved LV diastolic dysfunction. At present, cell therapy in patients with HFpEF is under investigation in 2 clinical studies (NCT02941705, NCT02923609). However, these studies do not aim to evaluate the clinical efficacy of cell therapy; therefore, further studies in this area of development are needed.

Treatment targeting cardiometabolic properties
Targeting mitochondria to preserve and restore mitochondrial function SS-31 (elamipretide) is a variant of Szeto-Schiller (SS) peptides, which act as cardioprotective antioxidants, reduce ROS production in mitochondria, and prevent maladaptive remodeling.[81] Results of 2 long-term phase II trials to evaluate the efficacy of elamipretide in HFpEF

are pending (NCT02814097, NCT02914665). Preclinical studies indicated that partial adenosine A1 receptor (A1R) agonists prevented mitochondrial dysfunction of cardiomyocytes under hypoxic conditions by mitochondrial permeability transition.[82] However, the partial A1R agonist neladenoson bialanate failed to improve exercise capacity, QOL, and NT-proBNP level.[82]

Targeting intramyocardial calcium homeostasis Levosimendan is a well-known inodilator in HFrEF that has a positive inotropic action on myocytes by calcium sensitization of troponin C and induces peripheral vasodilation by opening ATP-sensitive potassium channels on vascular smooth muscle cells.[83] It affects ATP-sensitive potassium channels on mitochondria and has cardioprotective[83] and phosphodiesterase-3 inhibition effects. In HFrEF, levosimendan has shown encouraging results in improving hemodynamics, cardiac reverse remodeling, and renal protection.[83–85] The NCT03541603 clinical study is underway to examine the effect of levosimendan on hemodynamics in patients with group 2 PH HFpEF; results will be reported in the future.

Prostacyclin analogue, iloprost
Iloprost, an inhaled synthetic prostacyclin analogue used for pulmonary arterial hypertension, mediates vasodilation of the systemic and pulmonary arteries leading to decreased pulmonary vascular resistance. It also prohibits the proliferation of vascular smooth muscle. The ILO-HOPE (Inhaled Iloprost and Exercise Hemodynamics and Ventricular Performance in Heart Failure with Preserved Ejection Fraction; NCT03620526) phase 2 trial has recruited patients with HFpEF and group 2 PH to investigate the therapeutic effect of iloprost. In the subgroup analysis of the ILO-HOPE trial, inhalation of iloprost before exercise improved subtle LV systolic function, such as global longitudinal strain, and LV diastolic parameters, including E/strain rate and estimated PA pressure.[86]

Sodium-glucose cotransporter-2 inhibitors
The sodium-glucose cotransporter-2 inhibitor empagliflozin (SGLT2 inhibitors: dapagliflozin, empagliflozin, and canagliflozin) has been reported to produce a significant reduction in HF hospitalization and mortality benefit in patients with type 2 diabetes and high CV risk.[87–89] In the DAPA-HF (Study to Evaluate the Effect of Dapagliflozin on the Incidence of Worsening Heart Failure or Cardiovascular Death in Patients With Chronic Heart Failure) trial, dapagliflozin significantly reduced worsening of HF or CV death in patients with HFrEF irrespective of the presence of diabetes.[90] The

beneficial effect of SGLT2 inhibitors might be derived from the decrease in intravascular volume via osmotic diuresis and natriuresis without RAAS activation and inhibition of the sodium-hydrogen exchanger in the heart and kidney.[91,92] This treatment might help relieve diuretic resistance in HF and prevent myocardial fibrosis, hypertrophy, and dysfunction.[92] Moreover, SGLT2 inhibitors improve myocardial energetics by enhancing metabolic efficiency and myocardial energy supply.[91] It was shown that SGLT2 inhibitors induce the decrease of oxidative stress, an increase of endothelial function, and vascular compliance.[93] These properties of SGLT2 inhibitors could be favorable for the treatment of HFpEF; however, their effectiveness in HFpEF is uncertain. Two ongoing large RCTs aim to elucidate the efficacy of SGLT2 inhibitors in reducing CV mortality and HF hospitalization in patients with HFpEF irrespective of diabetes (DELIVER [Dapagliflozin Evaluation to Improve the Lives of Patients with Preserved Ejection Fraction Heart Failure; NCT03619213] and EMPEROR-Preserved [Empagliflozin Outcome Trial in Patients with Chronic Heart Failure with Preserved Ejection Fraction; NCT03057951]). In contrast, EMPERIAL-preserved (Exercise Ability and Heart Failure Symptoms, in Patients with Chronic Heart Failure with Preserved Ejection Fraction; NCT03448406)[94] failed to show an effect of empagliflozin to improve exercise capacity in HFpEF and HFrEF. The PRESERVED-HF (Dapagliflozin in Preserved Ejection Fraction Heart Failure; NCT03030235) trial is ongoing and is expected to determine the effect of dapagliflozin treatment on exercise capacity.

Nonpharmacologic Treatment

Pressure monitoring
Increased LV filling pressure is a well-known pathophysiology of HFpEF symptoms and signs and is related to HF hospitalization and poor prognosis of HFpEF. A therapeutic strategy of hemodynamic monitoring with early therapeutic intervention could improve clinical outcomes in HFpEF as well as in HFrEF. The CardioMEMS heart sensor (Abbott, Sylmar, CA) is a wireless pressure sensor implanted in the PA that monitors PA pressure and heart rate. The CardioMEMS Heart Sensor Allows Monitoring of Pressure to Improve Outcomes in NYHA Class III Heart Failure Patients trial showed that PA pressure–guided pharmacologic therapy significantly reduced HF hospitalization regardless of LVEF.[95] The results of CardioMEMS postapproval study confirmed the beneficial effect of long-term hemodynamically guided therapy, showing that HF, as well as all-cause hospitalizations, was significantly reduced in patients treated with hemodynamically guided therapy.[96] These clinical benefits were reproduced in another RCT (MEMS-HF; CardioMEMS European Monitoring Study for Heart Failure).[97] A planned large RCT, GUIDE-HF (Hemodynamic-Guided Management of Heart Failure; NCT03387813) aims to confirm the reduced HF hospitalization, all-cause mortality, and intravenous diuretic visits over a 1-year duration.

Interatrial septal shunt
The interatrial septal shunt is targeted to reduce the high LV filling pressure and LA pressure. In the REDUCE LAP-HF I (Reduce Elevated Left Atrial Pressure in Patients with Heart Failure), 44 patients with HFpEF (LVEF ≥ 40%) were enrolled and randomized to an interatrial shunt device (DC Devices, Inc, Tewksbury, MA) or sham control.[98] An interatrial septal shunt was effective in decreasing pulmonary capillary wedge pressure (PCWP) during exercise for 1 month, and the efficacy lasted for long-term follow-up without significant complication.[98,99] The interatrial shunt is a potential therapeutic option for HFpEF with increased LA filling pressure caused by LA dysfunction, even though further studies to evaluate the long-term clinical efficacy are required. In this respect, the REDUCE LAP-HF II (NCT03088033) trial is currently underway to identify the effects of interatrial septal shunt on clinical outcomes including CV mortality, stroke, HF worsening and hospitalization, and QOL over 1 year.

Rate-adaptive pacing
Chronotropic incompetence plays a key role in impaired cardiac output reserve. Restoring the normal response of HR by pacemaker could provide a benefit to patients with HFpEF. Two clinical trials are currently testing the clinical and structural efficacy of rate-adaptive pacing (RAPID-HF [Efficacy Study of Pacemakers to Treat Slow Heart Rate in Patients with Heart Failure], NCT02145351, and PREFECTUS [Cardiac Resynchronization Therapy vs Rate-responsive Pacing in Heart Failure With Preserved Ejection Fraction], NCT03338374).

Cardiac contractility modulation
Cardiac contractility modulation (CCM) is a device therapy for HF that delivers an electrical signal to the RV septal wall in the absolute myocardial refractory period.[100] CCM signals induce mild augmentation of LV contractile strength via alteration of myocardial calcium handling and have some favorable biochemical and molecular effects irrespective of stimulation site.[101] In HFrEF, CCM has been shown to increase functional capacity and improve QOL.[101] The mechanism of action of CCM influences certain processes that are

also involved in the pathophysiology of HFpEF. At present, CCM-HFpEF (CCM in HF with Preserved Ejection Fraction) is investigating the effect of CCM on QOL in HFpEF (NCT03240237).

Cardiac resynchronization therapy

In HFpEF, LV dyssynchrony is associated with subtle LV systolic and diastolic functions and increased LV filling pressure.[102] Although limited consensus exists on LV dyssynchrony as one of the pathophysiologies of HFpEF,[103] the clinical role of cardiac resynchronization therapy in HFpEF is being evaluated in 2 ongoing clinical trials (NCT03338374 and NCT02145351).

Left atrial pacing

LA dysfunction is not just a bystander or by-product of increased LV filling pressure but is another key mechanism of HFpEF.[94] Patients with HFpEF have impaired LA systolic and diastolic functions and increased intra-atrial dyssynchrony.[104] Therefore, biatrial resynchronization could be a new treatment target of HFpEF.[105] In a pilot study of patients with symptomatic HFpEF and atrial dyssynchrony, LA pacing showed an improvement in symptoms and echocardiographic parameters.[106,107] The LEAD trial (Left Atrial Pacing in Diastolic Heart Failure; NCT01618981) for the evaluation of clinical efficacy of LA pacing has now been completed; results should be available soon.

Left ventricular expander

The CORolla device (Corassist Cardiovascular Ltd, Herzliya, Israel) is designed to increase LV diastolic volume and improve LV diastolic relaxation. The device, consisting of a wire with an elastic spring, is implanted in the LV, and it absorbs energy during systole and releases it during diastole to increase LV filling. The study to evaluate the safety and feasibility of the CORolla device in patients with NYHA III/IV HFpEF is currently ongoing (NCT 02499601).

Pericardiectomy

If cardiac volume increases and is greater than the reserve volume of pericardial space, the contact pressure by pericardial structure on the surface of the heart also increases. This constraint of the pericardial structure increases further and is transmitted to cardiac chambers, ultimately increasing intracavitary filling pressure.[108] In the experimental data, pericardiectomy was shown to improve diastolic compliance of LV[109] and to blunt the increment of LV filling pressure by volume loading.[110] Pericardiectomy had an impact in attenuating the increase in LV filling pressure in response to volume loading in a human pilot study.[111] The safety and long-term clinical efficacy of minimally invasive pericardiotomy are currently being investigated (NCT03923673).

Renal sympathetic denervation

Renal sympathetic denervation (RSDN) is radiofrequency catheter ablation of the renal sympathetic nerve and is used to treat malignant hypertension. Because RSDN leads to decreased LV mass and improved LV diastolic dysfunction,[112] a clinical trial to test the efficacy of RSDN in HFpEF was conducted.[113] This study was terminated early because of difficulty in recruitment and was underpowered to show the therapeutic value of RSDN. Further studies would be required to delineate the clinical impact of RSDN in HFpEF.

Lifestyle modification

In recent studies, physical inactivity, low fitness, and obesity have been identified as major risk factors for developing HFpEF, and these are potentially modifiable targets for the prevention and management of HFpEF.[114] Exercise including endurance and resistance training improved exercise capacity and QOL in patients with HFpEF.[115,116] Most patients with HFpEF are obese or overweight; the increased body adiposity triggers systemic inflammation and functional impairment of cardiac, vascular, and skeletal muscle.[4] In HFpEF, supervised exercise training was effective in improving exercise capacity and QOL but was ineffective for LV functional improvement.[117] The caloric reduction in older and obese patients with HFpEF significantly improved peak O_2 consumption, symptoms, and QOL, with an additive benefit from a combination of caloric restriction and exercise.[118] However, further investigations to validate the beneficial effect of lifestyle modification and explain their mechanism in HFpEF are required.

SUMMARY

HFpEF is the most common form of HF in an aging society with an unchanged worsening prognosis. Until now, there has been no promising therapy to improve clinical outcomes such as mortality. The results of clinical trials for numerous therapies have been neutral or less effective in meeting their primary outcomes. The limited effectiveness of therapy might be caused by an incomplete understanding of the heterogeneity of HFpEF, lack of universal diagnostic criteria for HFpEF, unconnected pathophysiologic mechanisms, and suboptimal trial designs for statistical power. Further research is required to understand and control the obvious but intricate HFpEF syndrome. Several clinical trials are ongoing to evaluate different therapeutic approaches. Prevention and management of comorbidities and risk factors of HFpEF are of great importance in the absence of proven therapies.

CLINICS CARE POINTS

- HFpEF is systemic disorder in which are intertwined various pathophysiology and multiple comorbidity. To date, neither pharmacologic nor nonpharmacologic treatment has been reported obviously to improve clinical outcomes.

- Although previous studies have not shown consistent results for the clinical efficacy of blockade of the RAAS, candesartan reduced HF hospitalization in the CHARM-preserved trial.

- In the TOPCAT trial, an aldosterone antagonist was effective to reduce heart failure hospitalization (HFH) in patients with increased natriuretic peptide levels at baseline. However, the cutoff value of LVEF was low (LVEF $\geq$ 40%).

- ARNI was effective to reduce mortality and HFH in female patients with HFpEF in the PARAGON-HF trial. In a recently reported meta-analysis, ARNI was superior to placebo or ARB to decrease HF hospitalization.

- Sodium-glucose cotransporter-2 inhibitor had been expected to be effective to reduce mortality and improve symptoms in patients with HFpEF because of its favorable effect on the pathophysiologic aspect of HFpEF. However, it was recently reported that empagliflozin failed to show efficacy in improving the clinical symptoms of HFpEF.

- In nonpharmacologic therapy, an interatrial shunt device was shown to improve symptoms of HFpEF and QOL. In addition, exercise (not only endurance but also resistance training) improves exercise capacity and QOL in HFpEF.

DISCLOSURE

None.

REFERENCES

1. Kitzman DW, Gardin JM, Gottdiener JS, et al. Importance of heart failure with preserved systolic function in patients > or = 65 years of age. CHS Research Group. Cardiovascular Health Study. Am J Cardiol 2001;87(4):413–9.

2. Heidenreich PA, Albert NM, Allen LA, et al. Forecasting the impact of heart failure in the United States: a policy statement from the American Heart Association. Circ Heart Fail 2013;6(3):606–19.

3. Roh J, Houstis N, Rosenzweig A. Why Don't we have proven treatments for HFpEF? Circ Res 2017;120(8):1243–5.

4. Shah SJ, Kitzman DW, Borlaug BA, et al. Phenotype-Specific treatment of heart failure with preserved ejection fraction: a multiorgan roadmap. Circulation 2016;134(1):73–90.

5. Kim MN, Park SM. Heart failure with preserved ejection fraction: insights from recent clinical researches. Korean J Intern Med 2020;35(4):1026.

6. Pfeffer MA, Shah AM, Borlaug BA. Heart failure with preserved ejection fraction in perspective. Circ Res 2019;124(11):1598–617.

7. Gevaert AB, Boen JRA, Segers VF, et al. Heart failure with preserved ejection fraction: a review of cardiac and noncardiac pathophysiology. Front Physiol 2019;10:638.

8. Vaduganathan M, Claggett BL, Desai AS, et al. Prior heart failure hospitalization, clinical outcomes, and response to Sacubitril/Valsartan compared with valsartan in HFpEF. J Am Coll Cardiol 2020; 75(3):245–54.

9. Franssen C, Chen S, Unger A, et al. Myocardial microvascular inflammatory endothelial activation in heart failure with preserved ejection fraction. JACC Heart Fail 2016;4(4):312–24.

10. Wintrich J, Kindermann I, Ukena C, et al. Therapeutic approaches in heart failure with preserved ejection fraction: past, present, and future. Clin Res Cardiol 2020;109(9):1079–98.

11. Suthahar N, Meijers WC, Silljé HHW, et al. Galectin-3 activation and inhibition in heart failure and cardiovascular disease: an update. Theranostics 2018;8(3):593–609.

12. Lam CSP, Voors AA, de Boer RA, et al. Heart failure with preserved ejection fraction: from mechanisms to therapies. Eur Heart J 2018;39(30):2780–92.

13. Ponikowski P, Voors AA, Anker SD, et al. 2016 ESC Guidelines for the diagnosis and treatment of acute and chronic heart failure: The Task Force for the diagnosis and treatment of acute and chronic heart failure of the European Society of Cardiology (ESC). Developed with the special contribution of the Heart Failure Association (HFA) of the ESC. Eur J Heart Fail 2016;18(8):891–975.

14. Yancy CW, Jessup M, Bozkurt B, et al. 2013 ACCF/AHA guideline for the management of heart failure: a report of the American College of Cardiology Foundation/American Heart Association Task Force on Practice Guidelines. J Am Coll Cardiol 2013; 62(16):e147–239.

15. Kim K-J, Cho H-J, Kim M-S, et al. Focused update of 2016 Korean Society of Heart Failure Guidelines

for the Management of Chronic Heart Failure. Int J Heart Fail 2019;1(1):4–24.

16. Abergel E, Lafitte S, Mansencal N. Evaluation of left ventricular filling pressure: Updated recommendations lack new evidence and have severe interpretation issues. Arch Cardiovasc Dis 2018;111(12):707–11.

17. Reddy YNV, Carter RE, Obokata M, et al. A simple, evidence-based approach to help guide diagnosis of heart failure with preserved ejection fraction. Circulation 2018;138(9):861–70.

18. Pieske B, Tschope C, de Boer RA, et al. How to diagnose heart failure with preserved ejection fraction: the HFA-PEFF diagnostic algorithm: a consensus recommendation from the Heart Failure Association (HFA) of the European Society of Cardiology (ESC). Eur Heart J 2019;40(40):3297–317.

19. Barandiaran Aizpurua A, Sanders-van Wijk S, Brunner-La Rocca HP, et al. Validation of the HFA-PEFF score for the diagnosis of heart failure with preserved ejection fraction. Eur J Heart Fail 2019. https://doi.org/10.1002/ejhf.1614.

20. Sueta D, Yamamoto E, Nishihara T, et al. H2FPEF score as a prognostic value in HFpEF patients. Am J Hypertens 2019;32(11):1082–90.

21. Kapłon-Cieślicka A, Kupczyńska K, Dobrowolski P, et al. On the search for the right definition of heart failure with preserved ejection fraction. Cardiol J 2020. https://doi.org/10.5603/CJ.a2020.0124.

22. Yancy CW, Januzzi JL Jr, Allen LA, et al. 2017 ACC expert consensus decision pathway for optimization of heart failure treatment: answers to 10 pivotal issues about heart failure with reduced ejection fraction: a report of the American College of Cardiology Task Force on expert consensus decision pathways. J Am Coll Cardiol 2018;71(2):201–30.

23. Jia G, Aroor AR, Hill MA, et al. Role of renin-angiotensin-aldosterone system activation in promoting cardiovascular fibrosis and stiffness. Hypertension 2018;72(3):537–48.

24. Pugliese NR, Masi S, Taddei S. The renin-angiotensin-aldosterone system: a crossroad from arterial hypertension to heart failure. Heart Fail Rev 2020;25(1):31–42.

25. Yusuf S, Pfeffer MA, Swedberg K, et al. Effects of candesartan in patients with chronic heart failure and preserved left-ventricular ejection fraction: the CHARM-Preserved Trial. Lancet 2003; 362(9386):777–81.

26. Cleland JG, Tendera M, Adamus J, et al. The perindopril in elderly people with chronic heart failure (PEP-CHF) study. Eur Heart J 2006;27(19):2338–45.

27. Massie BM, Carson PE, McMurray JJ, et al. Irbesartan in patients with heart failure and preserved ejection fraction. N Engl J Med 2008;359(23): 2456–67.

28. Rector TS, Carson PE, Anand IS, et al. Assessment of long-term effects of irbesartan on heart failure with preserved ejection fraction as measured by the minnesota living with heart failure questionnaire in the irbesartan in heart failure with preserved systolic function (I-PRESERVE) trial. Circ Heart Fail 2012;5(2):217–25.

29. Edelmann F, Wachter R, Schmidt AG, et al. Effect of spironolactone on diastolic function and exercise capacity in patients with heart failure with preserved ejection fraction: the Aldo-DHF randomized controlled trial. JAMA 2013;309(8):781–91.

30. Pitt B, Pfeffer MA, Assmann SF, et al. Spironolactone for heart failure with preserved ejection fraction. N Engl J Med 2014;370(15):1383–92.

31. Pfeffer MA, Claggett B, Assmann SF, et al. Regional variation in patients and outcomes in the Treatment of Preserved Cardiac Function Heart Failure With an Aldosterone Antagonist (TOPCAT) trial. Circulation 2015;131(1):34–42.

32. de Denus S, O'Meara E, Desai AS, et al. Spironolactone metabolites in TOPCAT - new insights into regional variation. N Engl J Med 2017;376(17): 1690–2. https://doi.org/10.1056/NEJMc1612601.

33. Greenberg B. Angiotensin Receptor-Neprilysin Inhibition (ARNI) in heart failure. Int J Heart Fail 2020;2(2):73–90.

34. Solomon SD, Zile M, Pieske B, et al. The angiotensin receptor neprilysin inhibitor LCZ696 in heart failure with preserved ejection fraction: a phase 2 double-blind randomised controlled trial. Lancet 2012;380(9851):1387–95.

35. Solomon SD, McMurray JJV, Anand IS, et al. Angiotensin-Neprilysin inhibition in heart failure with preserved ejection fraction. N Engl J Med 2019; 381(17):1609–20.

36. McMurray JJV, Jackson AM, Lam CSP, et al. Effects of Sacubitril-Valsartan versus valsartan in women compared with men with heart failure and preserved ejection fraction: insights from PARAGON-HF. Circulation 2020;141(5):338–51.

37. Regitz-Zagrosek V. Sex and gender differences in heart failure. Int J Heart Fail 2020;2(3):157–81.

38. McMurray JJ, Packer M, Desai AS, et al. Angiotensin-neprilysin inhibition versus enalapril in heart failure. N Engl J Med 2014;371(11):993–1004.

39. Solomon SD, Vaduganathan M, Brian LC, et al. Sacubitril/Valsartan across the spectrum of ejection fraction in heart failure. Circulation 2020;141(5): 352–61.

40. Martin N, Manoharan K, Thomas J, et al. Beta-blockers and inhibitors of the renin-angiotensin aldosterone system for chronic heart failure with preserved ejection fraction. Cochrane database Syst Rev 2018;6:Cd012721.

41. Kuno T, Ueyama H, Fujisaki T, et al. Meta-analysis evaluating the effects of renin-angiotensin-aldosterone system blockade on outcomes of heart failure with preserved ejection fraction. Am J

Cardiol 2020. https://doi.org/10.1016/j.amjcard.2020.01.009.

42. Simpson J, Castagno D, Doughty RN, et al. Is heart rate a risk marker in patients with chronic heart failure and concomitant atrial fibrillation? Results from the MAGGIC meta-analysis. Eur J Heart Fail Nov 2015;17(11):1182–91.

43. Yanagihara K, Kinugasa Y, Sugihara S, et al. Discharge use of carvedilol is associated with higher survival in Japanese elderly patients with heart failure regardless of left ventricular ejection fraction. J Cardiovasc Pharmacol 2013;62(5):485–90.

44. Gomez-Soto FM, Romero SP, Bernal JA, et al. Mortality and morbidity of newly diagnosed heart failure with preserved systolic function treated with beta-blockers: a propensity-adjusted case-control populational study. Int J Cardiol 2011;146(1):51–5.

45. van Veldhuisen DJ, Cohen-Solal A, Bohm M, et al. Beta-blockade with nebivolol in elderly heart failure patients with impaired and preserved left ventricular ejection fraction: Data From SENIORS (Study of Effects of Nebivolol Intervention on Outcomes and Rehospitalization in Seniors With Heart Failure). J Am Coll Cardiol 2009;53(23):2150–8.

46. Yamamoto K, Origasa H, Hori M. Effects of carvedilol on heart failure with preserved ejection fraction: the Japanese Diastolic Heart Failure Study (J-DHF). Eur J Heart Fail 2013;15(1):110–8.

47. Bavishi C, Chatterjee S, Ather S, et al. Beta-blockers in heart failure with preserved ejection fraction: a meta-analysis. Heart Fail Rev 2015;20(2):193–201.

48. Cleland JGF, Bunting KV, Flather MD, et al. Beta-blockers for heart failure with reduced, mid-range, and preserved ejection fraction: an individual patient-level analysis of double-blind randomized trials. Eur Heart J 2018;39(1):26–35.

49. Silverman DN, Plante TB, Infeld M, et al. Association of beta-blocker use with heart failure hospitalizations and cardiovascular disease mortality among patients with heart failure with a preserved ejection fraction: a secondary analysis of the TOPCAT trial. JAMA Netw Open 2019;2(12):e1916598.

50. Fukuta H, Goto T, Wakami K, et al. Effect of beta-blockers on heart failure severity in patients with heart failure with preserved ejection fraction: a meta-analysis of randomized controlled trials. Heart Fail Rev 2020. https://doi.org/10.1007/s10741-020-10013-5.

51. Cho JY. Beta-blockers in heart failure with preserved ejection fraction: could their use be vindicated as an acceptable option in the future treatment guideline? Korean Circ J 2019;49(3):249–51.

52. Komajda M, Isnard R, Cohen-Solal A, et al. Effect of ivabradine in patients with heart failure with preserved ejection fraction: the EDIFY randomized placebo-controlled trial. Eur J Heart Fail 2017;19(11):1495–503.

53. Conceição LSR, Gois C, Fernandes RES, et al. Effect of ivabradine on exercise capacity in individuals with heart failure with preserved ejection fraction. Heart Fail Rev 2020. https://doi.org/10.1007/s10741-020-10002-8.

54. Ahmed A, Rich MW, Fleg JL, et al. Effects of digoxin on morbidity and mortality in diastolic heart failure: the ancillary digitalis investigation group trial. Circulation 2006;114(5):397–403.

55. Park M, Sandner P, Krieg T. cGMP at the centre of attention: emerging strategies for activating the cardioprotective PKG pathway. Basic Res Cardiol 2018;113(4):24.

56. Redfield MM, Anstrom KJ, Levine JA, et al. Isosorbide mononitrate in heart failure with preserved ejection fraction. N Engl J Med 2015;373(24):2314–24.

57. Schwartzenberg S, Redfield MM, From AM, et al. Effects of vasodilation in heart failure with preserved or reduced ejection fraction implications of distinct pathophysiologies on response to therapy. J Am Coll Cardiol 2012;59(5):442–51.

58. Upadhya B, Haykowsky MJ, Kitzman DW. Therapy for heart failure with preserved ejection fraction: current status, unique challenges, and future directions. Heart Fail Rev 2018;23(5):609–29.

59. Chirinos JA, Zamani P. The Nitrate-Nitrite-NO pathway and its implications for heart failure and preserved ejection fraction. Curr Heart Fail Rep 2016;13(1):47–59.

60. Eggebeen J, Kim-Shapiro DB, Haykowsky M, et al. One week of daily dosing with beetroot juice improves submaximal endurance and blood pressure in older patients with heart failure and preserved ejection fraction. JACC Heart Fail 2016;4(6):428–37.

61. Shaltout HA, Eggebeen J, Marsh AP, et al. Effects of supervised exercise and dietary nitrate in older adults with controlled hypertension and/or heart failure with preserved ejection fraction. Nitric Oxide 2017;69:78–90.

62. Borlaug BA, Anstrom KJ, Lewis GD, et al. Effect of inorganic nitrite vs placebo on exercise capacity among patients with heart failure with preserved ejection fraction: the indie-hfpef randomized clinical trial. JAMA 2018;320(17):1764–73.

63. Guazzi M, Vicenzi M, Arena R. Phosphodiesterase 5 inhibition with sildenafil reverses exercise oscillatory breathing in chronic heart failure: a long-term cardiopulmonary exercise testing placebo-controlled study. Eur J Heart Fail 2012;14(1):82–90.

64. Guazzi M, Vicenzi M, Arena R, et al. Pulmonary hypertension in heart failure with preserved ejection

fraction: a target of phosphodiesterase-5 inhibition in a 1-year study. Circulation 2011;124(2):164–74.

65. Redfield MM, Chen HH, Borlaug BA, et al. Effect of Phosphodiesterase-5 inhibition on exercise capacity and clinical status in heart failure with preserved ejection fraction: a randomized clinical trial. JAMA 2013;309(12):1268–77.

66. Hoendermis ES, Liu LC, Hummel YM, et al. Effects of sildenafil on invasive haemodynamics and exercise capacity in heart failure patients with preserved ejection fraction and pulmonary hypertension: a randomized controlled trial. Eur Heart J 2015;36(38):2565–73.

67. Armstrong PW, Pieske B, Anstrom KJ, et al. Vericiguat in patients with heart failure and reduced ejection fraction. N Engl J Med 2020;382(20):1883–93.

68. Bonderman D, Pretsch I, Steringer-Mascherbauer R, et al. Acute hemodynamic effects of riociguat in patients with pulmonary hypertension associated with diastolic heart failure (DILATE-1): a randomized, double-blind, placebo-controlled, single-dose study. Chest 2014;146(5): 1274–85.

69. Pieske B, Maggioni AP, Lam CSP, et al. Vericiguat in patients with worsening chronic heart failure and preserved ejection fraction: results of the SOluble guanylate Cyclase stimulatoR in heArT failurE patientS with PRESERVED EF (SOCRATES-PRESERVED) study. Eur Heart J 2017;38(15):1119–27.

70. Udelson JE, Lewis GD, Shah SJ, et al. Effect of praliciguat on peak rate of oxygen consumption in patients with heart failure with preserved ejection fraction: the CAPACITY HFpEF Randomized Clinical Trial. JAMA 2020;324(15):1522–31.

71. Armstrong PW, Lam CSP, Anstrom KJ, et al. Effect of vericiguat vs placebo on quality of life in patients with heart failure and preserved ejection fraction: the VITALITY-HFpEF Randomized Clinical Trial. JAMA 2020;324(15):1512–21.

72. Szekely Y, Arbel Y. A review of Interleukin-1 in heart disease: where do we stand today? Cardiol Ther 2018;7(1):25–44.

73. Van Tassell BW, Arena R, Biondi-Zoccai G, et al. Effects of interleukin-1 blockade with anakinra on aerobic exercise capacity in patients with heart failure and preserved ejection fraction (from the D-HART pilot study). Am J Cardiol 2014;113(2):321–7.

74. Van Tassell BW, Buckley LF, Carbone S, et al. Interleukin-1 blockade in heart failure with preserved ejection fraction: rationale and design of the Diastolic Heart Failure Anakinra Response Trial 2 (D-HART2). Clin Cardiol 2017;40(9):626–32.

75. Ridker PM, Everett BM, Thuren T, et al. Antiinflammatory therapy with canakinumab for atherosclerotic disease. N Engl J Med 2017;377(12):1119–31.

76. Everett BM, Cornel JH, Lainscak M, et al. Anti-inflammatory therapy with canakinumab for the prevention of hospitalization for heart failure. Circulation 2019;139(10):1289–99.

77. Graziani F, Varone F, Crea F, et al. Treating heart failure with preserved ejection fraction: learning from pulmonary fibrosis. Eur J Heart Fail 2018; 20(10):1385–91.

78. King TE Jr, Bradford WZ, Castro-Bernardini S, et al. A phase 3 trial of pirfenidone in patients with idiopathic pulmonary fibrosis. N Engl J Med 2014; 370(22):2083–92.

79. Mirkovic S, Seymour AM, Fenning A, et al. Attenuation of cardiac fibrosis by pirfenidone and amiloride in DOCA-salt hypertensive rats. Br J Pharmacol 2002;135(4):961–8.

80. Hartog JW, Voors AA, Bakker SJ, et al. Advanced glycation end-products (AGEs) and heart failure: pathophysiology and clinical implications. Eur J Heart Fail 2007;9(12):1146–55.

81. Kumar AA, Kelly DP, Chirinos JA. Mitochondrial dysfunction in heart failure with preserved ejection fraction. Circulation 2019;139(11):1435–50.

82. Bertero E, Maack C. The Partial AdeNosine A1 receptor agonist in patients with Chronic Heart failure and preserved Ejection fraction (PANACHE) trial. Cardiovasc Res 2019;115(8):e71–3.

83. Cameli M, Incampo E, Navarri R, et al. Effects of levosimendan in heart failure: The role of echocardiography. Echocardiography 2019;36(8):1566–72.

84. Najjar E, Stålhberg M, Hage C, et al. Haemodynamic effects of levosimendan in advanced but stable chronic heart failure. ESC Heart Fail 2018; 5(3):302–8.

85. Lannemyr L, Ricksten SE, Rundqvist B, et al. Differential effects of Levosimendan and Dobutamine on glomerular filtration rate in patients with heart failure and renal impairment: a randomized double-blind controlled trial. J Am Heart Assoc 2018; 7(16):e008455.

86. Huang CY, Lee JK, Chen ZW, et al. Inhaled prostacyclin on exercise echocardiographic cardiac function in preserved ejection fraction heart failure. Med Sci Sports Exerc 2020;52(2):269–77.

87. Wiviott SD, Raz I, Bonaca MP, et al. Dapagliflozin and cardiovascular outcomes in Type 2 diabetes. N Engl J Med 2019;380(4):347–57.

88. Zinman B, Wanner C, Lachin JM, et al. Empagliflozin, cardiovascular outcomes, and mortality in Type 2 diabetes. N Engl J Med 2015;373(22):2117–28.

89. Neal B, Perkovic V, Mahaffey KW, et al. Canagliflozin and cardiovascular and renal events in Type 2 diabetes. N Engl J Med 2017;377(7):644–57.

90. McMurray JJV, Solomon SD, Inzucchi SE, et al. Dapagliflozin in patients with heart failure and reduced ejection fraction. N Engl J Med 2019; 381(21):1995–2008.

91. Lan NSR, Fegan PG, Yeap BB, et al. The effects of sodium-glucose cotransporter 2 inhibitors on left

ventricular function: current evidence and future directions. ESC Heart Fail 2019;6(5):927–35.

92. Packer M, Anker SD, Butler J, et al. Effects of Sodium-Glucose Cotransporter 2 inhibitors for the treatment of patients with heart failure: proposal of a novel mechanism of action. JAMA Cardiol 2017;2(9):1025–9.

93. Kato ET, Kimura T. Sodium-glucose Cotransporters-2 inhibitors and heart failure: state of the art review and future potentials. Int J Heart Fail 2020;2(1):12–22.

94. Obokata M, Borlaug BA. Left atrial dysfunction: the next key target in heart failure with preserved ejection fraction. Eur J Heart Fail 2019;21(4):506–8.

95. Abraham WT, Adamson PB, Bourge RC, et al. Wireless pulmonary artery haemodynamic monitoring in chronic heart failure: a randomised controlled trial. Lancet 2011;377(9766):658–66.

96. Shavelle DM, Desai AS, Abraham WT, et al. Lower rates of heart failure and all-cause hospitalizations during pulmonary artery pressure-guided therapy for ambulatory heart failure: one-year outcomes from the CardioMEMS post-approval study. Circ Heart Fail 2020;13(8):e006863.

97. Angermann CE, Assmus B, Anker SD, et al. Pulmonary artery pressure-guided therapy in ambulatory patients with symptomatic heart failure: the Cardio-MEMS European Monitoring Study for Heart Failure (MEMS-HF). Eur J Heart Fail 2020. https://doi.org/10.1002/ejhf.1943.

98. Feldman T, Mauri L, Kahwash R, et al. Transcatheter interatrial shunt device for the treatment of heart failure with preserved ejection fraction (REDUCE LAP-HF I [Reduce Elevated Left Atrial Pressure in Patients With Heart Failure]): a Phase 2, Randomized, Sham-Controlled Trial. Circulation 2018;137(4):364–75.

99. Shah SJ, Feldman T, Ricciardi MJ, et al. One-year safety and clinical outcomes of a transcatheter interatrial shunt device for the treatment of heart failure with preserved ejection fraction in the reduce elevated left atrial pressure in patients with heart failure (REDUCE LAP-HF I) trial: a randomized clinical trial. JAMA Cardiol 2018;3(10):968–77.

100. Borggrefe M, Mann DL. Cardiac contractility modulation in 2018. Circulation 2018;138(24):2738–40.

101. Tschöpe C, Kherad B, Klein O, et al. Cardiac contractility modulation: mechanisms of action in heart failure with reduced ejection fraction and beyond. Eur J Heart Fail 2019;21(1):14–22.

102. Santos AB, Kraigher-Krainer E, Bello N, et al. Left ventricular dyssynchrony in patients with heart failure and preserved ejection fraction. Eur Heart J 2014;35(1):42–7.

103. Biering-Sørensen T, Shah SJ, Anand I, et al. Prognostic importance of left ventricular mechanical dyssynchrony in heart failure with preserved ejection fraction. Eur J Heart Fail 2017;19(8):1043–52.

104. Liu S, Guan Z, Zheng X, et al. Impaired left atrial systolic function and inter-atrial dyssynchrony may contribute to symptoms of heart failure with preserved left ventricular ejection fraction: a comprehensive assessment by echocardiography. Int J Cardiol 2018;257:177–81.

105. Galderisi M, Santoro C, Esposito R. Left atrial function and dyssynchrony: Main characters and not actor appearances in heart failure with preserved ejection fraction. Int J Cardiol 2018;257:222–3.

106. Eicher JC, Laurent G, Mathé A, et al. Atrial dyssynchrony syndrome: an overlooked phenomenon and a potential cause of 'diastolic' heart failure. Eur J Heart Fail 2012;14(3):248–58.

107. Laurent G, Eicher JC, Mathe A, et al. Permanent left atrial pacing therapy may improve symptoms in heart failure patients with preserved ejection fraction and atrial dyssynchrony: a pilot study prior to a national clinical research programme. Eur J Heart Fail 2013;15(1):85–93.

108. LeWinter MM. Pericardiectomy to treat heart failure with preserved ejection fraction: unrestrained enthusiasm? Circ Heart Fail 2017;10(4):e003971.

109. LeWinter MM, Pavelec R. Influence of the pericardium on left ventricular end-diastolic pressure-segment relations during early and later stages of experimental chronic volume overload in dogs. Circ Res 1982;50(4):501–9.

110. Borlaug BA, Carter RE, Melenovsky V, et al. Percutaneous pericardial resection: a novel potential treatment for heart failure with preserved ejection fraction. Circ Heart Fail 2017;10(4):e003612.

111. Borlaug BA, Schaff HV, Pochettino A, et al. Pericardiotomy enhances left ventricular diastolic reserve with volume loading in humans. Circulation 2018;138(20):2295–7.

112. Brandt MC, Mahfoud F, Reda S, et al. Renal sympathetic denervation reduces left ventricular hypertrophy and improves cardiac function in patients with resistant hypertension. J Am Coll Cardiol 2012;59(10):901–9.

113. Patel HC, Rosen SD, Hayward C, et al. Renal denervation in heart failure with preserved ejection fraction (RDT-PEF): a randomized controlled trial. Eur J Heart Fail 2016;18(6):703–12.

114. Pandey A, Patel KV, Vaduganathan M, et al. Physical activity, fitness, and obesity in heart failure with preserved ejection fraction. JACC Heart Fail 2018;6(12):975–82.

115. Edelmann F, Gelbrich G, Dungen HD, et al. Exercise training improves exercise capacity and diastolic function in patients with heart failure with preserved ejection fraction: results of the Ex-DHF (Exercise training in Diastolic Heart Failure) pilot study. J Am Coll Cardiol 2011;58(17):1780–91.

116. Kitzman DW, Brubaker PH, Herrington DM, et al. Effect of endurance exercise training on endothelial function and arterial stiffness in older patients with heart failure and preserved ejection fraction: a randomized, controlled, single-blind trial. J Am Coll Cardiol 2013;62(7):584–92.

117. Fukuta H, Goto T, Wakami K, et al. Effects of exercise training on cardiac function, exercise capacity, and quality of life in heart failure with preserved ejection fraction: a meta-analysis of randomized controlled trials. Heart Fail Rev 2019;24(4):535–47.

118. Kitzman DW, Brubaker P, Morgan T, et al. Effect of caloric restriction or aerobic exercise training on peak oxygen consumption and quality of life in obese older patients with heart failure with preserved ejection fraction: a randomized clinical trial. JAMA 2016;315(1):36–46.

Clinical Phenogroups in Heart Failure with Preserved Ejection Fraction

Hidemi Sorimachi, MD, PhD, Kazunori Omote, MD, PhD,
Barry A. Borlaug, MD*

KEYWORDS

- HFpEF • Heart failure • Phenotype • Treatment

KEY POINTS

- Heart failure with preserved ejection fraction (HFpEF) accounts for more than one-half of patients with heart failure.
- Effective treatment of HFpEF has not been identified, likely in large part because of marked heterogeneity in the phenotypes of HFpEF.
- Categorizing patients with HFpEF based on pathophysiologic phenotype may provide more targeted and efficacious therapies.

INTRODUCTION

Heart failure (HF) is a major public health concern afflicting at least 6.2 million adults in the United States alone.[1] HF with preserved ejection fraction (HFpEF) accounts for more than one-half of all HF and is increasing in prevalence with the aging population and the burgeoning epidemics of obesity, hypertension, and diabetes mellitus.[2–5] The term HFpEF is often used as an all-encompassing term to describe a patient population that is heterogeneous in presentation and pathophysiology, and longitudinal studies are lacking.[6] Medications that improve outcomes in patients who have HF with reduced ejection fraction (HFrEF) have for the most part failed in HFpEF,[6,7] which may be explained by heterogeneity in the underlying pathophysiologic mechanisms in this population.[8] There is hope that management of HFpEF can be better individualized for each patient's phenotype, and that this will result in improved outcomes. This review focuses on various clinical phenotypes of HFpEF and possible therapies based on the current knowledge base.

Schemes for Phenotyping

Although the clinical need for improved phenotyping is generally well recognized, there is no consensus as to how to categorize patients with HFpEF into phenogroups. Possible metrics include the presence or absence of specific comorbidities that influence pathophysiology, imaging, hemodynamics, or other biomarkers (**Table 1**). Use of modern machine learning techniques may also hold promise and can incorporate each of these characteristics to cluster patients into specific phenogroups. Ultimately, the definition of specific phenogroups and metrics used to establish these definitions must be based on prospective studies that define natural history and response to treatment[5] (**Table 2**). Thus, in the current era, patients are categorized into specific clinical phenogroups, many of which overlap substantially with one another.

Department of Cardiovascular Medicine, Mayo Clinic, 200 First Street Southwest, Rochester, MN 55905, USA
* Corresponding author. Mayo Clinic and Foundation, 200 First Street Southwest, Rochester, MN 55905.
E-mail address: borlaug.barry@mayo.edu

Heart Failure Clin 17 (2021) 483–498
https://doi.org/10.1016/j.hfc.2021.02.009

Table 1
Clinical phenogroups of heart failure with preserved ejection fraction

Clinical Phenogroups	Pathophysiology	Definitions and Characteristics	Clinical Features
Obesity	Systemic inflammation Metabolic disorder Oxidative stress Endothelial dysfunction Coronary microvascular dysfunction Lipotoxicity Volume overload	High BMI (>30 kg/m^2) ↑Biventricular remodeling ↑RV dysfunction ↑Epicardial fat (EAT thickness) ↑Ventricular interaction ↑Visceral adiposity	Greater risk in women ↓Exercise capacity Hemodynamic derangements ↓Pulmonary vasodilation ↓QOL
LA myopathy	LV dysfunction LA remodeling LA dysfunction Electrical instability development of AF	↑LA volume (LA volume index) ↓LA reservoir strain ↑LA pressures	↑AF burden ↓Exercise capacity ↑HF hospitalization ↑Mortality

PH and RV dysfunction	Passive backward transmission of increased left-sided filling pressures
	Vasoconstriction and remodeling of the pulmonary arteries and veins
		Invasive evaluation
		  Mean PAP >20 mm Hg
		  PCWP>15 mm Hg
		  TPG>12 and PVR>3 WU
		Noninvasive evaluation
		  ↑E/e′, ↑RVSP
		  ↑RV enlargement
		  ↑RV systolic dysfunction (RV s′, TAPSE, FAC, RV strain)
			↓RV reserve
			↑AF burden
			↓Exercise capacity
			↑Mortality

Stiff artery	Aging Hormones/regulatory peptides Proinflammatory cytokines/chemokines Calcium deposition	↑Systemic vascular resistance ↑Backward wave amplitude ↓Arterial compliance ↓Vasodilatory reserve, ↓CO reserve ↑LV hypertrophy, ↑LV filling pressure	More common among older women and in patients with kidney disease
Ischemic phenogroup	Epicardial coronary disease and coronary microvascular dysfunction	Ischemia and cardiac injury ↑LV diastolic stiffness, ↓systolic function	↓Exercise capacity ↑Mortality
Diabetic phenogroup	Insulin resistance Hyperinsulinemia/hyperglycemia Inflammation Neurohormonal activation (RAAS system)	↑Diastolic dysfunction ↑LV filling pressure ↑LV hypertrophy	Severe HF-related symptoms ↓QOL ↑HF rehospitalization ↑Cardiovascular death

Abbreviations: AF, atrial fibrillation; BMI, body mass index; CO, cardiac output; EAT, epicardial adipose tissue; FAC, fractional area change; LA, left atrial; LV, left ventricle; PAP, pulmonary artery pressure; PCWP, pulmonary capillary wedge pressure; PH, pulmonary hypertension; PVR, pulmonary vascular resistance; QOL, quality of life; RAAS, renin-angiotensin-aldosterone system; RV, right ventricle; RVSP, right ventricular systolic pressure; TAPSE, tricuspid annular plane systolic exertion; TPG, transpulmonary pressure gradient; WU, Wood units.

The Obese Heart Failure with Preserved Ejection Fraction Phenogroup

Obesity is increasing at an alarming rate in the Western world. In 2015, a total of 603.7 million adults were obese.[9] Recent studies project that, by 2030, 1 in 2 adults in the United States will be obese.[10] Obesity is now recognized as the most common and clinically important phenotype of

Table 2
Potential treatment according to heart failure with preserved ejection fraction phenogroups

Clinical Phenogroups	Potential Intervention	Therapeutic Effect	Questions
Obesity	Bariatric Surgery	↓Body weight, new onset of HF ↓HF hospitalization	Obesity Paradox Negative effect of weight loss? Requires RCTs
	Pharmacologic weigh loss or Caloric restriction	↓Body weight, ↑Exercise capacity, ↓inflammation ↓RAP, ↓ PAP, ↓PCWP	
	Mineralocorticoid receptor antagonist	↓Plasma volume, ↓Sodium retention ↓Systemic inflammation	Not yet studied in obese phenotype specifically
	Neprilysin inhibitor	↓Plasma volume?	Not yet studied in obese phenotype specifically
	SGLT-2 inhibitor	↓Plasma volume, ↓Body weight, ↓Visceral adiposity ↓Systemic inflammation	Not yet studied in obese phenotype specifically
LA myopathy	ACE inhibitor/ ARB /Beta blocker	↓LA volume, ↓LV hypertrophy, ↓New onset AF ↓Mitral regurgitation	No benefit was observed in HFpEF patients
	Neprilysin inhibitor	↓NT-proBNP, ↓LA volume	Narrowly missed in improvement of HF hospitalization and cardiovascular death in HFpEF
	Interatrial shunt device (IASD)	Greater LA volume reduction was associated with higher LA compliance and RA reservoir strain	Cannot show the associations between the change in LA volume and clinical improvement
	SGLT-2 inhibitor	↓Incidence of AF	
	Sinus restoration	Improve QOL	Requires testing in randomized trials
PH and RV dysfunction	PDE5 inhibitor	↓PAP, ↓RAP, ↓PCWP, ↑RV function, ↑LV relaxation	Majority of trials failed to show benefit
	Inorganic nitrite	↓PCWP, ↓PAP, ↑PAC, ↓PVR, ↑CO reserve	No benefit in multicenter trial
	Albuterol	↓PVR during exercise, ↑CO reserve ↑RV-PA coupling, ↓RAP, ↓PAP, ↓PAC	Requires further study in longer term trials
	IASD	↑Qp, ↑Pulmonary artery O_2 content ↓PVR, ↑PAC, ↓PA-Ea	Patients with significant pulmonary vascular disease was not included
Stiff Artery	Inorganic sodium nitrite	↓Aortic wave reflections ↑TAC, ↓Ea, Improve central hemodynamics in HFpEF	
	Neprilysin inhibitor	Unclear effects on central aortic stiffness	Arterial effects not yet evaluated in HFpEF

(continued on next page)

Table 2
(continued)

Clinical Phenogroups	Potential Intervention	Therapeutic Effect	Questions
Ischemic Phenogroup	Revascularization	Less deterioration in LVEF Mortality	Has not yet been evaluated prospectively
	MPO inhibitor	Improve coronary microvascular function?	Under active investigation (NCT03611153)
Diabetic Phenogroup	Metformin	↓LV filling pressure, ↑Myocardial relaxation	
	SGLT-2 inhibitor	↓Hospitalization for HF ↓Cardiovascular death in HFrEF	Clinical trials are currently underway in HFpEF Benefits may not be specific to patients with diabetes

Abbreviations: ACE, angiotensin-converting enzyme; ARB, angiotensin II receptor blocker; Ea, arterial elastance; IASD, interatrial shunt device; LVEF, left ventricular ejection fraction; MPO, myeloperoxidase; NT-proBNP, N-terminal pro–B-type natriuretic peptide; PAC, pulmonary arterial compliance; PA-Ea, pulmonary artery elastance; PDE5, phosphodiesterase type 5; Qp, pulmonary flow; RAP, right atrial pressure; SGLT-2, sodium-glucose transporter-2; TAC, total arterial compliance.

HFpEF. In the United States and many Western countries, 60% to 80% of patients with HFpEF are obese, although this proportion is lower in countries with lower prevalence of obesity.[11] Within the broad spectrum of obesity-related HFpEF, there are likely additional subphenotypes; for example, patients with and without increased systemic inflammation.[5]

Obesity, defined as body mass index (BMI) greater than or equal to 30 kg/m^2, is a common and clinically important risk factor for HFpEF. The risk of HF in obese individuals is twice as high as in normal-weight persons. Although obesity often accompanies other established HF risk factors, such as coronary heart disease, hypertension, left ventricular hypertrophy, and diabetes mellitus (DM), the excess HF risk attributed to a high BMI is independent of these other risk factors, unlike other cardiovascular diseases such as coronary disease and stroke.[12] Moreover, the differential risk of HFpEF with obesity is more pronounced among women and may reflect sex differences in HF subtypes.[13]

Obesity may lead to HFpEF through several mechanisms, including systemic inflammation, alterations in metabolism and substrate use, oxidative stress, endothelial and coronary microvascular dysfunction, lipotoxicity and ectopic fat deposition, and pure volume overload.[14] Recent studies have shown that increases in visceral fat represent an important mediator of HFpEF.[15,16] Visceral fat may contribute to sodium retention and plasma volume expansion through the adipocyte-dependent elaboration of leptin, neprilysin, and aldosterone.[17] Moreover, abdominal visceral fat may secrete inflammatory mediators that either directly or indirectly influence cardiac function and hemodynamics, with origin either in adipocytes or macrophages[18,19] (**Fig. 1**).

Patients with obesity-related HFpEF show several distinct pathophysiologic features,[11,20] including greater biventricular remodeling, more severe volume overload, worse right ventricle (RV) dysfunction, increased epicardial fat thickness, greater ventricular interaction and pericardial restraint, and lower levels of natriuretic peptide secretion.[11] Patients with obesity-related HFpEF have more plasma volume expansion[21] but may be more reliant on volume expansion to maintain homeostasis, because they develop more impairment in renal function with decongestion compared with nonobese patients with HFpEF.[22] Compared with patients with nonobese HFpEF, those with the obese phenotype have poorer exercise capacity, more profound hemodynamic derangements, and impaired pulmonary vasodilation,[11] confirming that obesity should be considered as a specific HFpEF phenotype. The increase in body mass associated with obesity results in a higher metabolic cost for activity, with higher oxygen consumption relative to workload.[11,20] Compared with nonobese HFpEF, obese patients with HFpEF are nearly a decade younger than nonobese patients with HFpEF and they have a higher prevalence of metabolic disorders, including hypertension and DM.[20,23,24] Plasma

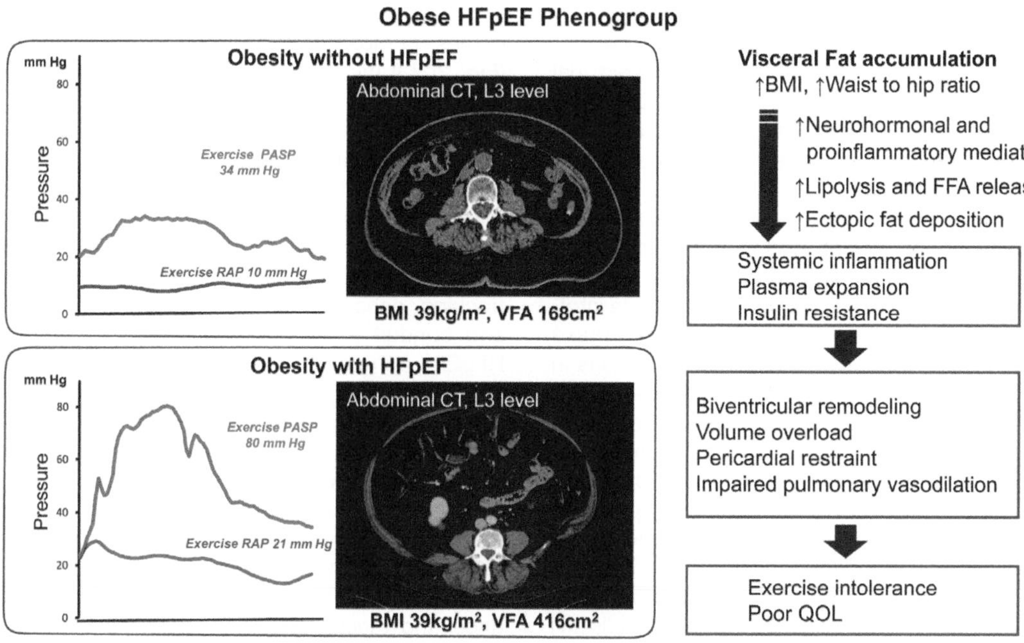

Fig. 1. Increase of visceral fat contributes to biventricular remodeling and dysfunction, which results in exercise intolerance and worse quality of life (QOL). CT, computed tomography; FFA, free fatty acid; PASP, pulmonary arterial systolic pressure; RAP, right atrial pressure; VFA, visceral fat area.

inflammatory markers are increased in obese compared with nonobese HFpEF. Moreover, obese patients with HFpEF have more severe symptoms and worse quality of life (QOL).[25]

Excess adipose content in specific locations, such as the visceral adipose tissue (VAT) and epicardial adipose tissue (EAT) depots, may be particularly detrimental by altering metabolic, inflammatory, and neuroendocrine pathways.[26,27] VAT has been suggested as a key risk factor for cardiovascular and metabolic diseases such as hypertension, coronary disease, diabetes, and hyperlipidemia, and the risk associated with VAT is greater in women. For example, there is a 3-fold greater risk of diabetes with increased VAT in women compared with men.[28] Recent data have shown that accumulation of excess VAT plays a distinct and important role in the pathophysiology of HFpEF preferentially in women. VAT was found to be significantly greater in women with HFpEF than in women without HFpEF. In contrast, no difference was observed in men. In addition to quantitative differences in VAT, there were qualitative differences in the relationship between VAT and hemodynamics. Increases in VAT among women were found to be directly related to pulmonary capillary wedge pressure (PCWP) increase during exercise, whereas there was no such relationship in men.[16] The

reasons for this sexual dimorphism in the effects of VAT remain as yet unexplained.

Other ectopic fat depots may also be involved. EAT is a different type of visceral fat that is increased in patients with HFpEF. Increases in EAT have been associated with higher right ventricular filling pressure.[29] Among patients with HFpEF with obesity, increased EAT is associated with more severe hemodynamic perturbations, both at rest and during exercise, and poorer exercise capacity.[30] In addition to the metabolic and inflammatory effects of EAT, it has been suggested to have direct effects on cardiac mechanics mediated by pericardial restraint and ventricular interdependence.[11,30] This finding suggests that excess EAT exacerbates ventricular interdependence in the setting of right HF, which is associated with poor outcomes in HFpEF.[31]

Treatment of the obese heart failure with preserved ejection fraction phenogroup

Exercise intolerance, the primary chronic symptom in HFpEF and a major contributor to reduced QOL, is significantly correlated with increased adiposity and skeletal muscle adipose infiltration.[11,32,33] Weight loss induced by bariatric surgery reduces new-onset HF, much of which is likely HFpEF.[34,35] In patients with established HF, weight loss induced by bariatric surgery may reduce HF hospitalizations.[36]

There is only one prospective randomized trial evaluating weight loss as a treatment of obese HFpEF. In the SECRET trial, Kitzman and colleagues[37] randomized patients with obesity and HFpEF to attention control, exercise training, weight loss induced by caloric restriction, or the combination of weight loss and training. Both diet-induced weight loss and aerobic exercise training resulted in improvements in exercise intolerance as measured by peak oxygen uptake (V$_{O_2}$).[37] There were also substantial reductions in VAT and decreases in inflammation measured by C-reactive protein. In a meta-analysis of obese patients without HF, weight loss was found to be associated with reductions in central venous pressure, PCWP, and mean pulmonary artery pressure (PAP), changes that would be expected to be beneficial in HFpEF.[38]

Although weight loss is associated with decreasing risk of development of HF, there is still concern about potential harm given the obesity paradox, an observation that lower body mass is associated with worse outcomes in several chronic diseases, including HF.[39,40] In addition to weight loss, there may be a role for treatments targeting the proinflammatory state and neurohormonal activation associated with obesity. Inhibitors of aldosterone, neprilysin, and sodium-glucose transporter-2 (SGLT-2) can ameliorate the plasma volume expansion and proinflammatory and profibrotic pathways, potentially opposing the action of diverse adipocytokines.[14]

The Left Atrial Myopathy Heart Failure with Preserved Ejection Fraction Phenotype

Left atrium (LA) remodeling and dysfunction are common in patients with HFpEF.[43]

Although HFpEF has traditionally been thought of as a disorder of the left ventricle (LV), abnormalities in the LA play an important role in the pathophysiology and disease progression of HFpEF.[41–47] The LA compensates for LV diastolic dysfunction through its reservoir and booster function, but, with prolonged LV dysfunction, there is LA remodeling, dysfunction, and electrical instability leading to development of paroxysmal and then permanent atrial fibrillation (AF).[41] This triad of remodeling, dysfunction, and electrical instability is collectively referred to as LA myopathy and is both common and associated with adverse outcomes in patients with HFpEF. Patients with HFpEF with AF show more severe LV diastolic dysfunction, more severe pulmonary vascular disease and right heart failure, more mitral and ease and right heart failure, more mitral and

tricuspid regurgitation, and worse clinical outcomes compared with those in sinus rhythm (**Fig. 2**). LA mechanical dysfunction is associated with increasing AF burden in HFpEF,[31,41,47] and AF is an independent predictor of HF hospitalization and mortality.[46,48,49]

Measurements of LA volume alone are important but insufficient to identify LA dysfunction. Recent studies have shown a potentially greater utility of LA deformation analyses using speckle-tracking echocardiography. LA reservoir strain and conduit strain are significantly impaired in HFpEF compared with noncardiac dyspnea (NCD).[50] Of all echocardiographic indices, LA reservoir strain discriminates HFpEF from NCD most effectively, outperforming E/e′, LA enlargement, tricuspid regurgitation velocity, LV hypertrophy, and LV global longitudinal strain. Indexing of the LA reservoir strain to estimate LA pressure (E/e′) as a surrogate for LA compliance further improves the diagnostic performance.[42] LA compliance and mechanics progressively decline with increasing AF burden in HFpEF, increasing the risk of new-onset AF and progressive AF.[41]

Treatment of the left atrial myopathy phenogroup

The effect of quinapril on LA size and function was examined in a double-blind, randomized controlled study that included patients with isolated diastolic dysfunction and a maximal LA volume of at least 32 mL/m^2. Patients receiving quinapril for 1 year showed an LA volume reduction, whereas the mean LA volume in the placebo group increased. There were similar findings in the LIFE (Losartan Intervention for Endpoint Reduction in Hypertension) trial,[51] in which reduction in LV mass was associated with a decrease in LA diameter and incidence of new-onset AF or mitral regurgitation (MR) during follow-up. However, neither of these studies were performed in patients with HFpEF, and, in large randomized trials evaluating angiotensin-converting enzyme inhibitor (ACEI) and angiotensin II receptor blockers (ARBs) in HFpEF, there has been no clinical benefit observed.[5]

Atrial natriuretic peptide (ANP) is synthesized in the myocytes of the atria and released in response to an increase in LA stretch,[52] and enhancing natriuretic peptide (NP) signaling is a rational treatment target in HF. Neprilysin plays a significant role in the degradation of the NPs, and the beneficial therapeutic effects of neprilysin inhibition may rely on ANP. The PARAMOUNT trial tested the effects of sacubitril/valsartan (LCZ696) compared with valsartan in patients with HFpEF, showing a greater decrease in N-terminal pro–B-type

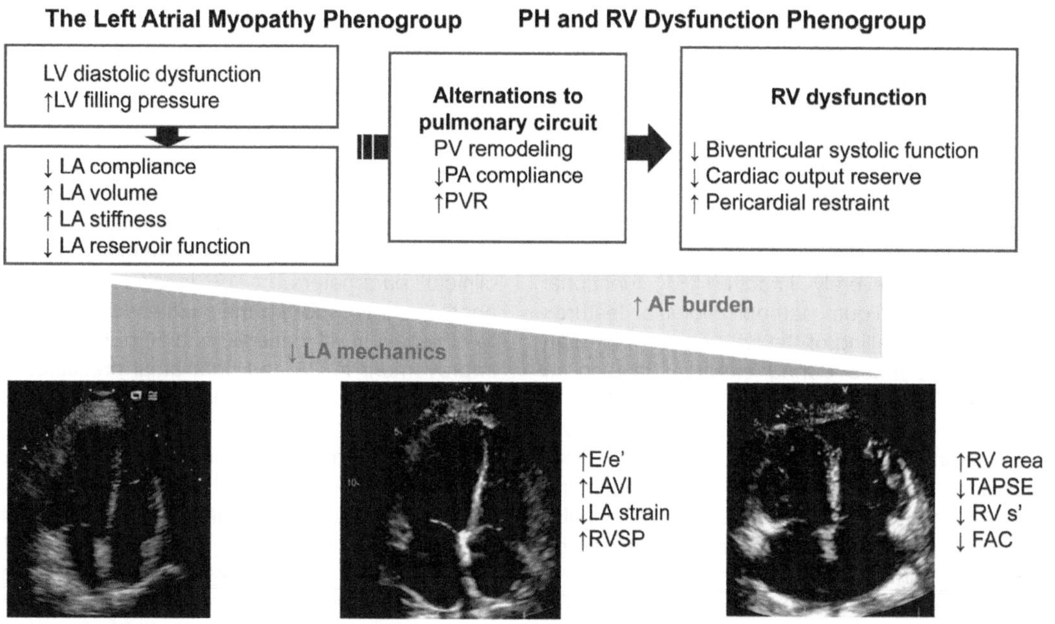

The Left Atrial Myopathy Phenogroup

PH and RV Dysfunction Phenogroup

LV diastolic dysfunction
↑LV filling pressure

↓ LA compliance
↑ LA volume
↑ LA stiffness
↓ LA reservoir function

Alternations to pulmonary circuit
PV remodeling
↓PA compliance
↑PVR

RV dysfunction

↓ Biventricular systolic function
↓ Cardiac output reserve
↑ Pericardial restraint

↑ AF burden

↓ LA mechanics

↑E/e'
↑LAVI
↓LA strain
↑RVSP

↑RV area
↓TAPSE
↓ RV s'
↓ FAC

Fig. 2. With prolonged LV dysfunction, there is LA remodeling and mechanical failure, which increase AF burden. Pulmonary hypertension (PH) related to HFpEF results from the passive backward transmission of increased left-sided filling pressure. It contributes to pathogenic alterations in the pulmonary circuit and right heart. FAC, fractional area change; LAVI, LV volume index; PA, pulmonary artery; PV, pulmonary vascular; RVSP, RV systolic pressure; TAPSE, tricuspid plane systolic exertion.

natriuretic peptide with LCZ696, which was associated with a greater reduction in LA volume index.[53] Despite this favorable effect in PARAMOUNT, LCZ696 narrowly missed in improving the primary end point of HF hospitalization and cardiovascular death in HFpEF in the pivotal PARAGON trial.[54]

In the REDUCE LAP-trial, a greater LA volume reduction following interatrial shunt device implantation was independently associated with higher LA compliance and right atrial reservoir strain, and there is hope that LA unloading with this therapy may improve LA myopathy in HFpEF.[55] DECLARE-TIMI 58 studied the cardiovascular efficacy of the sodium-glucose cotransporter 2 inhibitor (SGLT2i) dapagliflozin in patients with type 2 diabetes and either multiple risk factors for or established atherosclerotic cardiovascular disease.[56] In an interesting subanalysis, dapagliflozin was found to decrease the incidence of AF events in high-risk patients with type 2 diabetes, regardless of the patients' previous histories of AF, atherosclerotic cardiovascular disease, or HF. Considering the adverse functional and hemodynamic consequences of AF, restoration of sinus rhythm might improve clinical status,[57] but there is also concern for worsening hemodynamic and clinical status in patients in whom excessive atrial scarring develops.[58]

The Pulmonary Hypertension and Right Ventricle Dysfunction Phenogroup

Pulmonary hypertension (PH) and RV dysfunction are common in HFpEF[59] and are associated with poor prognosis.[60,61] PH is defined by a mean PAP greater than 20 mm Hg.[62] In postcapillary PH, the increase of pulmonary arterial wedge pressure (PAWP) leads to a proportionate increase in the mean PAP, maintaining a normal transpulmonary pressure gradient (TPG = mPAP − PAWP) less than 12 mm Hg and low pulmonary vascular resistance (PVR) less than 3 Wood units (WU). PH related to HFpEF primarily results from the passive backward transmission of increased left-sided filling pressures, which occur as a consequence of diastolic LV dysfunction.[63] As noted earlier, the presence of LA myopathy is strongly tied to PH in HFpEF. An increase in LA size, interstitial fibrosis causing LA stiffness, and reduced LA compliance, as well as impaired contractility, contribute to pathogenic alterations in the pulmonary circuit and right heart[41,64] (see **Fig. 2**). Although pulmonary venous hypertension contributes to PH, it does not fully account for the severity of PH in HFpEF, suggesting that a component of pulmonary arterial hypertension also contributes.[59]

The RV systolic pressure (RVSP) estimated by Doppler echocardiography is associated with an increased risk of death, independently of age, sex, comorbidities, ejection fraction, and diastolic function in patients with HF.[60,65] In a large cohort referred for invasive hemodynamic assessment, TPG, PVR, and diastolic pressure gradient were all predictors of mortality and cardiac hospitalizations in patients with HFpEF.[61] Patients with PH-HFpEF and increased PVR (combined precapillary and postcapillary PH) show poorer exercise capacity, more severely impaired RV functional reserve, and unique pathophysiologic features related to underfilling of the left heart owing to an inability to perfuse during exertion, leading to left-sided Frank-Starling failure.[66]

The presence of PH eventually leads to RV systolic dysfunction. The prevalence of RV dysfunction varies widely from 12% to 36%, depending on the characteristics of the study population.[31,67,68] RV systolic function is assessed by tricuspid annular plane systolic excursion (TAPSE), RV fractional area change (FAC), RV free-wall strain, and tricuspid annular systolic mitral annular tissue velocity (s′). Patients with HFpEF with RV dysfunction show clinical and echocardiographic evidence of more advanced HF, such as lower left ventricular ejection fraction (LVEF), worse diastolic dysfunction, lower blood pressure and cardiac output, higher pulmonary artery (PA) systolic pressure, and more severe RV enlargement and tricuspid valve regurgitation.[31,67,69] RV dysfunction assessed by either TAPSE or FAC is independently associated with higher all-cause mortality and cardiovascular mortality, and higher first and HF hospitalization rates.[31,67,69]

RV remodeling, indicated by increased RV wall thickness, is a strong predictor of adverse outcomes in patients with HFpEF.[70] Patients with HFpEF have more significant declines in RV systolic function over time compared with patients with LV systolic function. Moreover, development of RV dysfunction over time is independently associated with increased risk of death.[31] Recent data have shown that the response of the coupling of RV to PA is even more important, and that RV-PA coupling can then be assessed by the RV function/RVSP ratio. Abnormalities in RV-PA coupling during exercise are associated with greater increases in pulmonary congestion during exercise in HFpEF,[71] and lower TAPSE/RVSP ratios associated with adverse outcomes in HFpEF.[72,73]

Treatments targeting pulmonary hypertension and right ventricle dysfunction

Based on the prognostic impact of PH and RV dysfunction in HFpEF, treatment of PH in addition to established HF therapies seems to be a promising approach. The RELAX trial has shown that the phosphodiesterase type 5 inhibitor (PDE5i) sildenafil did not improve peak oxygen consumption and exercise capacity in patients with HFpEF in the absence of PH.[74] In a single-center, randomized, double-blind, placebo-controlled trial of 52 patients with PH in HFpEF, treatment with sildenafil did not reduce PAPs and did not improve other invasive hemodynamic or clinical parameters in 12 weeks.[75] However, another study reported the multifaceted response to sildenafil in 44 patients with HFpEF, including improvement in PA and right atrial pressure, RV function, LV relaxation, and PCWP in 1-year follow-up.[76]

Therapies targeting the nitric oxide–cyclic guanosine monophosphate pathway have been evaluated in HFpEF. Inorganic sodium nitrite in particular has been shown to reduce PCWP, PA pressure, and PVR while improving cardiac reserve in patients with HFpEF.[77–79] In a separate placebo-controlled trial, the inhaled beta-agonist albuterol was shown to improve cardiac output reserve and RV-PA coupling, reduce right atrium (RA) and PA pressures, and improve pulmonary arterial compliance (PAC) with no increase in PCWP.[80]

A novel transcatheter interatrial shunt device, developed as an investigational treatment of HF, increases Qp and PA O_2 content, which is associated with salutary effects on pulmonary vascular function, with improvements in PVR, PAC, and PA elastance without reductions in systemic blood flow or systemic O_2 delivery, but this study excluded patients with significant pulmonary vascular disease.[81] Other trials have been undertaken in HFpEF with PH, including studies evaluating pulmonary vasoactive agents, including endothelin antagonists (NCT03153111) and oral prostanoids (NCT03037580), but both of these have been stopped prematurely owing to slow enrollment.

The Stiff Artery Heart Failure with Preserved Ejection Fraction Phenotype

Most patients with HFpEF (80%–90%) have a history of hypertension. A smaller but still significant proportion of these patients have dramatic conduit vessel stiffening, which is further exacerbated during exercise, leading to increases in filling pressures.[82] Aging, hormones/regulatory peptides, proinflammatory cytokines/chemokines, and calcium deposition within the vasculature are recognized as mechanisms that contribute to the development of arterial stiffness.[83,84] Arterial stiffness augments the central aortic pressure wave and increases LV afterload through reductions in central aortic compliance and increases in wave reflection arriving in late systole, which may promote impaired diastolic function. Accordingly, the concept of abnormal ventricular-arterial coupling is a very important factor for understanding the pathophysiology of HFpEF.[85] Increased vascular stiffness increases LV afterload and unfavorably affects the loading sequence, contributing to impaired LV function, early relaxation and contractile function, LV hypertrophy, and subsequent risk of incident HF[85–87] (**Fig. 3**).

Although patients with HFpEF have similar indices of arterial afterload to hypertensive control patients without HF at rest, exercise unmasks significant limitations in arterial compliance and vasodilatory reserve that are correlated with increased ventricular filling pressures and inadequate cardiac output.[82] In a multiethnic study, systemic vascular resistance, total arterial compliance, and reflected and forward wave amplitude were significant independent predictors of LV hypertrophy.[88] Progressive hypertrophy and fibrotic changes in the heart lead to progressive diastolic dysfunction, ultimately leading to increased left-sided filling pressures and diastolic HF.

Treatments for the stiff artery heart failure with preserved ejection fraction phenotype

Ventricular-vascular stiffening can be treated with agents that acutely modulate ventricular systolic and diastolic performance, vascular smooth muscle tone, and endothelial function. Treatment of isolated hypertension with calcium channel blockers or ACEIs was shown to be effective for prevention of the development of HF,[89,90] even among patients aged 80 years or older.[91] Acute intravenous verapamil reduces vascular and ventricular stiffness and improves aerobic exercise performance, anaerobic threshold, oxygen consumption, and total exercise duration in healthy aged individuals.[92] In patients with HFpEF, arterial stiffening at rest and with exercise is partially reversed with inorganic sodium nitrite, a novel nitric oxide–providing therapy, and this is coupled with favorable improvements in central hemodynamics.[82] Inorganic nitrates have also been shown to cause aortic wave reflection with less effect on cerebral dilation and blood pressure in HFpEF.[93] However, inhaled sodium nitrite was not found to improve exercise capacity or QOL in the INDIE trial.[94] Dual angiotensin neprilysin inhibitor therapy failed to reduce aortic characteristic impedance in

The Stiff Artery HFpEF Phenogroup

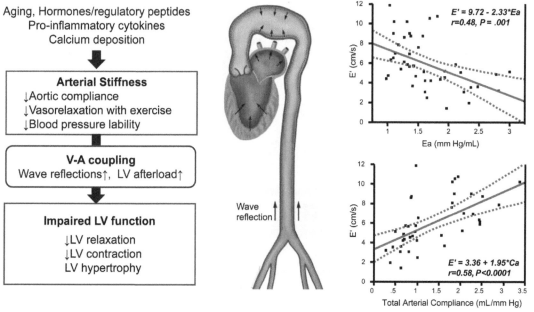

Fig. 3. Increased vascular stiffness increases LV afterload, which contributes to impaired LV, early relaxation, impaired contractile function, and LV hypertrophy. LV relaxation (E′) is inversely correlated with afterload and directly with arterial compliance. Ea, arterial elastance; V-A, ventricular-arterial. (*Adapted from* Reddy YNV, Andersen MJ, Obokata M et al. Arterial Stiffening with Exercise in Patients With Heart Failure and Preserved Ejection Fraction. J Am Coll Cardiol 2017;70(2):136-148 and Borlaug BA, Melenovsky V, Redfield MM et al. Impact of arterial load and loading sequence on left ventricular tissue velocities in humans. J Am Coll Cardiol. 2007;16;50(16):1570-7; with permission.)

patients with HFrEF, but this has not yet been evaluated in HFpEF.[95]

Ischemic Heart Failure with Preserved Ejection Fraction Phenotype

The prevalence of epicardial coronary artery disease (CAD) in HFpEF ranges from 0% to 67% depending on the characteristics of the populations and the definitions used.[96–98] Ischemic stress imaging, including echocardiography, is less accurate in patients with HFpEF, with higher rates of false-negative and false-positive results in the absence of epicardial stenosis, although the latter likely often relate to microvascular disease.[97] Coronary microvascular disease is also very common in HFpEF, observed in roughly 75% of patients.[99,100] This condition is caused by both endothelium-dependent and endothelium-independent processes, and the degree of coronary microvascular dysfunction is related to AF, microalbuminuria, right ventricular dysfunction, and greater increase in filling pressures.[99,100] There are also structural changes that develop in HFpEF that predispose to ischemia, including microvascular rarefaction, which is related to the magnitude of tissue fibrosis.[98] In addition to epicardial and microvascular dysfunction, patients with HFpEF may also develop ischemia and cardiac injury during exercise because of supply-demand mismatch. This condition is caused by systemic hypertension, which increases myocardial workload, and increases in LV diastolic filling pressure, which reduce the coronary perfusion gradient. Recent studies in animal models suggest that chronic, repeated exposure to pressure overload leads to cardiac injury and may induce increased diastolic stiffness as a means to reduce this injury.[101,102] Obokata and colleagues[103] recently showed myocardial injury increases acutely during exercise in HFpEF, and the degree of injury present is correlated with myocardial dysfunction, altered hemodynamics, and impairment in aerobic capacity.

Treatment of the ischemic heart failure with preserved ejection fraction phenotype

Patients with HFpEF with CAD have greater deterioration in ejection fraction and increased mortality compared with patients without CAD[97] (**Fig. 4**). Another study reported that CAD was independently associated with sudden death in patients with HFpEF.[104] Revascularization is associated with less deterioration in LVEF and lower mortality compared with patients who are not completely revascularized, independent of other predictors[97] (see **Fig. 4**). The systematic evaluation and management of CAD in HFpEF may lead to improved outcomes for this challenging clinical

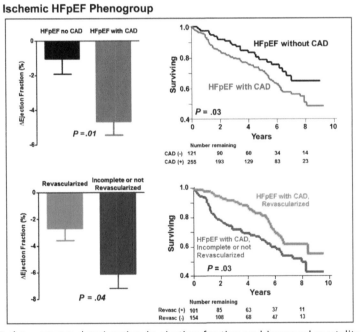

Fig. 4. Patients with HFpEF with CAD show greater deterioration in ejection fraction and increased mortality compared with patients without CAD. Complete revascularization is associated with less deterioration in LVEF and lower mortality compared with patients who are not completely revascularized. (*Adapted from* Hwang SJ, Melenovsky V, Borlaug BA. Implications of coronary artery disease in heart failure with preserved ejection fraction. J Am Coll Cardiol. 2014;63(25 Pt A):2817-27; with permission.)

syndrome, but this has not yet been evaluated prospectively. At present there is no treatment of coronary microvascular dysfunction, but drugs targeting this pathway are under active investigation (NCT03611153).

The Diabetic Heart Failure with Preserved Ejection Fraction Phenogroup

Like obesity, there is currently a worldwide epidemic of type 2 DM. In 2000, the World Health Organization estimated that more than 170 million people worldwide had DM, and the prevalence was projected to double by 2030.[105] The coexistence of DM and HF is common (30%–40% of patients).[106,107] Although the pathophysiologic mechanisms underlying diabetes-related cardiac dysfunction are not identical, the combination of insulin resistance, hyperinsulinemia, and hyperglycemia leads to inflammation, neurohormonal activation of the renin-angiotensin-aldosterone system, and eventual myocardial structural and functional changes.[108]

HF associated with diabetes is a condition often characterized by a restrictive phenotype with severe diastolic dysfunction,[109] high LV filling pressure (E/e′ ratio), and often concentric LV hypertrophy.[107] Patients with DM and HFpEF have worse New York Heart Association functional classes, more systemic inflammation and neurohormonal activation, more severe HF-related symptoms, and poorer QOL compared with patients without DM.[107,110] HFpEF with DM is associated with poor outcomes such as HF rehospitalization and cardiovascular death.[107,111]

Treatment of the diabetic heart failure with preserved ejection fraction phenogroup

Metformin is a first-line therapy for DM, and several studies suggest that metformin could be a beneficial treatment of patients with HFpEF or at risk of HFpEF.[112] Metformin therapy is associated with improvements in LV filling pressures and myocardial relaxation.[113] Interesting data for the prevention of HF in patients with DM come from the results of clinical studies of SGLT-2 inhibitors. The EMPA-REG OUTCOME trial showed that treatment with empagliflozin reduced hospitalization for HF in patients with DM at high cardiovascular risk and that this effect was independent of the presence of HF at baseline.[114,115] In the DAPA-HF and EMPEROR-REDUCED trials, treatment with SGLT2 inhibitors reduced the combined end point of HF hospitalization and cardiovascular death in patients with HFrEF. Several clinical trials are currently underway testing the effects of SGLT2 inhibitors in HFpEF, with results that are eagerly awaited.[116–118] Notably, these trials are not restricted to patients with diabetes, and it is thought that benefits may be independent of diabetic status.

SUMMARY

Effective pharmacologic treatment of HFpEF has not been established outside of diuretics. The lack of therapeutic options is largely related to the complexities and heterogeneity in the phenotypes of HFpEF, making it difficult to apply unified treatment approaches to patients with HFpEF. Categorization of patients based on underlying clinical and pathophysiologic phenotypes holds promise for improving outcomes by delivering the right therapies to the right patients. This review describes currently recognized HFpEF phenogroups and potential treatment strategies. Further study is required to define the optimal methods to phenotype patients and identify effective treatments in randomized controlled trials targeting specific phenogroups.

CLINICS CARE POINTS

- Identify the phenotypes of HFpEF based on clinical presentation, clinical history, characteristic changes in cardiac structures and function, hemodynamic signatures, exercise capacity, or presence of comorbidities.

- In addition to chest radiography, electrocardiogram, echocardiogram, and natriuretic peptide testing, invasive hemodynamic assessment provides useful findings for diagnose and phenotyping HFpEF.

- Some patients with HFpEF have normal resting hemodynamics but abnormal responses on exercise.

- Many clinical phenogroups overlap with one another, and some of the apparent differences in phenotypes could simply be related to the timing in the natural history.

- Control of hypervolemia with diuretics.

- Lifestyle interventions, such as exercise training and caloric restriction, improve functional capacity and should be encouraged.

- Therapies based on underlying clinical and pathophysiologic phenogroups hold promise for improving outcomes and require further evaluation in prospective trials.

SOURCES OF FUNDING

B.A. Borlaug is supported by R01 HL128526.

ACKNOWLEDGMENTS

None.

DISCLOSURE

None.

REFERENCES

1. Virani SS, Alonso A, Benjamin EJ, et al. Heart disease and stroke statistics-2020 update: a report from the American Heart Association. Circulation 2020;141(9):e139–596.

2. Borlaug BA, Paulus WJ. Heart failure with preserved ejection fraction: pathophysiology, diagnosis, and treatment. Eur Heart J 2011;32(6):670–9.

3. Owan TE, Hodge DO, Herges RM, et al. Trends in prevalence and outcome of heart failure with preserved ejection fraction. N Engl J Med 2006;355(3):251–9.

4. Borlaug BA. The pathophysiology of heart failure with preserved ejection fraction. Nat Rev Cardiol 2014;11(9):507–15.

5. Borlaug BA. Evaluation and management of heart failure with preserved ejection fraction. Nat Rev Cardiol 2020;17(9):559–73.

6. Yancy CW, Jessup M, Bozkurt B, et al. 2013 ACCF/AHA guideline for the management of heart failure: executive summary: a report of the American College of Cardiology Foundation/American Heart Association Task Force on practice guidelines. Circulation 2013;128(16):1810–52.

7. Pitt B, Pfeffer MA, Assmann SF, et al. Spironolactone for heart failure with preserved ejection fraction. N Engl J Med 2014;370(15):1383–92.

8. Redfield MM. Heart failure with preserved ejection fraction. N Engl J Med 2016;375(19):1868–77.

9. Afshin A, Forouzanfar MH, Reitsma MB, et al. Health effects of overweight and obesity in 195 countries over 25 years. N Engl J Med 2017;377(1):13–27.

10. Ward ZJ, Bleich SN, Cradock AL, et al. Projected U.S. state-level prevalence of adult obesity and severe obesity. N Engl J Med 2019;381(25):2440–50.

11. Obokata M, Reddy YNV, Pislaru SV, et al. Evidence supporting the existence of a distinct obese phenotype of heart failure with preserved ejection fraction. Circulation 2017;136(1):6–19.

12. Ndumele CE, Matsushita K, Lazo M, et al. Obesity and subtypes of incident cardiovascular disease. J Am Heart Assoc 2016;5(8). https://doi.org/10.1161/jaha.116.003921.

13. Savji N, Meijers WC, Bartz TM, et al. The association of obesity and cardiometabolic traits with incident HFpEF and HFrEF. JACC Heart Fail 2018;6(8):701–9.

14. Packer M, Lam CSP, Lund LH, et al. Characterization of the inflammatory-metabolic phenotype of heart failure with a preserved ejection fraction: a hypothesis to explain influence of sex on the evolution and potential treatment of the disease. Eur J Heart Fail 2020;22(9):1551–67.

15. Rao VN, Zhao D, Allison MA, et al. Adiposity and incident heart failure and its subtypes: MESA (Multi-Ethnic Study of Atherosclerosis). JACC Heart Fail 2018;6(12):999–1007.

16. Sorimachi H, Obokata M, Takahashi N, et al. Pathophysiologic importance of visceral adipose tissue in women with heart failure and preserved ejection fraction. Eur Heart J 2020. https://doi.org/10.1093/eurheartj/ehaa823.

17. Packer M. Leptin-aldosterone-neprilysin axis: identification of its distinctive role in the pathogenesis of the three phenotypes of heart failure in people with obesity. Circulation 2018;137(15):1614–31.

18. Paulus WJ, Tschöpe C. A novel paradigm for heart failure with preserved ejection fraction: comorbidities drive myocardial dysfunction and remodeling through coronary microvascular endothelial inflammation. J Am Coll Cardiol 2013;62(4):263–71.

19. Fontana L, Eagon JC, Trujillo ME, et al. Visceral fat adipokine secretion is associated with systemic inflammation in obese humans. Diabetes 2007;56(4):1010–3.

20. Reddy YNV, Lewis GD, Shah SJ, et al. Characterization of the obese phenotype of heart failure with preserved ejection fraction: a RELAX trial ancillary study. Mayo Clin Proc 2019;94(7):1199–209.

21. Miller WL, Borlaug BA. Impact of obesity on volume status in patients with ambulatory chronic heart failure. J Card Fail 2020;26(2):112–7.

22. Reddy YNV, Obokata M, Testani JM, et al. Adverse renal response to decongestion in the obese phenotype of heart failure with preserved ejection fraction. J Card Fail 2020;26(2):101–7.

23. Tromp J, Shen L, Jhund PS, et al. Age-related characteristics and outcomes of patients with heart failure with preserved ejection fraction. J Am Coll Cardiol 2019;74(5):601–12.

24. Tromp J, MacDonald MR, Tay WT, et al. Heart failure with preserved ejection fraction in the young. Circulation 2018;138(24):2763–73.

25. Reddy YNV, Rikhi A, Obokata M, et al. Quality of life in heart failure with preserved ejection fraction: importance of obesity, functional capacity, and physical inactivity. Eur J Heart Fail 2020;22(6):1009–18.

26. Packer M. Derangements in adrenergic-adipokine signalling establish a neurohormonal basis for obesity-related heart failure with a preserved ejection fraction. Eur J Heart Fail 2018;20(5):873–8.

27. Packer M. Epicardial adipose tissue may mediate deleterious effects of obesity and inflammation on the myocardium. J Am Coll Cardiol 2018;71(20):2360–72.

28. Karlsson T, Rask-Andersen M, Pan G, et al. Contribution of genetics to visceral adiposity and its relation to cardiovascular and metabolic disease. Nat Med 2019;25(9):1390–5.

29. Gorter TM, van Woerden G, Rienstra M, et al. Epicardial adipose tissue and invasive hemodynamics in heart failure with preserved ejection fraction. JACC Heart Fail 2020;8(8):667–76.

30. Koepp KE, Obokata M, Reddy YNV, et al. Hemodynamic and functional impact of epicardial adipose tissue in heart failure with preserved ejection fraction. JACC Heart Fail 2020;8(8):657–66.

31. Obokata M, Reddy YNV, Melenovsky V, et al. Deterioration in right ventricular structure and function over time in patients with heart failure and preserved ejection fraction. Eur Heart J 2019;40(8):689–97.

32. Haykowsky MJ, Brubaker PH, Morgan TM, et al. Impaired aerobic capacity and physical functional performance in older heart failure patients with preserved ejection fraction: role of lean body mass. JGerontol A Biol Sci Med Sci 2013;68(8):968–75.

33. Haykowsky MJ, Kouba EJ, Brubaker PH, et al. Skeletal muscle composition and its relation to exercise intolerance in older patients with heart failure and preserved ejection fraction. Am J Cardiol 2014;113(7):1211–6.

34. Sundström J, Bruze G, Ottosson J, et al. Weight loss and heart failure: a nationwide study of gastric bypass surgery versus intensive lifestyle treatment. Circulation 2017;135(17):1577–85.

35. Moussa O, Ardissino M, Heaton T, et al. Effect of bariatric surgery on long-term cardiovascular outcomes: a nationwide nested cohort study. Eur Heart J 2020;41(28):2660–7.

36. Shimada YJ, Tsugawa Y, Brown DFM, et al. Bariatric surgery and emergency department visits and hospitalizations for heart failure exacerbation: population-based, self-controlled series. J Am Coll Cardiol 2016;67(8):895–903.

37. Kitzman DW, Brubaker P, Morgan T, et al. Effect of caloric restriction or aerobic exercise training on peak oxygen consumption and quality of life in obese older patients with heart failure with preserved ejection fraction: a randomized clinical trial. JAMA 2016;315(1):36–46.

38. Reddy YNV, Anantha-Narayanan M, Obokata M, et al. Hemodynamic effects of weight loss in obesity: a systematic review and meta-analysis. JACC Heart Fail 2019;7(8):678–87.

39. Zhang J, Begley A, Jackson R, et al. Body mass index and all-cause mortality in heart failure patients with normal and reduced ventricular ejection fraction: a dose-response meta-analysis. Clin Res Cardiol 2019;108(2):119–32.

40. Horwich TB, Fonarow GC, Clark AL. Obesity and the obesity paradox in heart failure. Prog Cardiovasc Dis 2018;61(2):151–6.

41. Reddy YNV, Obokata M, Verbrugge FH, et al. Atrial dysfunction in patients with heart failure with preserved ejection fraction and atrial fibrillation. J Am Coll Cardiol 2020;76(9):1051–64.

42. Reddy YNV, Obokata M, Egbe A, et al. Left atrial strain and compliance in the diagnostic evaluation of heart failure with preserved ejection fraction. Eur J Heart Fail 2019;21(7):891–900.

43. Melenovsky V, Hwang SJ, Redfield MM, et al. Left atrial remodeling and function in advanced heart failure with preserved or reduced ejection fraction. Circ Heart Fail 2015;8(2):295–303.

44. Khan MS, Memon MM, Murad MH, et al. Left atrial function in heart failure with preserved ejection fraction: a systematic review and meta-analysis. Eur J Heart Fail 2020;22(3):472–85.

45. Patel RB, Shah SJ. Therapeutic targeting of left atrial myopathy in atrial fibrillation and heart failure with preserved ejection fraction. JAMA Cardiol 2020;5(5):497–9.

46. Freed BH, Daruwalla V, Cheng JY, et al. Prognostic utility and clinical significance of cardiac mechanics in heart failure with preserved ejection fraction: importance of left atrial strain. Circ Cardiovasc Imaging 2016;9(3). https://doi.org/10.1161/circimaging.115.003754.

47. Tamargo M, Obokata M, Reddy YNV, et al. Functional mitral regurgitation and left atrial myopathy in heart failure with preserved ejection fraction. Eur J Heart Fail 2020;22(3):489–98.

48. Zakeri R, Chamberlain AM, Roger VL, et al. Temporal relationship and prognostic significance of atrial fibrillation in heart failure patients with preserved ejection fraction: a community-based study. Circulation 2013;128(10):1085–93.

49. Melenovsky V, Kotrc M, Borlaug BA, et al. Relationships between right ventricular function, body composition, and prognosis in advanced heart failure. J Am Coll Cardiol 2013;62(18):1660–70.

50. Santos AB, Kraigher-Krainer E, Gupta DK, et al. Impaired left atrial function in heart failure with preserved ejection fraction. Eur J Heart Fail 2014;16(10):1096–103.

51. Gerdts E, Wachtell K, Omvik P, et al. Left atrial size and risk of major cardiovascular events during antihypertensive treatment: losartan intervention for endpoint reduction in hypertension trial. Hypertension 2007;49(2):311–6.

52. Nishikimi T, Kuwahara K, Nakao K. Current biochemistry, molecular biology, and clinical relevance of natriuretic peptides. J Cardiol 2011;57(2):131–40.

53. Solomon SD, Zile M, Pieske B, et al. The angiotensin receptor neprilysin inhibitor LCZ696 in heart

failure with preserved ejection fraction: a phase 2 double-blind randomised controlled trial. Lancet 2012;380(9851):1387–95.

54. Solomon SD, McMurray JJV, Anand IS, et al. Angiotensin-neprilysin inhibition in heart failure with preserved ejection fraction. N Engl J Med 2019; 381(17):1609–20.

55. Hanff TC, Kaye DM, Hayward CS, et al. Assessment of predictors of left atrial volume response to a transcatheter interatrial shunt device (from the REDUCE LAP-HF Trial). Am J Cardiol 2019; 124(12):1912–7.

56. Zelniker TA, Bonaca MP, Furtado RHM, et al. Effect of dapagliflozin on atrial fibrillation in patients with type 2 diabetes mellitus: insights from the DECLARE-TIMI 58 trial. Circulation 2020;141(15): 1227–34.

57. Mark DB, Anstrom KJ, Sheng S, et al. Effect of catheter ablation vs medical therapy on quality of life among patients with atrial fibrillation: the CABANA randomized clinical trial. JAMA 2019; 321(13):1275–85.

58. Packer M. Effect of catheter ablation on preexisting abnormalities of left atrial systolic, diastolic, and neurohormonal functions in patients with chronic heart failure and atrial fibrillation. Eur Heart J 2019;40(23):1873–9.

59. Lam CS, Roger VL, Rodeheffer RJ, et al. Pulmonary hypertension in heart failure with preserved ejection fraction: a community-based study. J Am Coll Cardiol 2009;53(13):1119–26.

60. Bursi F, McNallan SM, Redfield MM, et al. Pulmonary pressures and death in heart failure: a community study. J Am Coll Cardiol 2012;59(3):222–31.

61. Vanderpool RR, Saul M, Nouraie M, et al. Association between hemodynamic markers of pulmonary hypertension and outcomes in heart failure with preserved ejection fraction. JAMA Cardiol 2018; 3(4):298–306.

62. Simonneau G, Montani D, Celermajer DS, et al. Haemodynamic definitions and updated clinical classification of pulmonary hypertension. Eur Respir J 2019;53(1). https://doi.org/10.1183/13993003.01913-2018.

63. Vachiéry JL, Adir Y, Barberà JA, et al. Pulmonary hypertension due to left heart diseases. J Am Coll Cardiol 2013;62(25 Suppl):D100–8.

64. Rosenkranz S, Gibbs JS, Wachter R, et al. Left ventricular heart failure and pulmonary hypertension. Eur Heart J 2016;37(12):942–54.

65. Omote K, Nagai T, Kamiya K, et al. Long-term prognostic significance of admission tricuspid regurgitation pressure gradient in hospitalized patients with heart failure with preserved ejection fraction: a report from the japanese real-world multicenter registry. J Card Fail 2019;25(12): 978–85.

66. Gorter TM, Obokata M, Reddy YNV, et al. Exercise unmasks distinct pathophysiologic features in heart failure with preserved ejection fraction and pulmonary vascular disease. Eur Heart J 2018; 39(30):2825–35.

67. Melenovsky V, Hwang SJ, Lin G, et al. Right heart dysfunction in heart failure with preserved ejection fraction. Eur Heart J 2014;35(48):3452–62.

68. Shah AM, Shah SJ, Anand IS, et al. Cardiac structure and function in heart failure with preserved ejection fraction: baseline findings from the echocardiographic study of the Treatment of Preserved Cardiac Function Heart Failure with an Aldosterone Antagonist trial. Circ Heart Fail 2014;7(1):104–15.

69. Mohammed SF, Hussain I, AbouEzzeddine OF, et al. Right ventricular function in heart failure with preserved ejection fraction: a community-based study. Circulation 2014;130(25):2310–20.

70. Burke MA, Katz DH, Beussink L, et al. Prognostic importance of pathophysiologic markers in patients with heart failure and preserved ejection fraction. Circ Heart Fail 2014;7(2):288–99.

71. Reddy YNV, Obokata M, Wiley B, et al. The haemodynamic basis of lung congestion during exercise in heart failure with preserved ejection fraction. Eur Heart J 2019;40(45):3721–30.

72. Guazzi M, Bandera F, Pelissero G, et al. Tricuspid annular plane systolic excursion and pulmonary arterial systolic pressure relationship in heart failure: an index of right ventricular contractile function and prognosis. Am J Physiol Heart Circ Physiol 2013;305(9):H1373–81.

73. Hussain I, Mohammed SF, Forfia PR, et al. Impaired right ventricular-pulmonary arterial coupling and effect of sildenafil in heart failure with preserved ejection fraction: an ancillary analysis from the phosphodiesterase-5 inhibition to improve clinical status and exercise capacity in diastolic heart failure (RELAX) trial. Circ Heart Fail 2016;9(4):e002729.

74. Redfield MM, Chen HH, Borlaug BA, et al. Effect of phosphodiesterase-5 inhibition on exercise capacity and clinical status in heart failure with preserved ejection fraction: a randomized clinical trial. JAMA 2013;309(12):1268–77.

75. Hoendermis ES, Liu LC, Hummel YM, et al. Effects of sildenafil on invasive haemodynamics and exercise capacity in heart failure patients with preserved ejection fraction and pulmonary hypertension: a randomized controlled trial. Eur Heart J 2015;36(38): 2565–73.

76. Guazzi M, Vicenzi M, Arena R, et al. Pulmonary hypertension in heart failure with preserved ejection fraction: a target of phosphodiesterase-5 inhibition in a 1-year study. Circulation 2011;124(2):164–74.

77. Borlaug BA, Koepp KE, Melenovsky V. Sodium nitrite improves exercise hemodynamics and ventricular performance in heart failure with preserved

ejection fraction. J Am Coll Cardiol 2015;66(15):1672–82.

78. Borlaug BA, Melenovsky V, Koepp KE. Inhaled sodium nitrite improves rest and exercise hemodynamics in heart failure with preserved ejection fraction. Circ Res 2016;119(7):880–6.

79. Simon MA, Vanderpool RR, Nouraie M, et al. Acute hemodynamic effects of inhaled sodium nitrite in pulmonary hypertension associated with heart failure with preserved ejection fraction. JCI Insight 2016;1(18):e89620.

80. Reddy YNV, Obokata M, Koepp KE, et al. The β-adrenergic agonist albuterol improves pulmonary vascular reserve in heart failure with preserved ejection fraction. Circ Res 2019;124(2):306–14.

81. Obokata M, Reddy YNV, Shah SJ, et al. Effects of interatrial shunt on pulmonary vascular function in heart failure with preserved ejection fraction. J Am Coll Cardiol 2019;74(21):2539–50.

82. Reddy YNV, Andersen MJ, Obokata M, et al. Arterial stiffening with exercise in patients with heart failure and preserved ejection fraction. J Am Coll Cardiol 2017;70(2):136–48.

83. Chirinos JA, Segers P, Hughes T, et al. Large-artery stiffness in health and disease: JACC state-of-the-art review. J Am Coll Cardiol 2019;74(9):1237–63.

84. Weber T, Chirinos JA. Pulsatile arterial haemodynamics in heart failure. Eur Heart J 2018;39(43):3847–54.

85. Borlaug BA, Kass DA. Ventricular-vascular interaction in heart failure. Cardiol Clin 2011;29(3):447–59.

86. Chirinos JA, Kips JG, Jacobs DR Jr, et al. Arterial wave reflections and incident cardiovascular events and heart failure: MESA (Multiethnic Study of Atherosclerosis). J Am Coll Cardiol 2012;60(21):2170–7.

87. Borlaug BA, Melenovsky V, Redfield MM, et al. Impact of arterial load and loading sequence on left ventricular tissue velocities in humans. J Am Coll Cardiol 2007;50(16):1570–7.

88. Zamani P, Bluemke DA, Jacobs DR Jr, et al. Resistive and pulsatile arterial load as predictors of left ventricular mass and geometry: the multi-ethnic study of atherosclerosis. Hypertension 2015;65(1):85–92.

89. Staessen JA, Fagard R, Thijs L, et al. Randomised double-blind comparison of placebo and active treatment for older patients with isolated systolic hypertension. The Systolic Hypertension in Europe (Syst-Eur) Trial Investigators. Lancet 1997;350(9080):757–64.

90. Prevention of stroke by antihypertensive drug treatment in older persons with isolated systolic hypertension. Final results of the Systolic Hypertension in the Elderly Program (SHEP). SHEP Cooperative Research Group. JAMA 1991;265(24):3255–64.

91. Beckett NS, Peters R, Fletcher AE, et al. Treatment of hypertension in patients 80 years of age or older. N Engl J Med 2008;358(18):1887–98.

92. Chen CH, Nakayama M, Talbot M, et al. Verapamil acutely reduces ventricular-vascular stiffening and improves aerobic exercise performance in elderly individuals. J Am Coll Cardiol 1999;33(6):1602–9.

93. Chirinos JA, Londono-Hoyos F, Zamani P, et al. Effects of organic and inorganic nitrate on aortic and carotid haemodynamics in heart failure with preserved ejection fraction. Eur J Heart Fail 2017;19(11):1507–15.

94. Borlaug BA, Anstrom KJ, Lewis GD, et al. Effect of inorganic nitrite vs placebo on exercise capacity among patients with heart failure with preserved ejection fraction: the INDIE-HFpEF randomized clinical trial. JAMA 2018;320(17):1764–73.

95. Desai AS, Solomon SD, Shah AM, et al. Effect of sacubitril-valsartan vs enalapril on aortic stiffness in patients with heart failure and reduced ejection fraction: a randomized clinical trial. JAMA 2019;322(11):1–10.

96. Rusinaru D, Houpe D, Szymanski C, et al. Coronary artery disease and 10-year outcome after hospital admission for heart failure with preserved and with reduced ejection fraction. Eur J Heart Fail 2014;16(9):967–76.

97. Hwang SJ, Melenovsky V, Borlaug BA. Implications of coronary artery disease in heart failure with preserved ejection fraction. J Am Coll Cardiol 2014;63(25 Pt A):2817–27.

98. Mohammed SF, Hussain S, Mirzoyev SA, et al. Coronary microvascular rarefaction and myocardial fibrosis in heart failure with preserved ejection fraction. Circulation 2015;131(6):550–9.

99. Yang JH, Obokata M, Reddy YNV, et al. Endothelium-dependent and independent coronary microvascular dysfunction in patients with heart failure with preserved ejection fraction. Eur J Heart Fail 2020;22(3):432–41.

100. Shah SJ, Lam CSP, Svedlund S, et al. Prevalence and correlates of coronary microvascular dysfunction in heart failure with preserved ejection fraction: PROMIS-HFpEF. Eur Heart J 2018;39(37):3439–50.

101. Weil BR, Techiryan G, Suzuki G, et al. Adaptive reductions in left ventricular diastolic compliance protect the heart from stretch-induced stunning. JACC Basic Transl Sci 2019;4(4):527–41.

102. Weil BR, Suzuki G, Young RF, et al. Troponin release and reversible left ventricular dysfunction after transient pressure overload. J Am Coll Cardiol 2018;71(25):2906–16.

103. Obokata M, Reddy YNV, Melenovsky V, et al. Myocardial injury and cardiac reserve in patients with heart failure and preserved ejection fraction. J Am Coll Cardiol 2018;72(1):29–40.

104. Choudhury L, Gheorghiade M, Bonow RO. Coronary artery disease in patients with heart failure and preserved systolic function. Am J Cardiol 2002;89(6):719–22.

105. Wild S, Roglic G, Green A, et al. Global prevalence of diabetes: estimates for the year 2000 and projections for 2030. Diabetes care 2004;27(5):1047–53.

106. Seferović PM, Petrie MC, Filippatos GS, et al. Type 2 diabetes mellitus and heart failure: a position statement from the Heart Failure Association of the European Society of Cardiology. Eur J Heart Fail 2018;20(5):853–72.

107. Yap J, Tay WT, Teng TK, et al. Association of diabetes mellitus on cardiac remodeling, quality of life, and clinical outcomes in heart failure with reduced and preserved ejection fraction. J Am Heart Assoc 2019;8(17):e013114.

108. Paolillo S, Marsico F, Prastaro M, et al. Diabetic cardiomyopathy: definition, diagnosis, and therapeutic implications. Heart Fail Clin 2019;15(3):341–7.

109. Seferović PM, Paulus WJ. Clinical diabetic cardiomyopathy: a two-faced disease with restrictive and dilated phenotypes. Eur Heart J 2015;36(27):1718–27, 1727a-1727c.

110. Lindman BR, Dávila-Román VG, Mann DL, et al. Cardiovascular phenotype in HFpEF patients with or without diabetes: a RELAX trial ancillary study. J Am Coll Cardiol 2014;64(6):541–9.

111. Cavender MA, Steg PG, Smith SC Jr, et al. Impact of diabetes mellitus on hospitalization for heart failure, cardiovascular events, and death: outcomes at 4 years from the Reduction of Atherothrombosis for Continued Health (REACH) Registry. Circulation 2015;132(10):923–31.

112. Miles JM, Rule AD, Borlaug BA. Use of metformin in diseases of aging. Curr Diabetes Rep 2014;14(6):490.

113. Halabi A, Yang H, Wright L, et al. Evolution of myocardial dysfunction in asymptomatic patients at risk of heart failure. JACC Cardiovasc Imaging 2020. https://doi.org/10.1016/j.jcmg.2020.09.032.

114. Zinman B, Wanner C, Lachin JM, et al. Empagliflozin, cardiovascular outcomes, and mortality in type 2 diabetes. N Engl J Med 2015;373(22):2117–28.

115. Fitchett D, Zinman B, Wanner C, et al. Heart failure outcomes with empagliflozin in patients with type 2 diabetes at high cardiovascular risk: results of the EMPA-REG OUTCOME® trial. Eur Heart J 2016;37(19):1526–34.

116. Anker SD, Butler J, Filippatos G, et al. Baseline characteristics of patients with heart failure with preserved ejection fraction in the EMPEROR-preserved trial. Eur J Heart Fail 2020. https://doi.org/10.1002/ejhf.2064.

117. Anker SD, Butler J, Filippatos GS, et al. Evaluation of the effects of sodium-glucose co-transporter 2 inhibition with empagliflozin on morbidity and mortality in patients with chronic heart failure and a preserved ejection fraction: rationale for and design of the EMPEROR-preserved trial. Eur J Heart Fail 2019;21(10):1279–87.

118. Williams DM, Evans M. Dapagliflozin for heart failure with preserved ejection fraction: will the DELIVER study deliver? Diabetes Ther 2020;11(10):2207–19.

Phenomapping Heart Failure with Preserved Ejection Fraction Using Machine Learning Cluster Analysis
Prognostic and Therapeutic Implications

Elena Galli, MD, PhD[a], Corentin Bourg, MD[a], Wojciech Kosmala, MD, PhD[b], Emmanuel Oger, MD, PhD[c], Erwan Donal, MD, PhD[a],*

KEYWORDS

- Heart failure with preserved ejection fraction • Machine learning • Phenomapping • Prognosis
- Precision medicine • Targeted treatment

KEY POINTS

- Heart failure represents one of the main causes of morbidity and mortality worldwide.
- Heart failure with preserved ejection fraction (HFpEF) is a specific entity characterized by complex pathophysiology and high heterogeneity of clinical presentations.
- The application of phenomapping to a huge amount of data can disclose the intrinsic complexity of HFpEF and allows the identification of specific phenogroups of patients.
- The lack of a successful therapeutic strategy for HFpEF might be strictly linked with the intrinsic complexity and heterogeneity of the disease.
- Phenomapping might represent a step toward personalized medicine in HFpEF, permitting the identification of the best therapeutic options for specific phenogroups of patients.

INTRODUCTION

Heart failure (HF) is a growing public health pandemic, with a preva lence of 1% to 2% in the adult populations of developed countries, rising to 10% in the eldest,[1] and nearly 40 million individuals affected worldwide.[2]

According to the 2016 recommendations of the European Society of Cardiology, the diagnosis of HF is based on (1) the presence of clinical sign and symptoms of the disease; (2) the elevation in natriuretic peptides, and (3) the evidence of cardiac structural abnormalities (eg, left atrial [LA] dilatation and/or left ventricle [LV] hypertrophy) and/or diastolic dysfunction.[3]

About 50% of patients with HF exhibit a left ventricle ejection fraction (LVEF) ≥50%, the so-called heart failure with preserved ejection fraction (HFpEF). Despite initially considered a relatively benign form of HF, HFpEF is characterized by a high rate of hospitalization and mortality (84% and 76% at 5 years, respectively), which are similar to those observed for heart failure with

No conflicts of interest for this article, and nothing to disclose for any of the authors.
Funded by: FRENCH.
[a] University of Rennes, CHU Rennes, INSERM, LTSI–UMR 1099, Rennes F-35000, France; [b] Cardiology Department, Wroclaw Medical University, Wroclaw, Poland; [c] University of Rennes, EA 7449 REPERES [Pharmacoepidemiology and Health Services Research], Rennes, France
* Corresponding author. Service de Cardiologie, Hôpital Pontchaillou, CHU Rennes, Rennes F-35033, France.
E-mail address: erwan.donal@chu-rennes.fr

Heart Failure Clin 17 (2021) 499–518
https://doi.org/10.1016/j.hfc.2021.02.010
1551-7136/21/© 2021 Elsevier Inc. All rights reserved.

reduced ejection fraction (HFrEF).[4] These epidemiologic data claim for the development of specific and innovative therapies to reduce the burden of morbidity and mortality associated with this disease.

One of the main problems with HFpEF relates to the definition and identification of this entity. In a recent article, Ho and colleagues[5] have shown that the diagnostic algorithms for HFpEF proposed by the American and European scientific societies identify different clinical profiles of patients, and this heterogeneity is mirrored by diverging clinical outcomes. Moreover, restrictive definitions have poor sensitivity for the detection of patients who have no or mild physiologic alteration at rest and significant alterations during exercise, supporting the importance of exercise test in patients with HFpEF.[5] Accordingly, the latest diagnostic strategy provided by the Heart Failure Association of the European Society of Cardiology included exercise echocardiography as a relevant step in the recognition of HFpEF.[6]

PATHOPHYSIOLOGY OF HEART FAILURE WITH PRESERVED EJECTION FRACTION

Compared with HFrEF, which is due to a primary myocardial damage (eg ischemia, cardiomyopathies, toxicity) and associated with significant neurohormonal activation, HFpEF is characterized by a heterogeneous etiologic background. Initially referred to as "diastolic heart failure," HFpEF is typified by a constellation of LV systolic and diastolic abnormalities, LA stiffness, pulmonary artery hypertension (PAH), vascular stiffness, impaired vasodilatation, and skeletal muscle abnormalities.[7] Some of these derangements, such as the impairment in LV contractile reserve and heart rate reserve, or PAH may become evident only during exertion, which is a significant diagnostic and therapeutic challenge.[6,8]

Patients with HFpEF are often older, with several comorbidities and cardiovascular (CV) risk factors, such as ischemic heart disease (IHD), diabetes mellitus (DM), obesity, arterial hypertension (HTN), chronic obstructive pulmonary disease (COPD), obstructive sleep apnea syndrome (OSAS), and kidney failure (chronic kidney disease [CKD]). According to the proposed hypothesis, these pathologic conditions are triggers for chronic systemic inflammation,[9] which causes endothelial dysfunction and myocardial microvascular endothelial activation,[10] promoting myocyte hypertrophy and interstitial fibrosis. After the initial CV involvement, the next step in the progression of the disease is multiorgan involvement with development/worsening of ventriculoatrial coupling,

PAH, CKD, and skeletal muscle abnormalities[11] (**Fig. 1**).

The complex pathophysiology of HFpEF coupled with its highly heterogenous phenotypical presentations is the main cause of the lack of effective therapeutic strategies and of the disappointing results of recent randomized trials (eg, CHARM-Preserved,[12] I-PRESERVE,[13] RELAX,[14] NEAT,[15] PARAGON-HF[16]). The inhibition of the neurohumoral burden that is effective in improving the quality of life and in reducing the morbidity and mortality in HFrEF does not provide equivalent benefits in patients with HFpEF. The development of dedicated therapeutic strategies for HFpEF is therefore the main aim of the research in this field.

PHENOMAPPING IN HEART FAILURE WITH PRESERVED EJECTION FRACTION

Machine learning (ML) is focused on the application of computational algorithms to huge amounts of data to identify patterns between variables that are not disclosed by the application of standard statistical methods.[17] Phenomapping is a particular kind of unsupervised ML that is applied to data without a priori knowledge of the outcomes to uncover mathematical relationships between data and to cluster patients into different and mutually exclusive groups.[17]

The application of phenomapping to dense multidimensional data (clinical and biohumoral data, imaging-derived features, hemodynamics variables) obtained from patients with HFpEF seems particularly attractive, because it might solve the intrinsic heterogeneity of the syndrome, generate new pathophysiologic hypothesis, and prompt the application of tailored therapeutic strategies[18]

In 2014, Shah and colleagues[19] published the first article applying unbiased clustering to 397 patients with HFpEF.

After the exploitation of a phenotypic domain consisting of 67 continuous clinical, laboratory, electrocardiographic, echocardiographic, and hemodynamic variables, the authors were able to identify 3 separate clusters of patients with different prognosis. Interestingly, the 3 clusters corresponded to 3 potential archetypes of HFpEF, which exhibited also significantly different prognoses: the natriuretic peptide deficiency syndrome (cluster 1); the obesity/cardiometabolic phenotype (cluster 2); and the right ventricular (RV) failure/cardiorenal phenotype (cluster 3).[19] After this landmark work,[19] an increasing number of studies have been published on the application of phenomapping to different cohorts of patients with HFpEF (**Table 1**).[19–27]

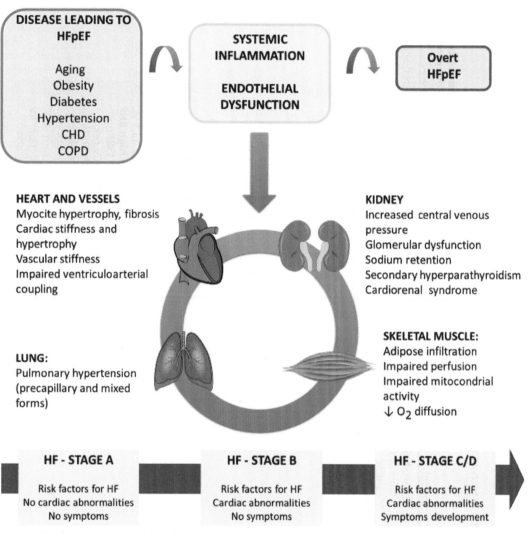

Fig. 1. Pathophysiologic mechanisms for HFpEF. CHD, coronary heart disease.

Depending on the set of input variables, various pathophysiologic profiles were identified, the prognosis of which could not be effectively predicted relying exclusively on conventional risk stratification approaches.

The main issue emerging from the comparison of the different cohorts is the large heterogeneity of the included patients, with a significant difference in mean age (from 65 years in the study of Shah and colleagues[19] to 78 years in the study of Hedman and colleagues[25]), sex, clinical status, and prevalence of comorbidities. Several differences can also be found in the quality and number of selected features, which can vary from 11 to nearly 100 descriptors: some studies focused only on clinical and laboratory parameters[20,27]; others included echocardiographic parameters obtained at rest.[19,23,25,26] Only a small amount of

studies dealt with echocardiographic data obtained at rest and during submaximal exercise, including the evaluation of LV deformation.[21,22] Although the assessment of LV performance during exercise is still underused, the analysis of exercise data might provide important information. It seems particularly valuable in specific subsets of patients who have mild symptoms and modest cardiac abnormalities at rest, but might develop significant impairment of LV systolic and diastolic function and PAH during exercise.[6] The evaluation under an exercise load can also verify the asymptomatic status of patients categorized as stage A and B HF.

The current HFA-PEFF diagnostic algorithm underscores the importance of performing cardiac catheterization for the diagnosis of HFpEF.[6] Nevertheless, only 1 ML study included

Table 1
Main studies applying phenomapping to heart failure with preserved ejection fraction

Authors	Population	Clustering	Variables	Endpoints	Clusters	Prognosis (Better to Worst)
Shah et al,[19] *Circulation*, 2015	397 patients Prospective study Mean age: 64.7 ± 13 y; Female: 63% Black: 39% LVEF: 61% ± 7% Validation cohort: 107 pts	Penalized model-based clustering	46 variables: clinical, laboratory, EKG, TTE, cardiac catheterization	Primary endpoint: CV hospitalization or death Secondary endpoint: HF hospitalization	1. Younger (60.7 ± 13.6 y), lower BNP (72 [26–161] pg/mL). Main CV risk factors: obesity (51%). less electric (AF, 13%) and myocardial remodeling, no hemodynamic derangement 2. Intermediate age (65.7 ± 11.3 y). Several CV risk factors: obesity (84%), DM (52%), HTN (90%), OSAS (50%). Worst LV relaxation, highest PCWP (24.6 ± 8.3 mm Hg) and PVR (2.8 ± 4.6 WU) 3. Older (67.3 ± 13.1 y), CKD (53%), high BNP (607 [329–1138] pg/mL). Main CV risk factors: HTN (75%). More severe electric (AF 43%) and LV remodeling, overt diastolic dysfunction, RV remodeling, and dysfunction	1 (ref) > 2 > 3 for both the endpoints

| Kao et al,[20] *Eur J Heart Fail,* 2015 | 4113 pts from the I-PRESERVED cohort Retrospective analysis Age: >60 y Female: 60% LVEF: 59% (52%–65%) Validation cohort: 3203 pts from the CHARM-Preserved cohort | Latent class analysis | 11 variables: clinical, EKG No imaging data | Primary endpoint: all-cause mortality or CV hospitalization Secondary endpoint: HF hospitalization or cardiac death | A. Median age: 65 y, males: 100% B. Median age: 65 y, females: 96% A and B. Younger patients, few CV risk factors, and less electrical remodeling (AF 18% and 5%, respectively). C. Median age: 70 y, males: 59%. Higher prevalence of CV risk factors: obesity (75%), DM (100%), IHD (66%), CKD (63%). Moderate electrical remodeling (AF 33%) D. Median age: 73 y, females: 100% women. Intermediate prevalence of CV risk factors: obesity (46%); DM (23%), CKD (36%). Moderate electrical remodeling (AF 32%) E. Older (median age: 75 y), males 100%. Main CV risk factor: IHD (62%). Significant electrical remodeling (AF 44%) F. Median age: 82%, females: 78%. Lower BMI, high prevalence of CKD (80%). Marked electrical remodeling (AF 51%) | B > A (ref) > D > E > C > F |

(continued on next page)

Table 1
(continued)

Authors	Population	Clustering	Variables	Endpoints	Clusters	Prognosis (Better to Worst)
Sanchez-Martinez et al,[21] *Circ Cardiovasc Imaging,* 2018	156 pts (testing: 72 HFpEF, 33 healthy subjects; validation: 24 HTN, 27 with noncardiac dyspnea) from the MEDIA cohort Mean age: >60 y Females: 65% LVEF: 62.3% ± 6.7%	Agglomerative hierarchical clustering	22 variables from LV velocity traces acquired at rest and during exercise echocardiography	Discriminate between healthy and HFpEF subjects and identify new descriptors to characterize HFpEF	1. "Healthy cluster" 2. "HFpEF": Older (mean age: 71 y), higher NTproBNP, BMI, impaired exercise tolerance at 6-MWT, LV hypertrophy, higher E/e′ ratio. Absence of significant differences in exercise-echo derived parameters	—
Przewlocka-Kosmala et al,[22] *J Am Soc Echocardiogr,* 2019	228 patients (177 HFpEF, 51 asymptomatic controls) Prospective study Females: 71% LVEF: >60%	Automated hierarchical clustering	Variables: clinical, laboratory, rest and exercise, TTE, CPET	Primary endpoint: CV hospitalization or death	1. *Normal CR/DR:* mean age: 62.2 ± 7.9 y; normal increase in HR and diastolic function during exercise 2. *Altered CR/DR:* mean age: 63.9 ± 7.9 y; decreased exercise tolerance at CPET; chronotropic incompetence and diastolic dysfunction on exercise (higher E/e′ ratio and lower LA strain values)	Normal CR/DR group > abnormal CR/DR group

| Segar et al,[23] *Eur J Heart Fail,* 2020 | 654 pts from the TOPCAT cohort Retrospective analysis Age: 71.2 ± 9.9 y Females: 49% Blacks: 19.4% Internal validation cohort: 1113 from the TOPCAT trial External validation cohort: 198 pts from the RELAX trial | Finite mixture model-based clustering | 61 variables: clinical, laboratory, EKG, TTE | Primary endpoint: HF hospitalization or cardiac death Secondary endpoint: all-cause death, all-cause hospitalization, HF hospitalization, MACEs (myocardial infarction, stroke, or CV death) | 1. Older: 73 y; males: 76%. Several CV risk factors: obesity; DM (74%), HTN (91%), worse renal function. Significant LV concentric remodeling, LA dilatation, diastolic dysfunction 2. Median age: 71 y; males 51%. Low prevalence of CV risk factors. Moderate LV concentric remodeling. Moderate LA dilatation and higher prevalence of moderate MR (24%) 3. Median age: 71 y; males 52%. Intermediate burden of CV risk factors, mainly DM (44%) and HTN (91%). Moderate LV concentric remodeling and LA dilatation | 3 > 2 > 1 |

(continued on next page)

Table 1
(continued)

Authors	Population	Clustering	Variables	Endpoints	Clusters	Prognosis (Better to Worst)
Cohen et al,[24] *JACC Heart Fail,* 2020	3442 pts from the TOPCAT cohort Retrospective analysis Mean age: 69 ± 10 y Females: 52% LVEF ≥45%	Latent class analysis	Variables: clinical, laboratory, TTE, arterial tonometry	Primary endpoint: CV death, HF hospitalization, aborted cardiac arrest	1. Younger (61 ± 6 y), relatively preserved functional class, main CV risk factor: smoking (24%). Low prevalence of diabetes (9%). Low prevalence of CKD (15%). Normal LV geometry 2. Older age (77 ± 5 y), females: 56%, moderate electrical remodeling: AF 49%, high prevalence of CKD (58%), main CV risk factor: obesity (37%). Low prevalence of diabetes (17%). LV concentric remodeling. High arterial stiffness, elevated NTproBNP 3. Intermediate age (66 ± 8 y), females: 46%. Several CV risk factors: diabetes (88%), obesity (98%). High prevalence of CKD (57%), impaired functional class, high prevalence of depression (36%). LV concentric hypertrophy	1 > 2 > 3

et al,[25] *Eur J Heart Fail,* 2020	cohort Retrospective analysis Mean age: 75.9 ± 9.2 y Females: 55.6% LVEF: 62.3% ± 6.7% No validation cohort	based clustering	laboratory, TTE echocardiogram + 92 plasma proteins analysis in 76 patients	cause death and HF hospitalization	5–4 > 3

females: 50%. Several CV risk factors: HTN (100%), IHD (47%), DM (53%), and CKD (67%). Marked LV concentric remodeling, modest electric remodeling (AF 37%)

2. Older age: 78.0 ± 8 y; females: 45%. Main CV risk factor: HTN (83%). Significant LA dilatation and higher prevalence of RV failure. Severe electric remodeling (AF 85%)

3. Younger (71.6 ± 11.5 y); females: 44%. Main CV risk factor: HTN (75%). Modest LV remodeling and electric remodeling (AF 48%)

4. Age: 74.4 ± 8.0 y; females: 44%. Main CV risk factor: HTN (75%). Significant LV and atrial remodeling, highest electrical remodeling (AF 90%)

5. Age: 77.5 ± 8.5 y; female 66%. Main CV risk factor: HTN (75%), IHD (40%). Moderate LV remodeling, moderate electrical remodeling (AF 43%)

(continued on next page)

Table 1
(continued)

Authors	Population	Clustering	Variables	Endpoints	Clusters	Prognosis (Better to Worst)
					6. Age: 77.6 ± 7.2 y; females: 69%; low BMI (27.0 ± 5.2). Main CV risk factor: HTN (79%). Severe LA remodeling, RV dysfunction; significant electric remodeling (AF 96%)	
Schrub et al,[26] *Arch Cardiovasc Dis*, 2020	356 pts from the KaRen cohort Retrospective analysis Mean age: 76.1 ± 9.3 y; Female: 56.5% LVEF >45% No validation cohort	Hierarchical cluster analysis	55 variables: clinical, laboratory, EKG, TTE	Primary endpoint: all-cause death or HF hospitalization Secondary endpoint: all-cause death	1. Younger (73.8 ± 10.3 y): males: 60%. Several CV risk factors: HTN (89%), DM (60%), obesity (BMI: 31 ± 7 kg/m²), CKD (60%). Less electric remodeling, LV hypertrophy, lowest rate of severe MR (2%) 2. Intermediate age (76.7 ± 9.4 y); females: 69%. Main CV risk factor: HTN (73%). Less LV remodeling, but significant LA atrial dilatation and higher severe MR rate (6%)	No statistical difference between the 3 clusters Tendency toward a higher long-term all-cause mortality for cluster 2 and 3 vs cluster 1

Source	Population	Method	Variables	Endpoints	Clusters/Results
Gu et al,[27] Int J Cardiol, 2020	970 pts Prospective study Mean age: 70.0 ± 6.5 y Female: 42% LVEF >50% Validation cohort: 290 pts	Hierarchical cluster analysis	11 variables: clinical, laboratory, EKG, TTE	Primary endpoint: all-cause death Secondary endpoint: all-cause death or HF hospitalization	1. Younger (69.3 ± 6.7 y); males: 59%. Main CV risk factor: HTN (72%). Less electric remodeling (AF 37%) and myocardial remodeling 2. Older (70.9 ± 6.7 y); females: 50%. Main CV risk factor: HTN (74%). Moderate LV hypertrophy and diastolic dysfunction, and moderate electrical remodeling (AF 47%) 3. Age: (70.3 ± 6.1 y), males: 62%. Several CV risk factors: obesity, IHD (48%), DM (39%). Less electric remodeling (AF 36%), worse LV remodeling and diastolic dysfunction 3. Oldest (78.3 ± 6.9 y); females: 62%. Severe electrical remodeling (AF 87%), severe LA dilatation, higher prevalence of severe MR (11%) 1 > 2 > 3 for both the endpoints

Abbreviations: 6-MWT, 6-minute walking test; CPET, cardiopulmonary exercise test; CR, chronotropic reserve; DR, diastolic reserve; EKG, electrocardiogram; LA, left atrium; MACEs, major adverse cardiovascular events; NTproBNP, N-terminal pro brain natriuretic peptide; pts, patients; PVR, pulmonary vascular resistance; TTE, transthoracic echocardiography.

hemodynamics parameters in the phenomapping algorithm.[19] Cardiac catheterization is complicated to implement in the daily routine practice of these comorbid patients. It should be emphasized that only 4 studies among those listed in **Table 1** have a validation cohort.[19,20,23,27] The presence of an external frame of reference is fundamental in the process of strengthening and verification of ML-derived algorithms and has pivotal importance for their validation and future application in clinical practice.

PHENOGROUPS IN HEART FAILURE WITH PRESERVED EJECTION FRACTION

The heterogeneity of the investigated HFpEF populations as well as of the applied phenotyping approaches is the reason for inconsistencies in the phenomapping outcomes, with the identified clusters differing from 1 study to another. Despite this variety, some phenotypes share similar characteristics and prognosis across different cohorts of patients and merit specific consideration.

Different Archetypes of Heart Failure with Preserved Ejection Fraction

Phenogroup 1 includes younger, often overweight, or obese patients, with low brain natriuretic peptide (BNP), exercise deconditioning, few signs of LV remodeling, and favorable diastolic profile.

Phenogroup 2 includes patients with several longstanding CV risk factors (such as DM, HTN, obesity, dyslipidemia), severe LV myocardial remodeling (LV hypertrophy, LV longitudinal impairment, and diastolic dysfunction), without significant right heart alterations.

Phenogroup 3 includes patients with several longstanding CV risk factors often associated with pulmonary disease (eg, COPD or OSAS), biventricular remodeling with PAH, and CKD.

Phenogroup 4 includes patients with few CV risk factors, lower body mass index (BMI), high prevalence of atrial fibrillation (AF), significant LA dilatation, but modest LV remodeling.

Phenogroup 5 includes older patients, most often women, with lower BMI, high prevalence of AF, severe LA dilatation, high prevalence of mitral regurgitation (MR), PAH, RV dysfunction, and CKD.

If the first 3 groups correspond to the classification already proposed by Shah and colleagues,[19] the last 2 have been described in some other studies,[20,25–27] which included oldest patients and considered age and AF important factors of discrimination between phenogroups.

PATHOPHYSIOLOGY AND TREATMENT ACROSS THE PROPOSED HEART FAILURE WITH PRESERVED EJECTION FRACTION PHENOGROUPS

According to the simplified classification proposed above, some pathophysiologic hypotheses and specific therapeutic approaches can be proposed (**Figs. 2** and **3**).

Phenogroup 1: The Natriuretic Peptide Deficiency Syndrome

Phenogroup 1 corresponds to the "natriuretic peptide deficiency syndrome" already described in the literature.[19,28] In these patients, the combination of overweight/obesity and insulin resistance triggers the production of adipocyte-derived cell signaling molecules, which increase the activity of neprilysin and aldosterone.[29,30] The increased BNP clearance and reduced BNP production[31] are responsible for the reduced BNP plasma levels, whereas the elevation in aldosterone level contributes to the aggravated sodium retention and liquid expansion. These patients often have few or no symptoms at rest, but they might develop dyspnea, LV longitudinal dysfunction, and eventually overt signs of cardiac dysfunction during exercise.[22] In this subset, weight loss and aerobic training with subsequent improvement in insulin resistance might signify a pillar of the treatment. Interestingly, the reduction of obesity by either behavioral intervention or bariatric surgery is associated with significant cardiac reverse remodeling, improvement of symptoms, and an increase in BNP plasma levels, which might have beneficial effects on natriuresis.[32,33]

The role of pharmacologic treatment to improve symptoms and the progression of the disease in these patients is an object of debate, particularly because patients in phenogroup 1 are commonly excluded from trials on HFpEF because of their low BNP levels. Nevertheless, the increased aldosterone levels observed in obese patients might explain why in the TOPCAT trial, patients with the lowest BNP levels seemed to benefit more from spironolactone.[34] For similar reasons, the neprilysin inhibitor Sacubitril, which has not shown benefit in an unselected HFpEF population in the PARAGON trial,[16] might prove beneficial in this specific subset of patients with HFpEF who have increased neprilysin activity. Neprilysin inhibitors might have a direct natriuretic effect, but they also have pleiotropic effects by suppressing the secretion and antagonizing the effect of aldosterone,[35] and by having a lipolytic and anti-inflammatory action.[30,36]

The sodium-glucose type 2 (sodium-glucose transport protein-2, SGLT-2) inhibitors might

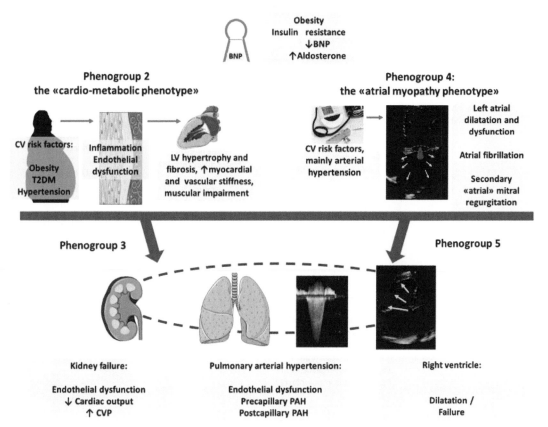

Fig. 2. Main HFpEF clusters identified across the different studies. CVP, central venous pressure; T2DM, type 2 diabetes mellitus.

represent another therapeutic option in obese patients with HFpEF. Particularly, the SGLT-2 inhibitor empagliflozin has been reported to have favorable effects on vascular resistance[37] and visceral adiposity,[38] and to reduce HF hospitalization in diabetic patients.[39] In the EMPEROR-HF trial, patients with HF and reduced LVEF taking empagliflozin 10 mg/d on top of their medical treatment have experienced a significant reduction in HF hospitalization and death and less renal function deterioration.[40] Despite the absence of specific studies in HFpEF, empagliflozin might counterbalance the oxidative and metabolic derangements and the sodium retention observed in obese patients with HFpEF, potentially disrupting the development of the obesity-HFpEF phenotype.[41]

Phenogroups 2 and 3: The Cardiometabolic Phenotype and its Evolution

These 2 phenogroups include patients with several CV risk factors but at different stages of the disease.

Phenogroup 2 comprises the "cardiometabolic phenotype." This group exemplifies the effect of longstanding CV risk factors on myocyte and cardiac microcirculatory function. As well described by Paulus and Tschöpe,[42] the proinflammatory state caused by multiple CV risk factors is responsible for the coronary microvascular endothelial inflammation and dysfunction, reduced nitric oxide (NO) bioavailability, and impaired protein kinase G activity (PKG).[43] This process causes T-tubule disruption in the cardiomyocytes, with a subsequent imbalance in calcium handling and impaired LV relaxation.[44]

Another factor contributing to myocardial stiffness and diastolic dysfunction is the increase in collagen deposition and the proliferation of myocardial fibroblasts resulting in interstitial myocardial fibrosis.[45]

The mechanisms provoking myocardial remodeling and dysfunction are also responsible for the development of arterial stiffness at rest[43,46] and altered ventriculoatrial coupling during exercise.[47]

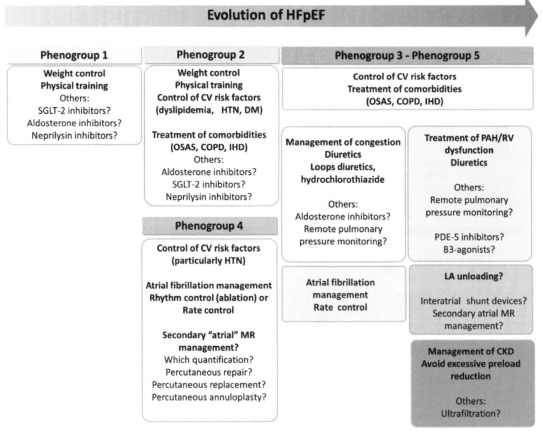

Fig. 3. Current proposed therapeutic approaches for the management of HFpEF according to phenogroups. PDE-5, phosphodiesterase-5.

From a therapeutic point of view, the first approach to patients in phenogroup 2 is the management of CV risk factors. Normalization of blood pressure, calories restriction, and careful control of DM might be the key to preventing the progression of the disease. According to previous data and to a post hoc analysis of the TOPCAT trial,[24,48] the administration of spironolactone to patients belonging to phenogroup 2 might be considered to improve exercise tolerance[48] and survival.[24] SGLT-2 inhibitors, given their potential to target specific pathogenetic mechanisms in HFpEF and beneficial effects found in HFrEF, might also be a useful treatment option[41]; however, more clinical evidence is needed. Other potential disease-modifying strategies in these patients might include drugs targeting the NO-PKG axis. Direct NO donors, such as isosorbide dinitrate, have already been tested in HFpEF and have proven no benefit in terms of quality-of-life improvement and exercise tolerance compared with placebo.[15] Nevertheless, in a small pilot study, intravenous administration of sodium nitrite, which is

converted to NO in vivo, has been shown to decrease pulmonary capillary wedge pressure (PCWP) at rest and during exercise in patients with HFpEF.[49]

Phenogroup 3 corresponds to patients with longstanding CV risk factors and elevated filling pressure, who develop PAH, RV dysfunction, and kidney failure.

The appearance of PAH and subsequent RV dysfunction represents a landmark in the evolution of HFpEF, because it is associated with increased hospitalization rate and poor prognosis.[50]

In patients with HF, the impaired LV relaxation and chronic elevation in LV filling pressure are always the primum movens for the development of PAH, because it causes an elevation in LA pressure, which is transmitted back to the pulmonary circulation, causing postcapillary PAH. Importantly, nearly 12% of patients with HFpEF develop concomitant precapillary PAH (cpc-PAH). It is a consequence of a process involving endothelial dysfunction, smooth muscle cell proliferation, and extensive remodeling of the pulmonary veins and arteries. This process is driven by the same mechanisms that are responsible for endothelial dysfunction in other vascular districts in patients with HFpEF.[51]

The development of PAH is often accompanied by the development of RV dysfunction, which is a predictor of poor prognosis. Nevertheless, PAH is not the only mechanism for RV impairment in HFpEF. Some recent studies have shown that in HFpEF, the RV undergoes a process of hypertrophy and fibrosis, which is like that observed in the LV. After the development of RV diastolic dysfunction, the next step in the progression of RV disease is the development of RV dilatation and systolic dysfunction.[52]

All these pathophysiologic observations might have important therapeutic implications. On one hand, patients with isolated postcapillary PAH might benefit from titration of diuretics to reduce filling pressure and PAH. The use of remote pulmonary pressure monitoring systems, such as the CardioMEMs, might be useful in patients with frequent HF hospitalization and/or persisting symptoms to optimize diuretics therapy and reduce hospitalization rate.[53]

On the other hand, patients with a predominant cpc-PAH might eventually benefit from a careful administration of pulmonary vasodilators. Despite the results of a preliminary trial showing that the inclusion of Sildenafil 50 mg thrice a day in patients with HFpEF and PAH was able to reduce PAH and improve RV dysfunction,[54] the multicentric RELAX trial failed to demonstrate the benefit of sildenafil on the clinical status and exercise capacity of patients with HFpEF.[14] A potential explication for these findings is that the study included patients with PAH irrespective of the evaluation of the precapillary or postcapillary component. One of the goals of current research in this field is therefore to improve the phenotyping of PAH in patients with HFpEF.[55] Other potential therapeutic strategies may arise from new medications. For instance, the SPHERE-HF trial, a phase 2 study, has the objective to verify the effect of mirabegron, a β3-agonist, on the pulmonary hemodynamics, clinical, biochemical, and imaging parameters in patients with HF and cpc-PAH.

Another finding of phenogroup 3 is the development of kidney failure, which is a well-known predictor of poor prognosis in HF patients.[56] The main pathophysiologic mechanism for the development of renal dysfunction in HFpEF is the increase in central venous pressure with a subsequent increase in renal venous pressure, which causes a substantial decrease in the glomerular pressure gradient and glomerular filtration rate, elevation in plasma renin and aldosterone activity, and reduced urine output.[57] CKD alters the metabolism of phosphates, causing secondary hyperparathyroidism, which might lead to increased calcium level, pulmonary vessels vasoconstriction, and ectopic calcification, thus contributing to PAH and RV failure.[58]

Preventing the onset and/or worsening of renal failure in HFpEF patients is fundamental to improve survival. Nevertheless, few studies have specifically addressed this issue in patients with HFpEF. The CARESS-HF trial, including patients with all EF categories, has shown the benefit of stepped diuretic treatment over ultrafiltration in acute decompensated HF.[59] Regarding the use of inhibitors of the renin-angiotensin-aldosterone systems, both the TOPCAT trial[34] and the I-PRESERVE trial have shown the detrimental effect of antialdosterone drugs and irbesartan on renal function in patients with HFpEF.[13] It might be because all drugs acting on the renin-angiotensin-aldosterone axis cause a significant reduction in preload. Patients with HFpEF are sensitive to preload modification because of the steep relationship between LV pressure and volume, and decreased venous return might lead to a reduction in cardiac output and contribute to a deterioration of renal function.

Phenogroup 4 and 5: The Atrial Myopathy Phenotype and its Evolution

Phenogroup 4 corresponds to the recently described "atrial fibrillation/atrial myopathy" phenotype of HFpEF. Analogous to phenogroups 2 and 3, phenogroups 4 and 5 probably represent 2 different phases of the same disease pathway.

Phenogroup 4 includes patients having HTN as a main CV risk factor, LA dilatation, and a high prevalence of AF. From a pathophysiologic point of view, in patients with HFrEF, atrial dilatation and dysfunction are phenomena that are related to the progressive increase in LA pressure. It pushes for the development of functional MR. In patients with HFpEF, the LA has been initially considered a simple bystander of the progressive exacerbation of LV stiffness and dysfunction. Nevertheless, von Roeder and colleagues[60] elegantly showed that the deterioration of LA reservoir and conduit function is already evident in the initial phases of HFpEF. Interestingly, in a canine model of early HFpEF, Zakeri and colleagues[61] demonstrated that renal-induced HTN and aldosterone excess are associated with the development of atrial myocyte hypertrophy, titin hyperphosphorylation, and microvascular dysfunction, supporting the hypothesis that a common pathophysiologic process acts in all myocardial chambers. From a functional point of view, these structural alterations are responsible for the development of impaired atrial function and associated with an impaired atrioventricular coupling.[61]

There are 2 important consequences of the LA myopathy observed in HFpEF: the development of AF and the appearance of MR. The occurrence of AF can predate the diagnosis of HFpEF in 29% of patients. AF can be observed in up to 75% of patients with HFpEF in the advanced phases of the disease and is a strong predictor of morbidity and mortality.[62] Interestingly, in the Rochester Epidemiology Project, age and HTN were the main independent predictors of AF in patients with HFpEF, which exactly mirrors the clinical characteristics observed in patients belonging to phenogroup 4.

Mild to moderate MR is a frequent finding in patients with HFpEF and was initially considered an innocent bystander. Nevertheless, Tamargo and colleagues[63] have shown that patients with HFpEF and mild to moderate MR have a higher prevalence of AF, more advanced diastolic dysfunction, LA functional impairment, more dilated RV, and a higher prevalence of PAH and RV dysfunction as compared with patients with HFpEF and no MR. All these abnormalities result in the alteration of the RV–pulmonary artery coupling and culminate in substantial impairment in cardiac output reserve with exercise.

Interestingly, Tamargo and colleagues[63] also showed that mitral annulus dilatation and LA dilatation were the major determinants of MR in multivariable analysis. Despite that it is quite difficult to establish a clear causality or sequentiality between AF and MR in HFpEF, the mutual relationship between these 2 entities might create a vicious circle and further promote atrial remodeling and dysfunction.

The mechanisms described above are responsible for the development of a specific, distinct cause of MR, recently referred to as "atrial functional mitral regurgitation."[64] Up to 57% of patients with HFpEF might present with mild to moderate MR.[63,64]

Phenotype 5 represents the natural and progressive evolution of phenotype 4.

With the ongoing disease, the severity of MR increases, and patients develop PAH, overt RV dysfunction, and CKD, all of which are typical for HFpEF phenotype 5 and are associated with a very poor outcome.[20,26,65]

The management of patients with HFpEF belonging to phenogroups 4 and 5 is not established. The control of CV risk factors, particularly HTN, which is very frequent in patients from phenotype 4, should be obtained. The inhibitors of the renin-angiotensin-aldosterone system have proven to reduce the burden of new AF episodes in patients with HFrEF, but they have not shown similar efficacy in HFpEF.[66] The ongoing IMPRESS-AF trial is investigating the effect of spironolactone on the quality of life and exercise tolerance in patients with AF and HFpEF.[67]

In patients with AF, the maintenance of sinus rhythm through medical therapy or transcatheter ablation could be discussed. The AFFIRM (Atrial Fibrillation Follow-up Investigation of Rhythm Management) trial showed that the restoration of sinus rhythm did not outperform heart rate control in terms of survival and adverse CV events. Nevertheless, the benefit of rhythm control will probably be more evident in patients in the initial phase of the disease, with mild to moderate MR and less pronounced LA remodeling.[68]

All interventions aimed at reducing the load of the left atrium are also important in these patients. In addition to the optimization of diuretic therapy to reduce LA and LV pressure, MR and LA remodeling, another potential option is represented by percutaneous atrial septostomy. The initial results of the REDUCE LAP-HF I trial have shown the safety of the implantation of an interatrial shunt device in patients with HFpEF in New York Heart Association class II and III.[69] Nevertheless, the effect of this intervention on LA size seems more evident in patients with higher LA compliance and right atrial reservoir function, which probably correspond to less advanced atrial disease.[70] On the other hand, the benefit of LA unloading following the placement of a left-to-right shunt should be supported by the absence of a detrimental effect on the right heart function and on PAH, which is expected to be evidenced in future studies.

The current definitions of MR severity rely on patients with typical primary or secondary MR, with no recommendations for atrial functional MR. In a cohort of patients with severe MR undergoing surgery, Pimor and colleagues[71] have shown that patients having atrial functional MR have the poorest outcome. It is probable that in patients with HFpEF and noncompliant LV and atria, a moderate degree of MR might be sufficient to cause detrimental effects on the LA and the downstream pulmonary circulation. The optimal timing and modality of intervention for atrial functional MR (surgical mitral valve replacement/repair vs percutaneous mitral edge-to-edge mitral valve repair/percutaneous annuloplasty) are fundamental issues, which need to be clarified in specifically designed studies.

Prognosis Across Heart Failure with Preserved Ejection Fraction Phenogroups

All the studies on phenomapping in HFpEF consider all-cause mortality and a composite of mortality and HF hospitalization as endpoints. The intrinsic heterogeneity of the populations enrolled in the studies cited in **Table 1** makes the generalization of the prognostic stratification of patients uncertain. Nevertheless, looking at the phenogroups' classification proposed above, patients in phenogroup 1 can be identified as a "low-risk" group. Patients belonging to phenogroup 3 and 5, who often have RV dysfunction, PAH, and kidney failure, have the poorest prognosis and represent a "high-risk" group.[20,25,26] Finally, patients in phenogroups 2 and 4 belong to an "intermediate" risk category, who can eventually progress into a higher risk group.

SUMMARY

Medicine will experience many changes in the future because of the availability of an increasing amount of digitalized data coming from electronic health records, genomic databases, medical imaging, lifestyle datasets, and wearable devices. The availability of computational tools that can deal with these records will improve the characterization of patients and allow proposing specific and personalized diagnostic and therapeutic strategies, which can change current health care systems. The striking novelty of this approach is evident by the interest developed in this field by several political and health care institutions, such as the National Institute of Health in the United States,[72] or the European Union.[73]

HFpEF appears to be an ideal field for the application of personalized medicine, given its heterogeneity and lack of specific therapeutic management. This individualized, high-technology–based strategy might facilitate the identification of patients who can benefit from specific therapies, reduce the risk of drug side effects,[74] and finally, improve the quality of life and survival.

Nevertheless, several points need improvements to attend these ambitious goals:

1. Collection of data relying on reliable registries and focused research trials
2. Development of validation cohorts to allow the verification of the algorithms proposed through different ML approaches
3. Design of multicenter studies to verify the efficacy of specific therapeutic strategies in distinct patient categories.

Because ML-based clustering does not supply specific thresholds for phenotypic data, a framework for the introduction of patient categorization into clinical practice should be developed.

CLINICS CARE POINTS

- Description of the phenotypes and hypothesis-driven proposals for a best management and control of symptoms.
- There are comorbidities that one looks for and that helps in defining the risk of a patients. These co-morbidities should be treated and considered seriously for decreasing the risk of cardiovascular event in the follow-up. A clear understanding of these phenogroups and of the component of them is important for all the physicians who care about heart failure.

REFERENCES

1. Mosterd A, Hoes AW. Clinical epidemiology of heart failure. Heart 2007;93(9):1137–46.
2. Vos T, Flaxman AD, Naghavi M, et al. Years lived with disability (YLDs) for 1160 sequelae of 289 diseases and injuries 1990–2010: a systematic analysis for the Global Burden of Disease Study 2010. Lancet 2012; 380(9859):2163–96.
3. Ponikowski P, Voors AA, Anker SD, et al. 2016 ESC Guidelines for the diagnosis and treatment of acute and chronic heart failure: the Task Force for the Diagnosis and Treatment of Acute and Chronic Heart Failure of the European Society of Cardiology (ESC) developed with the special contribution of the Heart Failure Association (HFA) of the ESC. Eur Heart J 2016;37(27):2129–200.
4. Shah KS, Xu H, Matsouaka RA, et al. Heart failure with preserved, borderline, and reduced ejection fraction: 5-year outcomes. J Am Coll Cardiol 2017; 70(20):2476–86.
5. Ho JE, Zern EK, Wooster L, et al. Differential clinical profiles, exercise responses, and outcomes associated with existing HFpEF definitions. Circulation 2019;140(5):353–65.
6. Pieske B, Tschöpe C, de Boer RA, et al. How to diagnose heart failure with preserved ejection fraction: the HFA–PEFF diagnostic algorithm: a consensus recommendation from the Heart Failure Association (HFA) of the European Society of Cardiology (ESC). Eur Heart J 2019;40(40):3297–317.
7. Borlaug BA. The pathophysiology of heart failure with preserved ejection fraction. Nat Rev Cardiol 2014;11(9):507–15.
8. Obokata M, Kane GC, Reddy YNV, et al. Role of diastolic stress testing in the evaluation for heart failure with preserved ejection fraction: a simultaneous invasive-echocardiographic study. Circulation 2017;135(9):825–38.

9. Sanders-van Wijk S, van Empel V, Davarzani N, et al. Circulating biomarkers of distinct pathophysiological pathways in heart failure with preserved vs. reduced left ventricular ejection fraction: biomarkers in heart failure with preserved vs. reduced EF. Eur J Heart Fail 2015;17(10):1006–14.

10. Franssen C, Chen S, Unger A, et al. Myocardial microvascular inflammatory endothelial activation in heart failure with preserved ejection fraction. JACC Heart Fail 2016;4(4):312–24.

11. Shah SJ, Kitzman DW, Borlaug BA, et al. Phenotype-specific treatment of heart failure with preserved ejection fraction: a multiorgan roadmap. Circulation 2016;134(1):73–90.

12. Yusuf S, Pfeffer MA, Swedberg K, et al. Effects of candesartan in patients with chronic heart failure and preserved left-ventricular ejection fraction: the CHARM-Preserved Trial. Lancet 2003;362(9386): 777–81.

13. Massie BM, Carson PE, McMurray JJ, et al. Irbesartan in patients with heart failure and preserved ejection fraction. N Engl J Med 2008;359(23):2456–67.

14. Redfield MM, Chen HH, Borlaug BA, et al. Effect of phosphodiesterase-5 inhibition on exercise capacity and clinical status in heart failure with preserved ejection fraction: a randomized clinical trial. JAMA 2013;309(12):1268.

15. Redfield MM, Anstrom KJ, Levine JA, et al. Isosorbide mononitrate in heart failure with preserved ejection fraction. N Engl J Med 2015;373(24):2314–24.

16. Solomon SD, McMurray JJV, Anand IS, et al. Angiotensin–neprilysin inhibition in heart failure with preserved ejection fraction. N Engl J Med 2019; 381(17):1609–20.

17. Krittanawong C, Zhang H, Wang Z, et al. Artificial intelligence in precision cardiovascular medicine. J Am Coll Cardiol 2017;69(21):2657–64.

18. Shah SJ. Precision medicine for heart failure with preserved ejection fraction: an overview. J Cardiovasc Transl Res 2017;10(3):233–44.

19. Shah SJ, Katz DH, Selvaraj S, et al. Phenomapping for novel classification of heart failure with preserved ejection fraction. Circulation 2015;131(3):269–79.

20. Kao DP, Lewsey JD, Anand IS, et al. Characterization of subgroups of heart failure patients with preserved ejection fraction with possible implications for prognosis and treatment response: HFpEF subtypes-prognosis and treatment response. Eur J Heart Fail 2015;17(9):925–35.

21. Sanchez-Martinez S, Duchateau N, Erdei T, et al. Machine learning analysis of left ventricular function to characterize heart failure with preserved ejection fraction. Circ Cardiovasc Imaging 2018;11(4): e007138.

22. Przewlocka-Kosmala M, Marwick TH, Dabrowski A, et al. Contribution of cardiovascular reserve to prognostic categories of heart failure with preserved ejection fraction: a

classification based on machine learning. J Am Soc Echocardiogr 2019;32(5):604–15.e6.

23. Segar MW, Patel KV, Ayers C, et al. Phenomapping of patients with heart failure with preserved ejection fraction using machine learning-based unsupervised cluster analysis. Eur J Heart Fail 2020;22(1):148–58.

24. Cohen JB, Schrauben SJ, Zhao L, et al. Clinical phenogroups in heart failure with preserved ejection fraction: detailed phenotypes, prognosis, and response to spironolactone. JACC Heart Fail 2020; 8(3):172–84.

25. Hedman ÅK, Hage C, Sharma A, et al. Identification of novel pheno-groups in heart failure with preserved ejection fraction using machine learning. Heart 2020;106(5):342–9.

26. Schrub F, Oger E, Bidaut A, et al. Heart failure with preserved ejection fraction: a clustering approach to a heterogenous syndrome. Arch Cardiovasc Dis 2020;113(6–7):381–90.

27. Gu J, Pan J, Lin H, et al. Characteristics, prognosis and treatment response in distinct phenogroups of heart failure with preserved ejection fraction. Int J Cardiol 2020. https://doi.org/10.1016/j.ijcard.2020.08.065.

28. Anjan VY, Loftus TM, Burke MA, et al. Prevalence, clinical phenotype, and outcomes associated with normal B-type natriuretic peptide levels in heart failure with preserved ejection fraction. Am J Cardiol 2012;110(6):870–6.

29. Standeven KF, Hess K, Carter AM, et al. Neprilysin, obesity and the metabolic syndrome. Int J Obes 2011;35(8):1031–40.

30. Packer M, Kitzman DW. Obesity-related heart failure with a preserved ejection fraction. JACC Heart Fail 2018;6(8):633–9.

31. Gupta DK, Wang TJ. Natriuretic peptides and cardiometabolic health. Circ J 2015;79(8):1647–55.

32. Chen-Tournoux A, Khan AM, Baggish AL, et al. Effect of weight loss after weight loss surgery on plasma N-terminal pro-B-type natriuretic peptide levels. Am J Cardiol 2010;106(10):1450–5.

33. Arora P, Reingold J, Baggish A, et al. Weight loss, saline loading, and the natriuretic peptide system. J Am Heart Assoc 2015;4(1):e001265.

34. Anand IS, Claggett B, Liu J, et al. Interaction between spironolactone and natriuretic peptides in patients with heart failure and preserved ejection fraction: from the TOPCAT trial. JACC Heart Fail 2017;5(4):241–52.

35. Nakagawa H, Oberwinkler H, Nikolaev VO, et al. Atrial natriuretic peptide locally counteracts the deleterious effects of cardiomyocyte mineralocorticoid receptor activation. Circ Heart Fail 2014;7(5): 814–21.

36. Polak J, Kotrc M, Wedellova Z, et al. Lipolytic effects of B-type natriuretic peptide 1–32 in adipose tissue of heart failure patients compared with healthy controls. J Am Coll Cardiol 2011;58(11):1119–25.

37. Chilton R, Tikkanen I, Cannon CP, et al. Effects of empagliflozin on blood pressure and markers of arterial stiffness and vascular resistance in patients with type 2 diabetes. Diabetes Obes Metab 2015; 17(12):1180–93.

38. Ridderstråle M, Andersen KR, Zeller C, et al. Comparison of empagliflozin and glimepiride as add-on to metformin in patients with type 2 diabetes: a 104-week randomised, active-controlled, double-blind, phase 3 trial. Lancet Diabetes Endocrinol 2014;2(9):691–700.

39. Zinman B, Wanner C, Lachin JM, et al. Empagliflozin, cardiovascular outcomes, and mortality in type 2 diabetes. N Engl J Med 2015;373(22):2117–28.

40. Packer M, Anker SD, Butler J, et al. Cardiovascular and renal outcomes with empagliflozin in heart failure. N Engl J Med 2020;383(15):1413–24.

41. Hallow KM, Helmlinger G, Greasley PJ, et al. Why do SGLT2 inhibitors reduce heart failure hospitalization? A differential volume regulation hypothesis. Diabetes Obes Metab 2018;20(3):479–87.

42. Shah SJ, Lam CSP, Svedlund S, et al. Prevalence and correlates of coronary microvascular dysfunction in heart failure with preserved ejection fraction: PROMIS-HFpEF. Eur Heart J 2018;39(37):3439–50.

43. Paulus WJ, Tschöpe C. A novel paradigm for heart failure with preserved ejection fraction. J Am Coll Cardiol 2013;62(4):263–71.

44. Shah SJ, Aistrup GL, Gupta DK, et al. Ultrastructural and cellular basis for the development of abnormal myocardial mechanics during the transition from hypertension to heart failure. Am J Physiol Heart Circ Physiol 2014;306(1):H88–100.

45. Mohammed SF, Hussain S, Mirzoyev SA, et al. Coronary microvascular rarefaction and myocardial fibrosis in heart failure with preserved ejection fraction. Circulation 2015;131(6):550–9.

46. Desai AS, Mitchell GF, Fang JC, et al. Central aortic stiffness is increased in patients with heart failure and preserved ejection fraction. J Card Fail 2009; 15(8):658–64.

47. Reddy YNV, Andersen MJ, Obokata M, et al. Arterial stiffening with exercise in patients with heart failure and preserved ejection fraction. J Am Coll Cardiol 2017;70(2):136–48.

48. Kosmala W, Rojek A, Przewlocka-Kosmala M, et al. Effect of aldosterone antagonism on exercise tolerance in heart failure with preserved ejection fraction. J Am Coll Cardiol 2016;68(17):1823–34.

49. Borlaug BA, Koepp KE, Melenovsky V. Sodium nitrite improves exercise hemodynamics and ventricular performance in heart failure with preserved ejection fraction. J Am Coll Cardiol 2015;66(15): 1672–82.

50. Vanderpool RR, Saul M, Nouraie M, et al. Association between hemodynamic markers of pulmonary hypertension and outcomes in heart failure with preserved ejection fraction. JAMA Cardiol 2018; 3(4):298–306.

51. Ranchoux B, Nadeau V, Bourgeois A, et al. Metabolic syndrome exacerbates pulmonary hypertension due to left heart disease. Circ Res 2019; 125(4):449–66.

52. Obokata M, Reddy YNV, Melenovsky V, et al. Deterioration in right ventricular structure and function over time in patients with heart failure and preserved ejection fraction. Eur Heart J 2019;40(8):689–97.

53. Adamson PB, Abraham WT, Bourge RC, et al. Wireless pulmonary artery pressure monitoring guides management to reduce decompensation in heart failure with preserved ejection fraction. Circ Heart Fail 2014;7(6):935–44.

54. Guazzi M, Vicenzi M, Arena R, et al. Pulmonary hypertension in heart failure with preserved ejection fraction: a target of phosphodiesterase-5 inhibition in a 1-year study. Circulation 2011;124(2):164–74.

55. Hoeper MM, Lam CSP, Vachiery J-L, et al. Pulmonary hypertension in heart failure with preserved ejection fraction: a plea for proper phenotyping and further research. Eur Heart J 2016;ehw597.

56. Bock JS, Gottlieb SS. Cardiorenal syndrome: new perspectives. Circulation 2010;121(23):2592–600.

57. Damman K, Testani JM. The kidney in heart failure: an update. Eur Heart J 2015;36(23):1437–44.

58. Anastasia Mouratoglou S, Giannakoulas G, Defteres S, et al. Intra- and intercellular calcium handling in pulmonary arterial hypertension. Med Chem 2016;12(2):162–9.

59. Bart BA, Goldsmith SR, Lee KL, et al. Ultrafiltration in decompensated heart failure with cardiorenal syndrome. N Engl J Med 2012;367(24):2296–304.

60. von Roeder M, Rommel K-P, Kowallick JT, et al. Influence of left atrial function on exercise capacity and left ventricular function in patients with heart failure and preserved ejection fraction. Circ Cardiovasc Imaging 2017;10(4):e005467.

61. Zakeri R, Moulay G, Chai Q, et al. Left atrial remodeling and atrioventricular coupling in a canine model of early heart failure with preserved ejection fraction. Circ Heart Fail 2016;9(10):e003238.

62. Zakeri R, Chamberlain AM, Roger VL, et al. Temporal relationship and prognostic significance of atrial fibrillation in heart failure patients with preserved ejection fraction: a community-based study. Circulation 2013;128(10):1085–93.

63. Tamargo M, Obokata M, Reddy YNV, et al. Functional mitral regurgitation and left atrial myopathy in heart failure with preserved ejection fraction. Eur J Heart Fail 2020;22(3):489–98.

64. Deferm S, Bertrand PB, Verbrugge FH, et al. Atrial functional mitral regurgitation. J Am Coll Cardiol 2019;73(19):2465–76.

65. Kajimoto K, Sato N, Takano T, et al. Functional mitral regurgitation at discharge and outcomes in patients

hospitalized for acute decompensated heart failure with a preserved or reduced ejection fraction. Eur J Heart Fail 2016;18(8):1051–9.

66. Olsson LG, Swedberg K, Ducharme A, et al. Atrial fibrillation and risk of clinical events in chronic heart failure with and without left ventricular systolic dysfunction: results from the Candesartan in Heart failure-Assessment of Reduction in Mortality and morbidity (CHARM) program. J Am Coll Cardiol 2006;47(10):1997–2004.

67. Shantsila E, Haynes R, Calvert M, et al. IMproved exercise tolerance in patients with PReserved Ejection fraction by Spironolactone on myocardial fibrosiS in Atrial Fibrillation rationale and design of the IMPRESS-AF randomised controlled trial. BMJ Open 2016;6(10):e012241.

68. Gertz ZM, Raina A, Saghy L, et al. Evidence of atrial functional mitral regurgitation due to atrial fibrillation. J Am Coll Cardiol 2011;58(14):1474–81.

69. Obokata M, Reddy YNV, Shah SJ, et al. Effects of interatrial shunt on pulmonary vascular function in heart failure with preserved ejection fraction. J Am Coll Cardiol 2019;74(21):2539–50.

70. Hanff TC, Kaye DM, Hayward CS, et al. Assessment of predictors of left atrial volume response to a transcatheter interatrial shunt device (from the REDUCE LAP-HF Trial). Am J Cardiol 2019;124(12):1912–7.

71. Pimor A, Galli E, Vitel E, et al. Predictors of postoperative cardiovascular events, focused on atrial fibrillation, after valve surgery for primary mitral regurgitation. Eur Heart J Cardiovasc Imaging 2018;20(2):177–84.

72. Collins FS, Varmus H. A new initiative on precision medicine. N Engl J Med 2015;372(9):793–5.

73. Nimmesgern E, Norstedt I, Draghia-Akli R. Enabling personalized medicine in Europe by the European Commission's funding activities. Per Med 2017 14(4):355–65.

74. Pedrós C, Formiga F, Corbella X, et al. Adverse drug reactions leading to urgent hospital admission in an elderly population: prevalence and main features. Eur J Clin Pharmacol 2016;72(2):219–26.

Moving?

Make sure your subscription moves with you!

To notify us of your new address, find your **Clinics Account Number** (located on your mailing label above your name), and contact customer service at:

Email: journalscustomerservice-usa@elsevier.com

800-654-2452 (subscribers in the U.S. & Canada)
314-447-8871 (subscribers outside of the U.S. & Canada)

Fax number: 314-447-8029

Elsevier Health Sciences Division
Subscription Customer Service
3251 Riverport Lane
Maryland Heights, MO 63043

*To ensure uninterrupted delivery of your subscription, please notify us at least 4 weeks in advance of move.